Neurological Disorders in Women: from Epidemiology to Outcome

Editor

RIMA M. DAFER

NEUROLOGIC CLINICS

www.neurologic.theclinics.com

Consulting Editor
RANDOLPH W. EVANS

May 2023 • Volume 41 • Number 2

ELSEVIER

1600 John F. Kennedy Boulevard • Suite 1800 • Philadelphia, Pennsylvania, 19103-2899

http://www.theclinics.com

NEUROLOGIC CLINICS Volume 41, Number 2
May 2023 ISSN 0733-8619, ISBN-13: 978-0-323-98691-5

Editor: Stacy Eastman
Developmental Editor: Hannah Almira Lopez

Neurologic Clinics (ISSN 0733-8619) is published quarterly by Elsevier Inc., 360 Park Avenue South, New York, NY 10010–1710. Months of issue are February, May, August, and November. Periodicals postage paid at New York, NY, and additional mailing offices. Subscription prices are $353.00 per year for US individuals, $809.00 per year for US institutions, $100.00 per year for US students, $433.00 per year for Canadian individuals, $980.00 per year for Canadian institutions, $489.00 per year for international individuals, $980.00 per year for international institutions, $210.00 for foreign students/residents, and $100.00 for Canadian students/residents. To receive student/resident rate, orders must be accompanied by name of affiliated institution, date of term, and the *signature* of program/residency coordinator on institution letterhead. Orders will be billed at individual rate until proof of status is received. Foreign air speed delivery is included in all *Clinics* subscription prices. All prices are subject to change without notice. **POSTMASTER:** Send address changes to *Neurologic Clinics*, Elsevier Health Sciences Division, Subscription Customer Service, 3251 Riverport Lane, Maryland Heights, MO 63043. **Customer Service: Telephone: 1-800-654-2452 (U.S. and Canada); 314-447-8871 (outside U.S. and Canada). Fax: 314-447-8029. E-mail: journalscustomerservice-usa@elsevier.com (for print support); journalsonlinesupport-usa@elsevier.com (for online support).**

Reprints. For copies of 100 or more of articles in this publication, please contact the Commercial Reprints Department, Elsevier Inc., 360 Park Avenue South, New York, New York, 10010-1710; Tel.: +1-212-633-3874; Fax: +1-212-633-3820, and E-mail: reprints@elsevier.com.

Neurologic Clinics is also published in Spanish by Nueva Editorial Interamericana S.A., Mexico City, Mexico.

Neurologic Clinics is covered in *Current Contents/Clinical Medicine, MEDLINE/PubMed (Index Medicus), EMBASE/Excerpta Medica, and PsycINFO, and ISI/BIOMED.*

Contributors

CONSULTING EDITOR

RANDOLPH W. EVANS, MD
Clinical Professor, Department of Neurology, Baylor College of Medicine, Houston, Texas

EDITOR

RIMA M. DAFER, MD, MPH
Professor, Department of Neurological Sciences, Rush University Medical Center, Chicago, Illinois

AUTHORS

NEELUM T. AGGARWAL, MD
Professor of Neurological Sciences, Department of Neurological Sciences, Rush Alzheimer's Disease Center, Rush University Medical Center, Chicago, Illinois

SHARLET A. ANDERSON, PhD
Assistant Professor, Department of Neurological Sciences, Rush University Medical Center, Chicago, Illinois

ZACHARY B. BULWA, MD
Department of Neurology, NorthShore University HealthSystem, Evanston, Illinois

LAUREL CHERIAN, MD, MS
Associate Professor, Division Chief, Cerebrovascular Diseases, Director of Research, Cerebrovascular Diseases, Assistant Dean, Medical Student Affairs, Rush University Medical Center, Chicago, Illinois

EMILY F. DILLON, PhD
Rush University Medical Center, Chicago, Illinois

FATEN EL AMMAR, MD
Neurosciences Intensive Care Unit, Department of Neurology, University of Illinois Chicago, Chicago, Illinois

EDITH L. GRAHAM, MD
Assistant Professor of Neurology, Department of Neurology, Division of Neuroimmunology, Northwestern University, Chicago, Illinois

FARAH KHAN, MD
Loyola University Medical Center, Maywood, Illinois

KATIE KOMPOLITI, MD
Professor of Neurological Sciences, Rush University Medical Center, Chicago, Illinois

PRIYA KUMTHEKAR, MD
Department of Neurology, Malnati Brain Tumor Institute at the Robert H. Lurie Comprehensive Cancer Center, Feinberg School of Medicine, Northwestern University, Chicago, Illinois

BRIDGET A. MAKOL, PhD
Rush University Medical Center, Chicago, Illinois

MAGGIE L. McNULTY, MD
Assistant Professor, Department of Neurology, Rush University Medical Center, Chicago, Illinois

MICHELLE M. MIELKE, PhD
Professor of Epidemiology and Prevention, Professor of Gerontology and Geriatric Medicine, Department of Epidemiology and Prevention, Wake Forest University School of Medicine, Wake Forest, North Carolina

RACHEL ELANA NORRIS, MA, MD
Imagine Healthcare, PLLC, Chicago, Illinois

CESAR OCHOA-LUBINOFF, MD, MPH
Rush University Medical Center, Chicago, Illinois

NICHOLAS DYKMAN OSTERAAS, MD, MS
Department of Neurological Sciences, Division of Cerebrovascular Diseases, Rush University Medical Center, Chicago, Illinois

ROSHNI PATEL, MD, MS
Assistant Professor of Neurological Sciences, Jesse Brown VA Medical Center, Rush University, Chicago, Illinois

DITTE PRIMDAHL, MD
Department of Neurology, Malnati Brain Tumor Institute at the Robert H. Lurie Comprehensive Cancer Center, Feinberg School of Medicine, Northwestern University, Chicago, Illinois

ASHLEY RAEDY, DO
Loyola University Medical Center, Maywood, Illinois

INDIA C. RANGEL, BS
Mayo Clinic Alix School of Medicine, Scottsdale, Arizona

MARIA A. ROSSETTI, PhD
Assistant Professor, Department of Neurology, University of Virginia School of Medicine, Charlottesville, Virginia

STASIA ROUSE, MBChB
Medical Director of Epilepsy, Advocate Lutheran General Hospital, Park Ridge, Illinois

FIDAA SHAIB, MD, FCCP, FAASM
Associate Professor, Medical Director, Baylor Medicine Sleep Center, Department of Medicine, Section of Pulmonary, Critical Care, and Sleep Medicine, Baylor College of Medicine, Houston, Texas

LAUREN SINGER, MD
Department of Neurology, Malnati Brain Tumor Institute at the Robert H. Lurie Comprehensive Cancer Center, Feinberg School of Medicine, Northwestern University, Chicago, Illinois

AMAAL J. STARLING, MD
Associate Professor, Department of Neurology, Mayo Clinic, Scottsdale, Arizona

AIMEN VANOOD, MD
Department of Neurology, Mayo Clinic, Scottsdale, Arizona

Contents

Gender Differences in Intracerebral Hemorrhage 283

Nicholas Dykman Osteraas

Differences exist between genders in intracerebral hemorrhage cause, epidemiology, and outcomes. These gender differences are in part attributable to physiologic differences; however, demographic, social/behavioral risk factors, along with health care system variation and potential family and/or clinician bias play a role as well. These factors vary from region to region and interact, making comprehensive and definitive conclusions regarding sex differences a challenging task. Differences between the genders in intracerebral hemorrhage epidemiology and extensive differences in underlying pathophysiology, intervention, risk factors, and outcome are all discussed.

Neurologic Disorders in Women and Sleep 297

Fidaa Shaib

Sleep disorders in women remain underrecognized and underdiagnosed mainly because of gender bias in researching and characterizing sleep disorders in women. Symptoms of common sleep disorders are frequently missed in the general female population and are expected to be further overlooked because of overlapping symptoms in women with neurologic disorders. Given the bidirectional relationship with sleep and neurologic disorders, it remains critical to be aware of the presentation and impact of sleep disorders in this patient population. This article reviews available data on sleep disorders in women with neurologic disorders and discusses their distinctive features.

Neuroimmunological Disorders: The Gender Effect 315

Edith L. Graham

Multiple sclerosis is a disease that tends to affect women during their childbearing years. Although relapse risk decreases during pregnancy, patients should still be optimized on disease-modifying therapy before and after pregnancy to minimize gaps in treatment. Certain disease-modifying therapies are considered to be safe while breastfeeding. Treatments for other neuroimmunologic disorders such as neuromyelitis optica spectrum disorder, myelin oligodendrocyte glycoprotein antibody-associated disease, neurosarcoidosis, and central nervous system vasculitis may require rituximab before and prednisone or intravenous immunoglobulin therapy during pregnancy.

Neuro-Oncology in Women: Clinical Considerations 331

Lauren Singer, Ditte Primdahl, and Priya Kumthekar

Sex differences play a large role in oncology. It has long been discussed that the incidence of different types of tumors varies by sex, and this holds in neuro-oncology. There are also profound survival sex differences, biologic factors, and treatment effects. This review aims to summarize some of the main sex differences observed in primary brain tumors and goes on to focus specifically on gliomas and meningiomas, as these are two commonly encountered primary brain tumors in clinical practice. Additionally, considerations unique to female individuals, including pregnancy

and breastfeeding, are explored. This review sheds light on many of the unique attributes that must be considered when diagnosing and treating female patients with primary brain tumors in clinical practice.

Sex Differences in Alzheimer's Disease **343**

Neelum T. Aggarwal and Michelle M. Mielke

Reviewing the research presented in this article, it is evident that from an epidemiological perspective, it is important to evaluate the extent to which findings of sex and gender differences in Alzheimer's dementia (AD) are due to differences in longevity, survival bias, and comorbidities. Medical, genetic, psychosocial, and behavioral factors, in addition to hormonal factors, can differentially affect the risk and progression of AD in women versus men. Further, evaluation of sex differences in AD progression and the trajectory of change in cognitive function, neuroimaging, cerebrospinal fluid (CSF), and blood-based biomarkers of AD is needed. Finally, identifying sex differences in AD biomarkers and change across the lifespan is critical for the planning of prevention trials to reduce the risk of developing AD.

Sex-Specific Neurocognitive Impairment **359**

Sharlet A. Anderson and Maria A. Rossetti

This article explores sex-specific neurocognitive impairment. It first defines relevant terms such as gender and sex. Next, it describes the nature of the problem including under-representation of women and other gender and sexual minorities in neuroscience research, including cognitive studies. A biopsychosocial framework is employed to account for structural and social determinants of health in sex/gender-specific neurocognitive impairment. Issues in assessment including the use of gender/sex-specific normative data are also discussed. Lastly, the article covers the current state of research as it relates to sex/gender-specific neurocognitive impairment across a range of medical conditions including neurodegenerative diseases and coronavirus disease-2019.

Sex and Gender Differences in Parkinson's Disease **371**

Roshni Patel and Katie Kompoliti

The lower prevalence of Parkinson disease (PD) in females is not well understood but may be partially explained by sex differences in nigrostriatal circuitry and possible neuroprotective effects of estrogen. PD motor and nonmotor symptoms differ between sexes, and women experience disparities in care including undertreatment with DBS and less access to caregiving. Our knowledge about PD in gender diverse individuals is limited. Future studies should improve our understanding of the role of hormone replacement therapy in PD, address gender-based inequities in PD care and expand our understanding of PD in SGM and marginalized communities.

NEUROLOGIC CLINICS

FORTHCOMING ISSUES

August 2023
Medicolegal Issues in Neurology
Joseph S. Kass and Michael A. Rubin, *Editors*

November 2023
Functional Neurological Disorders
David L. Perez and Sara A. Finkelstein, *Editors*

February 2024
Multiple Sclerosis
Carrie M. Hersh, *Editor*

RECENT ISSUES

February 2023
Outpatient Neurology
Everton A. Edmondson and Doris H. Kung, *Editors*

November 2022
Epilepsy
Steven C. Schachter, *Editor*

August 2022
Imaging of Headache
Sangam Kanekar, *Editor*

ISSUES OF RELATED INTEREST

Neurosurgery Clinics
https://www.neurosurgery.theclinics.com/
Neuroimaging Clinics
https://www.neuroimaging.theclinics.com/
Psychiatric Clinics
https://www.psych.theclinics.com/
Child and Adolescent Psychiatric Clinics
https://www.childpsych.theclinics.com/

Preface

Current State of Sex and Gender Influence in Neurology

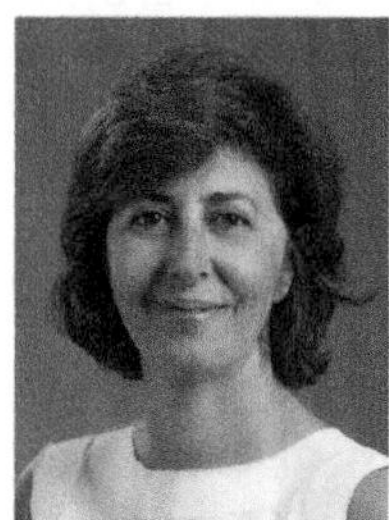

Rima M. Dafer, MD, MPH
Editor

Sex and gender disparities in health care are frequently encountered.[1] The understanding of neurophysiologic differences between men and women and the emerging role of sex-related effect on brain structure and function are very intriguing, and both sex and gender independently play an important role in the prevalence and natural course of common neurologic diseases. Several neurologic conditions affect women differently than men, based on disease susceptibility, prevalence, pathophysiology, as well as clinical symptoms and disease severity. The response to treatment modalities may also differ among sexes, and tailored precision medicine may be necessary to halt disease progression and improve outcome. Despite these known distinctions, the sex effect on various neurologic conditions in women remains poorly studied, and clinical trials do not take into consideration the sex disparities, or the treatment response based on gender.

For instance, differences in symptoms, semiology, risk factors, as well as treatment and outcome have extensively been described in vascular neurologic disorders.[2,3] Certain causes of ischemic strokes are specific to women, with unique risk factors, such as pregnancy and puerperium.[4] Hormonal contraception can also impact the risk of ischemic stroke.[5] Women also have higher risk of aneurysmal subarachnoid hemorrhage compared to men, and poorer outcome after major ischemic strokes.[3]

Also, many neurologic conditions are more prevalent in women, including migraine, multiple sclerosis, and Alzheimer disease (AD). The mechanism behind these differences is complex, varying from the molecular level to the role that sex hormones may play in women.

Migraine is two to three times more prevalent in women than in men and is more frequent and more disabling.[6] Women are likely to report more severe and longer migraine attacks, association with comorbid disorders, and higher burden of

Neurol Clin 41 (2023) xiii–xvi
https://doi.org/10.1016/j.ncl.2022.12.002

disability.[6] While the genetic role may be a major determinant in the sex disparities, such effect is not clearly understood. The disease expression during ovulation, menstruation, and pregnancy suggests that migraine in women may be in part driven by the effects of sex hormones.[7] Migraine treatments and prevention strategies should take into consideration such disease disparity and the role of the sex hormones in the disease symptoms.[8]

Similarly, multiple sclerosis and other autoimmune conditions are more prevalent in women, with variability in clinical presentations and fluctuation of clinical symptoms associated with sex hormones.[9] Management strategies of these neurologic conditions are complex around pregnancy, including risks of potential teratogenicity; therefore, family planning and counseling are important when treating patients with autoimmune conditions who wish to conceive.[10]

Sex dimorphism has also been identified in primary malignant brain neoplasm, which also affects management approaches and treatment outcome.[11]

AD is more prevalent in women, with sex differences in symptoms mainly cognitive and psychiatric symptoms and disease progression. These disparities are crucial for early disease detection and precision treatment implementation.[12]

There is also a growing recognition of sex and gender disparity in sleep-related disorders, with women reporting more sleep disruption,[13] while men have higher incidence of obstructive sleep apnea.[14] In addition, hormonal fluctuations may increase the incidence of sleep disorders during pregnancy, affecting the quality of life of the mother and endangering the fetus' development. These hormonal effects also affect the women's quality of life perimenopausally.

Other common neurologic conditions, such as Parkinson disease (PD) and autism, are less prevalent in women. Women have different semiology[15] and tend to experience more side effects to current PD medications.[16] Autism spectrum disorder disproportionally affects males, with differences in presentations and more camouflaging in females than males.[17] These gender variations in clinical presentation delay timely diagnosis of autism in females.[18]

Sex differences in seizure susceptibility are well known although poorly investigated, with higher susceptibility and incidence of epilepsy among men, and sex-specific epilepsy in women associated with menstruation, pregnancy, and menopause.[19] Clinicians should be cautious when treating women with seizure disorders, as several antiseizure drugs may interact with hormonal contraception, causing unplanned pregnancies and potential teratogenicity.

In this special issue, we intend to provide an up-to-date review of sex- and gender-related differences in the most common neurologic disorders, including migraine, autism, sleep disorder, epilepsy, stroke, multiple sclerosis and other autoimmune conditions, neuro-oncology, movement disorders, and neurodegenerative disorders. We also address gender disparities in neurology training, and specific challenges that women as caregivers face while caring for patients with a neurologic condition, whether in a professional setting, such as the challenges encountered during the COVID-19 pandemic, or in the personal setting, as caregivers to family members with disabling or progressive neurologic conditions. Despite the increased proportion of women in medicine over the past several decades, women physicians continue to face challenges during their medical training. Women neurologists constantly struggle with work-life balance, which was accentuated during the COVID-19 pandemic, when many women physicians had to adjust their work schedules to care for home-staying children and family members. Overall, the persistent disparities in career development significant impact the ability of women physicians to focus on scholarly activities, research projects, speakership engagements, and leadership opportunities.

In summary, in this special issue, we hope to highlight sex disparity in common neurologic conditions, and we review differences in epidemiology, pathophysiology, clinical presentation, disease progression, and response to treatment. We aim to increase awareness of sex- and gender-based variations in these disease courses. We recommend that clinical trials take into consideration sex- and gender-specific data to help guide clinicians toward precision medicine.

Rima M. Dafer, MD, MPH
Department of Neurological Sciences
Rush University Medical Center
1725 West Harrison Street, POB 1121
Chicago, IL 60612, USA

E-mail address:
Rima_dafer@rush.edu

REFERENCES

1. Mauvais-Jarvis F, Bairey Merz N, Barnes PJ, et al. Sex and gender: modifiers of health, disease, and medicine. Lancet 2020;396(10250):565–82. https://doi.org/10.1016/S0140-6736(20)31561-0.
2. Branyan TE, Sohrabji F. Sex differences in stroke co-morbidities. Exp Neurol 2020;332:113384. https://doi.org/10.1016/j.expneurol.2020.113384.
3. Bushnell CD, Chaturvedi S, Gage KR, et al. Sex differences in stroke: challenges and opportunities. J Cereb Blood Flow Metab 2018;38(12):2179–91. https://doi.org/10.1177/0271678X18793324.
4. Kapral MK, Bushnell C. Stroke in women. Stroke 2021;52(2):726–8. https://doi.org/10.1161/STROKEAHA.120.033233.
5. Christensen H, Bushnell C. Stroke in women. Continuum (Minneap Minn) 2020;26(2):363–85. https://doi.org/10.1212/CON.0000000000000836.
6. Vetvik KG, MacGregor EA. Sex differences in the epidemiology, clinical features, and pathophysiology of migraine. Lancet Neurol 2017;16(1):76–87. https://doi.org/10.1016/S1474-4422(16)30293-9.
7. Burch R. Epidemiology and treatment of menstrual migraine and migraine during pregnancy and lactation: a narrative review. Headache 2020;60(1):200–16. https://doi.org/10.1111/head.13665.
8. Rossi MF, Tumminello A, Marconi M, et al. Sex and gender differences in migraines: a narrative review. Neurol Sci 2022;43(9):5729–34. https://doi.org/10.1007/s10072-022-06178-6.
9. Angeloni B, Bigi R, Bellucci G, et al. A case of double standard: sex differences in multiple sclerosis risk factors. Int J Mol Sci 2021;22(7):3696–707.
10. Krysko KM, Graves JS, Dobson R, et al. Sex effects across the lifespan in women with multiple sclerosis. Ther Adv Neurol Disord 2020;13:1–30.
11. Carrano A, Juarez JJ, Incontri D, et al. Sex-specific differences in glioblastoma. Cells 2021;10(7):1783–805.
12. Nebel RA, Aggarwal NT, Barnes LL, et al. Understanding the impact of sex and gender in Alzheimer's disease: a call to action. Alzheimers Dement 2018;14(9):1171–83. https://doi.org/10.1016/j.jalz.2018.04.008.
13. Suh S, Cho N, Zhang J. Sex differences in insomnia: from epidemiology and etiology to intervention. Curr Psychiatry Rep 2018;20(9):69. https://doi.org/10.1007/s11920-018-0940-9.

14. Bonsignore MR, Saaresranta T, Riha RL. Sex differences in obstructive sleep apnoea. Eur Respir Rev 2019;28(154):154–65.
15. Crispino P, Gino M, Barbagelata E, et al. Gender differences and quality of life in Parkinson's disease. Int J Environ Res Public Health 2020;18(1):198–211.
16. Vaidya B, Dhamija K, Guru P, et al. Parkinson's disease in women: mechanisms underlying sex differences. Eur J Pharmacol 2021;895:173862. https://doi.org/10.1016/j.ejphar.2021.173862.
17. Ruigrok ANV, Lai MC. Sex/gender differences in neurology and psychiatry: autism. Handb Clin Neurol 2020;175:283–97. https://doi.org/10.1016/B978-0-444-64123-6.00020-5.
18. Lai MC, Szatmari P. Sex and gender impacts on the behavioural presentation and recognition of autism. Curr Opin Psychiatry 2020;33(2):117–23. https://doi.org/10.1097/YCO.0000000000000575.
19. Reddy DS. Brain structural and neuroendocrine basis of sex differences in epilepsy. Handb Clin Neurol 2020;175:223–33. https://doi.org/10.1016/B978-0-444-64123-6.00016-3.

Migraine and the Gender Divide

Aimen Vanood, MD[a,1], India C. Rangel, BS[b,1], Amaal J. Starling, MD[a,1,*]

KEYWORDS

• Migraine • Headache • Pain • Female

KEY POINTS

- Migraine is the leading cause of disability in woman under the age of 50. It is highly prevalent and disabling.
- Sex hormones play a prominent role in migraine pathophysiology and are likely one reason for sex differences in migraine prevalence, symptoms, and treatment response.
- The management of migraine includes risk reduction through modifications of daily activities, acute treatment for individual attacks, and preventive treatment to reduce attack frequency.
- Migraine prevention should be offered to patients experiencing four or more migraine headache days per month in efforts to improve function and reduce disability.
- Diseases that disproportionately affect women have higher levels of stigma. The reduction of stigma combined with therapeutic advancements will overcome barriers to care in migraine.

INTRODUCTION

Migraine affects more than 10% of the US population, with higher global prevalence estimates. Chronic migraine, defined as 15 or more headache days per month with at least 8 days with migraine features, impacts 1% to 2% of the world population.[1] Migraine is a leading cause of global disability[2] but also an invisible disease that disproportionately impacts women.[3] There is increasing evidence to suggest sex hormones play a role in migraine pathophysiology.[4] Sex differences have important implications in clinical care, from treatment to disease-related stigma.

EPIDEMIOLOGY

Incidence

The estimated migraine incidence is approximately 8.1 per 1000 person-years.[1,5,6] The estimated lifetime incidence of migraine by age of onset peaks later in women

[a] Department of Neurology, Mayo Clinic, Scottsdale, AZ, USA; [b] Mayo Clinic Alix School of Medicine, Scottsdale, AZ, USA
[1] Present address: 13400 East Shea Boulevard, Scottsdale, AZ 85259.
* Corresponding author.
E-mail address: starling.amaal@mayo.edu

Neurol Clin 41 (2023) 231–247
https://doi.org/10.1016/j.ncl.2023.01.002
0733-8619/23/

(20 to 24 years) at 18.2 per 1000 person-years, and earlier in men (15 to 19 years) at 6.2 per 1000 person-years. Studies have consistently shown a higher incidence in women compared with men.[7–9]

Prevalence

Twelve percent of the US population is affected by migraine (18% of women and 6% of men).[1] More recent estimates replicate these findings, suggesting US migraine prevalence has remained stable over the past three decades.[10,11] Worldwide, the highest prevalence was found in the European Union (35%) and the lowest in China (9%).[6] This range may have been observed because migraine diagnostic criteria varied across studies.

Global Burden

The Global Burden of Disease Study revealed that in terms of years lived with disability, migraine ranks second overall. In women under 50 years of age, however, migraine was the leading cause of disability.[12,13]

Migraine is often considered a women's disease, due to female predominance and because women may experience more debilitating symptoms.[3,14] Migraine attacks are longer for women, and associated symptoms, such as nausea and sensory sensitivities, are more commonly reported by women.[9] There is an association between migraine and menstruation, suggesting a connection between biological sex hormones and migraine.[9,15,16] Although it is clear that migraine has a higher incidence, prevalence, and burden in women, it remains poorly understood. A deeper understanding of the pathophysiology of migraine and the influence of sex hormones, genetics, and other internal and external factors will lead to these answers.

PATHOPHYSIOLOGY

Cortical Spreading Depression and Trigeminovascular System

Migraine physiology involves cortical spreading depression (CSD) and the trigeminovascular system (TVS). CSD is a self-propagating wave of hyperactivity (depolarization) followed by inhibition (depression) that is the neurophysiological correlate of migraine aura.[17] Migraine aura consists of fully reversible focal neurologic symptoms that typically precede the pain phase of a migraine attack. Symptoms are typically visual, sensory, or speech. CSD begins in a focal cortical area, typically corresponding to the localization of the aura symptoms, and spreads contiguously across the cortex. The trigger for the initiation of CSD is unclear.[18] This wave leads to the opening of various ion channels, releasing pro-inflammatory mediators, including kappa-B, nitrous oxide (NO), substance P, and calcitonin gene-related peptide (CGRP). These diffuse to the surface of the cortex, causing neurogenic inflammation, vasodilation, plasma cell extravasation, and mast cell degranulation. This stimulates trigeminal afferents to the trigeminal nucleus caudalis (TNC) which is particularly involved in nociception. Projections from this nucleus travel to the thalamus and sensory cortex, allowing one to perceive the "pain" of migraine. Stimulation of the trigeminal nerve causes further release of pro-inflammatory mediators, propagating nociception and creating a state of sensitization where the threshold for depolarization is lowered. This promotes the increased sensitivity to light, sound, and other sensory stimuli during a migraine attack. CGRP plays an important role in migraine pathophysiology through TVS sensitization and neurogenic inflammation.[19,20]

Hormonal Influences

Sex hormones play a prominent role in migraine pathophysiology and are likely one reason for sex differences in migraine prevalence, symptoms, and treatment response.[4]

- Ovarian hormone receptors are present in the TVS.[21]
- Estrogen lowers the threshold for CSD, promotes nociception at the level of the TNC, and modulates the release of CGRP.[22,23]
- Women have increased migraine incidence after menarche and during perimenopause, but the decreased incidence in premenarche and menopause.[21] Migraine attacks are less frequent during pregnancy.[24]
- Men with migraine have higher estradiol levels when compared with men without migraine.[25]
- Patients receiving estrogen therapy for male-to-female transition developed migraine attacks.[26] In another study of patients receiving androgen antagonists and estrogen, migraine prevalence was similar to women of the female sex at birth.[27]

Based on clinical observations and the aforementioned studies, estrogen and its associated fluctuations are a strong trigger for migraine. Conversely, progesterone serves as a protective factor.[28] Progesterone has no impact on the threshold for CSD and decreases TVS activation.[29]

One subtype of migraine observed exclusively in women is menstrual migraine (MM), either pure MM or menstrually related migraine. In this migraine subtype, recurrent attacks occur 2 days before or 3 days after the onset of menses.[30] If attacks occur only during that time of vulnerability, it is a pure MM. If it occurs around menses and at other times of the cycle, it is a menstrually related migraine. Symptoms are typically more painful and disabling than non-MM attacks.[31] Work-related disability is more common in MM.[32,33] Interestingly, the onset of MM attacks is triggered by the drop in estrogen during the luteal phase. Women with migraine were found to have a faster decline in estradiol during the luteal phase when compared with women without migraine. Thus, it is not low estrogen levels, but rather the abrupt withdrawal that is suspected to trigger MM attacks.[34] Intramuscular injections of estradiol during the late luteal phase delayed the onset of an MM attack by 3 to 9 days.[35] Surgical menopause is associated with worsening migraine, even with add-back hormones, although physiologic menopause otherwise yields improvement.[33] This is poorly understood.

Genetics

Migraine is commonly familial; however, genome-wide association studies have not discovered genetic differences with large effect sizes.[36] In population studies, about 38 genomic loci have been associated with migraine.[37] In addition, a few rare migraine syndromes, like familial hemiplegic migraine, are associated with single gene mutations that are helpful to understand the pathophysiology of migraine.[38] This type of genetic diversity speaks to the pathophysiologic diversity that is likely present in patients, providing a hypothetical reason for differences in the phenotypic presentation of migraine and treatment responsiveness.

Vascular Associations

Migraine is a vascular risk factor, particularly in women.[39,40] Migraine with aura (MwA) confers an increased risk of ischemic stroke (IS) in women.[41] According to the Women's Health Study, women with MwA have higher odds of cardiovascular disease (CVD) and myocardial infarction.[42,43] Smoking and estrogen-containing oral contraceptive pills (OCP) use increase IS and CVD risk by seven-fold in women with MwA.[44,45] On their own, combined OCPs increase the risk of IS by sixfold.[46] Estrogen has prothrombotic effects on the coagulation cascade[47] Thus, estrogen-containing

OCPs are typically not recommended in patients with MwA.[48] MwA patients also have a higher prevalence of patent foramen ovale (PFO); those with migraine without aura have a PFO prevalence similar to non-migraine patients. For young patients who suffer cryptogenic strokes, migraine is more common in those with PFO.[49]

Imaging Findings

A longitudinal study following patients with migraine-like symptoms for over two decades found that those with MwA are more likely to have infarct-like lesions on magnetic resonance imaging. In women specifically, when comparing those with MwA to those without migraine, cerebellar infarct-like lesions are more likely. This predilection is not observed in men.[50] In a prospective study that followed migraine patients with brain lesions over 9 years, a greater proportion of women had progression of deep white matter hyperintense lesions. In multivariate logistic regression analysis, migraine was independently associated with the progression of these lesions. Men did not have progression.[51] Compared with men, women with migraine are more likely to have a thicker posterior insula, an area involved in nociception and pain processing.[52] Although multiple sex differences in imaging have been identified, these are solely associations with minimal data regarding causality.

TREATMENT

Management of migraine includes risk reduction through modifications of daily activities, acute treatment for individual attacks, and preventive treatment to reduce attack frequency and severity.

Lifestyle changes or adjustments to daily habits can reduce migraine-related disability and improve function through reduced frequency and severity. Structured counseling using the mnemonic SEEDS (Sleep habits, Exercise weekly, Eat regularly, Diary maintenance, and Stress management) may be useful.[53] The overarching theme is to maintain consistency in sleep-wake timing, exercise, and meals. Stress management techniques including mindfulness and meditation may be helpful for overall well-being and migraine.[54] Behavioral techniques including biofeedback and cognitive behavioral therapy (CBT) are evidence-based preventive treatment options for migraine.[55,56]

Acute Treatment

Effective acute treatment reduces symptom burden and improves disability during an attack.[57] Acute treatment is more effective when used at the onset of a migraine attack. Ineffective treatment can lead to disease chronification and increased disability.[58]

Options for acute treatment (**Table 1**) include non-specific and migraine-specific medications. Non-specific medications include acetaminophen, nonsteroidal anti-inflammatory drugs (NSAIDs), and combination analgesics (acetaminophen-aspirin-caffeine-containing compounds). Migraine-specific medications include triptans, ergotamine derivatives, gepants, and lasmiditan. Non-specific acute treatment can be effective for some patients especially if attacks are mild to moderate in intensity. However, migraine-specific medications are associated with improved pain and function.[59] Triptans, $5HT_{1B/D/F}$ receptor agonists, include sumatriptan, almotriptan, eletriptan, frovatriptan, naratriptan, rizatriptan, and zolmitriptan.[60] Triptans are well tolerated, but for some patients they can be ineffective, poorly tolerated, or, due to vasoconstrictive properties, contraindicated in patients with severe vascular diseases.[61] Gepants are CGRP receptor antagonists (ubrogepant and rimegepant) found

Table 1
Acute migraine treatment of individual attacks

	Class	Medications
Non-specific acute treatment	Nonsteroidal anti-inflammatory drugs (NSAIDs)	Aspirin; diclofenac; ibuprofen; Naproxen sodium
	Non-NSAID analgesics	Acetaminophen
	Combination analgesics	Acetaminophen-aspirin-caffeine
	Anti-emetics	Metoclopramide; prochlorperazine; promethazine
Migraine-specific acute treatment	Triptans	Sumatriptan; almotriptan; eletriptan; frovatriptan; naratriptan; rizatriptan; zolmitriptan
	Ergot derivatives	Dihydroergotamine mesylate; ergotamine
	Gepants	Ubrogepant; rimegepant
	Ditans	Lasmiditan

Summary of medications used for the acute treatment of migraine attacks.

to be effective for acute treatment with good tolerability.[62] Lasmiditan is a 5 HT $_{1F}$ receptor agonist found to be effective for acute migraine treatment without any vasoconstrictive properties, although sedation is a potential side effect.[63] Dopaminergic antiemetics, including metoclopramide, prochlorperazine, chlorpromazine, and promethazine, are probably effective for the acute treatment of migraine.[64] These antiemetics can be used as a standalone treatment or combined with nonspecific or migraine-specific acute treatment for synergistic effects on pain and nausea. Opioids have limited evidence in acute migraine treatment.[59] In addition, there are several noninvasive neuromodulation devices, including external trigeminal nerve stimulation, supraorbital and occipital nerve stimulation, single-pulse transcranial magnetic stimulation, noninvasive vagus nerve stimulation, and conditioned pain modulation, that have shown efficacy, tolerability, and safety for the acute treatment of migraine.[65] Notably, overuse of most acute medications, defined as 10 to 15 or more days per month depending on the medication, may contribute to a complication of high-frequency migraine called medication overuse headache (MOH).[30] MOH is a secondary headache disorder associated with the overuse of acute medications. Initiating migraine prevention is essential in these cases.[66]

Preventive Treatment

Prevention reduces the frequency, severity, and duration of migraine attacks.[67] Migraine prevention should be offered to patients experiencing four or more migraine headache days per month with (1) functional impairment, (2) inefficacy or poor tolerability of acute treatment options, and/or (3) patient preference.

There are both nonspecific and migraine-specific preventive treatment options (**Table 2**). Nutraceuticals, including magnesium,[68] riboflavin, and coenzyme Q10 are well-tolerated supplements that can be used for prevention.[69] In terms of prescription oral medications, antihypertensives, antidepressants, and anticonvulsants have shown efficacy or were found to be probably effective (see **Table 2**). Start at a low dose and titrate slowly to the goal dose. Persistence at the goal dose for 8 to 12 weeks is necessary to determine the benefit. These oral medications can be effective for

Table 2
Preventive migraine treatment

	Class	Medications
Non-specific preventive treatment	Nutraceuticals	Magnesium; riboflavin; Coenzyme Q10; feverfew
	Antihypertensives: beta blockers	Metoprolol; propranolol
	Antihypertensives: other	Candesartan; lisinopril;
	Antidepressants	Amitriptyline; venlafaxine
	Anticonvulsants	Divalproex sodium; topiramate
	Neurotoxin	OnabotulinumtoxinA
	Other	Cyproheptadine
Migraine-specific preventive treatment	Gepants	Atogepant; rimegepant
	CGRP-targeting monoclonal antibodies	Erenumab; eptinezumab; Fremanezumab; galcanezumab

Summary of medications used for the prevention of migraine.

some patients. However, many discontinue these options within the first year of treatment, likely due to inefficacy or side effects.[70] In contrast, onabotulinumtoxinA injections for the preventive treatment of chronic migraine are effective, well-tolerated, and have high rates of adherence.[71]

Anti-CGRP medications are migraine-specific preventive treatment options including both the CGRP monoclonal antibodies and select gepants. For prevention, atogepant taken daily or rimegepant taken every other day is effective and typically well tolerated, except for potential constipation.[72,73] CGRP monoclonal antibodies are effective and well-tolerated for the preventive treatment of both episodic and chronic migraine.[74] Therapeutic monoclonal antibodies are highly specific, targeting either the CGRP ligand (galcanezumab, fremanezumab, and eptinezumab) or the CGRP receptor (erenumab). In addition, monoclonal antibodies have a long half-life, allowing for infrequent dosing. Frequency of administration depends on the medication, with subcutaneous injections monthly or every 3 months and intravenous infusions every 3 months. Likely due to target specificity, CGRP monoclonal antibodies had very low clinical trial dropout rates from adverse events, suggesting good tolerability. Side effect profiles are limited to constipation (erenumab) and injection site reactions with subcutaneous injections. Clinically, these treatment options have shown a robust response in a subset of patients, excellent tolerability, and reduced frequency of administration. CGRP monoclonal antibodies have higher rates of adherence compared with oral medications for the prevention of migraine.[75]

Various studies have evaluated sex differences in prescribing patterns. Mean annual costs of preventative medications were higher overall in women than men.[76] However, the MAST study showed that men are more likely than women to use prescription preventative medications (13.1% in men vs 10.6% in women).[77] Women are more likely to use complementary medicine, such as acupuncture, massage, or yoga, as adjuncts to management.[78] However, when preventive medications were used, a greater proportion of women required later lines of treatment when compared with men.[79]

Currently, no studies evaluate sex differences in efficacy and outcomes of anti-CGRP medications. Anti-CGRP medications hold a theoretic vascular risk; human studies are still pending to support this hypothesis.[21] It is important to note that the most common pathophysiological mechanism of myocardial infarction (MI) differs in men and women. In men, MI is most commonly from occlusion of the proximal coronary circulation. In women however, vasospasm of the smaller vessels within the coronary circulation is the most common cause of MI.[80] CGRP promotes vasodilation of these smaller vessels, which suggests medications that alter CGRP levels could pose different risks in men and women.[81] Some studies have investigated short-term vascular effects. One small study ($n = 7$) did not observe any change in cerebral blood flow or middle cerebral artery diameter 3 h after CGRP inhibitor infusion.[82] Another study evaluated the impact of erenumab on stable angina. Participants were randomized to placebo versus erenumab infusion and completed an exercise stress test 30 min after administration. There was no difference in time to exercise-induced angina or time to onset of ST depression between the erenumab and placebo cohorts.[83] However, these studies did not evaluate the long-term impact of anti-CGRP medications on vascular risk. This is still unknown.

Treatment of Menstrual Migraine

The acute treatment of MM is similar to non-MM migraine. Multiple studies have shown that sumatriptan, zolmitriptan, rizatriptan, and naratriptan confer immediate pain relief (within 24 h) in a greater proportion of MM patients when compared with placebo.[84,85] For more refractory attacks resistant to triptans alone, a combination of a triptan plus an NSAID or steroid or anti-emetic may be effective.[86–88]

Typical acute medications can also be used for short-term MM prevention. A 6-day regimen of frovatriptan 2.5 mg once daily or twice daily started 2 days before anticipated MM onset increased the number of headache-free perimenstrual periods and reduced the severity of breakthrough attacks compared with placebo.[89] A longer study spanning over 12 to 15 months found similar results with good tolerability and no medication overuse headache.[90] Sumatriptan 25 mg three times per day started 2 to 3 days before menses and continued 5 days after preventing MM attacks in 52.4% of 126 menstrual cycles.[91] Several other triptans have shown efficacy for short-term MM prevention using two or three times per day dosing started in the days before menses and continued for the next 5 to 7 days.[92–94] NSAIDs, such as naproxen, and supplements, such as magnesium, have also shown efficacy as short-term prevention in MM.[95–97] Hormonal interventions that reduce estrogen fluctuations have been effective in some studies. Estradiol gel, used as short-term prevention, can decrease the severity of MM attacks.[98,99] Extended cycle combination hormonal contraceptives may reduce the severity of MM.[100,101]

Pregnancy and Breastfeeding

New onset headache or significant worsening of preexisting headache disorder including migraine in the setting of pregnancy is a potential red flag due to an increased risk of a secondary headache disorder or pregnancy complication with headache as a symptom.[102] After a secondary headache has been ruled out, the management of migraine during pregnancy can be challenging, as many treatments are contraindicated or not studied in the setting of pregnancy and breastfeeding.[103] For this reason, nonpharmacological approaches, including acupuncture, biofeedback, and other behavioral interventions, are first-line options.[104] In addition, migraine often improves during the second and third trimester, limiting the need for pharmacologic intervention for many women.

Regarding acute pharmacologic management, acetaminophen is the safest option for acute migraine treatment during pregnancy. This can be combined with oral metoclopramide for a synergistic benefit. Intravenous metoclopramide 10 to 20 mg has been studied as a safe migraine adjunct during the first trimester and has shown efficacy in patients who do not respond to initial treatment with acetaminophen.[105] Triptans can be used for acute treatment. A meta-analysis of acute migraine treatments during pregnancy revealed that, when compared with the general population, triptan use in pregnancy was not associated with an increased risk of fetal malformations, low birth weight, or preterm birth.[106] NSAID use in the first and third trimesters is associated with adverse fetal outcomes. Aspirin confers greater risk when used in the third trimester.[107] Ergots are contraindicated due to teratogenicity.[107] Gepants and lasmiditan have limited data at present, and thus are not recommended in the setting of pregnancy. Lidocaine peripheral nerve blocks and neuromodulation devices are also well-tolerated, likely safe options in the setting of pregnancy. [33,104,108]

For prevention, supplements, including magnesium, riboflavin, and coenzyme Q10 can be taken.[104,109] Memantine has shown efficacy in migraine prevention and can be used safely during pregnancy.[16] Beta-blockers, particularly metoprolol, can be safely used for migraine prevention during pregnancy, but must be tapered off 2 to 3 days before delivery to reduce the risk of fetal hypoglycemia, bradycardia, and hypotension. Amitriptyline in doses less than 50 mg can also be taken; doses higher than this may be linked to fetal limb deformities. This needs to be tapered off 3 to 4 weeks before delivery, to reduce the risk of fetal hyperexcitability and difficulty suckling as a newborn.[110] Lidocaine peripheral nerve blocks may have particular utility in this patient population.[33] The safety of onabotulinumtoxinA during pregnancy was initially unclear. A 24-year retrospective review of onabotulinumtoxinA injections showed no significant increase in fetal malformations when compared with the general population, thus may be an option for some pregnant patients.[111] Owing to teratogenicity, topiramate and valproate are contraindicated.[112] In terms of the novel anti-CGRP medications, their safety during pregnancy is uncertain and, due to the long half-life, discontinuation is recommended 5 to 6 months before conception.[113]

Breastfeeding poses similar treatment considerations. Acetaminophen, ibuprofen, and diclofenac are considered safe acute treatment options. Aspirin is to be avoided due to concern for Reyes syndrome in the infant.[114] Triptans can be used for acute treatment; sumatriptan is most commonly used but eletriptan is more highly protein-bound and least likely to transfer to breast milk.[115] Metoclopramide is safe to use in breastfeeding patients and has the added benefit of stimulating milk production. Conversely, promethazine and diphenhydramine can decrease milk production. Prochlorperazine is avoided as it can cause infant apnea and sedation. Ergots are contraindicated. For prevention, propranolol is preferred because it has low circulating levels. Topiramate is generally well-tolerated.[104] Amitriptyline can be used for prevention but may cause infant sedation.[16] Zonisamide, atenolol, and tizanidine should be avoided. OnabotulinumtoxinA injections, nerve blocks, and neuromodulation devices are all effective and well-tolerated options during lactation.[109]

COMORBIDITIES

Migraine is associated with comorbidities that impact disease severity (**Table 3**). Psychiatric conditions, such as mood disorders, anxiety, and stress disorders (posttraumatic stress disorder and panic disorder) are often reported more in women with migraine.[116] Sleep disorders, including insomnia, obstructive sleep apnea (OSA), and restless leg syndrome (RLS) are also comorbid with migraine.[117] Of these, insomnia[118] and RLS[119] occur more commonly in women. CBT for insomnia has been shown to improve migraine frequency and intensity.[120]

Table 3
Migraine comorbidities

Migraine Comorbidity	More Common in Women
Psychiatric disorders	
Mood disorders Bipolar disorder Depression	X
Anxiety disorders	X
Stress disorders Posttraumatic stress disorder Panic disorder	X
Sleep disorders	
Insomnia	X
Obstructive sleep apnea (OSA)	
Restless leg syndrome (RLS)	X
Vascular disorders	
Myocardial infarction	
Stroke	
Obesity	
Raynaud's phenomenon	X
Chronic inflammatory disorders	
Multiple sclerosis	X
Rheumatoid arthritis	X
Systemic lupus erythematosus (SLE)	X
Chronic pain disorders	
Irritable bowel syndrome	X
Fibromyalgia	X
Temporomandibular joint dysfunction	X
Other	
Epilepsy	
Asthma	
Allergic rhinitis	

Commonly reported migraine comorbidities that are also more prevalent in women.

Migraine is also associated with chronic inflammatory conditions, such as multiple sclerosis (MS), rheumatoid arthritis, and Raynaud's phenomenon (RP), which are also more prevalent in women.[1,117,121–123] Low levels of CGRP are found in RP, and thus CGRP-inhibiting medications could worsen RP. In a recent study, out 169 patients started on CGRP monoclonal antibody, 5 patients experienced worsening of preexisting RP, and 4 developed new onset RP.[124] Another study reported 99 cases of RP after use of CGRP-targeting medications.[125] Thus, caution should be taken when prescribing anti-CGRP medications to patients with RP.

Other migraine comorbidities include chronic pain conditions, such as fibromyalgia,[126] temporomandibular joint disorder (TMD),[127] and irritable bowel syndrome (IBS),[128] all of which are more prevalent in women. Often optimization of one chronic pain condition can improve migraine outcomes.[129–132]

STIGMA AND ADVOCACY

Stigma is a major barrier to adequate funding, research, diagnosis, and treatment in migraine.[133,134] Diseases that affect women disproportionately often have higher levels of stigma. Stigma affects patient-doctor relationships and hinders research advancements by influencing funding and recruitment.[135,136] There are two types of stigma: internal and external. Internal stigma, occurring when patients believe outside stereotypes, can prevent patients from seeking treatment. People living with migraine are less likely to seek treatment due to a fear of stigmatization.[137] External stigma occurs when outside stereotypes change others' perception and treatment of those living with migraine. After a search of the top image-searching websites, migraine was most commonly depicted as a thin, white woman with her eyes closed in pain and hands on her temples.[138] Frailty and weakness are common themes in the public image of migraine, rather than being a resilient fighter of a chronic disease. In addition to images, language can also perpetuate stigma. Many chronic diseases have moved toward person-first language, so instead of "migraineur," saying person with migraine is less stigmatizing.[133] We need to reframe the disease of migraine, empower our patients living with migraine, use nonstigmatizing person-first language, and continue the work on legislative advocacy for policy and funding changes to improve patient care and reduce the burden of disease. Hopefully, the reduction of stigma combined with therapeutic advancements will help overcome barriers in migraine care including speaking with the clinician about migraine symptoms, getting the accurate diagnosis, and receiving evidence-based treatment.

SUMMARY

Migraine is a chronic neurologic disease that disproportionately impacts women in terms of symptom frequency and severity, associated disability, increased comorbidities, and disease-related stigma. Pathophysiologic discoveries have led to a recent expansion in our treatment toolbox for both acute and preventive treatment of migraine. However, the stigma of migraine is still a barrier to care. Advocacy can reframe the disease of migraine, reduce stigma, and increase access to evidence-based care.

CLINICS CARE POINTS

- Migraine pathophysiology is influenced by sex hormones, particularly changes in estrogen levels. In women, migraine onset and severity can correlate with the menstrual cycle, with migraine attacks declining during menopause.
- Optimization of the acute treatment of migraine reduces symptoms, relieves burden, and likely lowers the risk of migraine chronification.
- Have a low threshold to initiate migraine prevention to reduce the risk of migraine chronification. Migraine prevention should be offered to patients having 4 or more migraine days per month with some impairment of function.
- Novel treatment options including anti-calcitonin gene-related peptide medications have shown good efficacy and tolerability with minimal side effects, however, long-term effects is an area of ongoing research.

DISCLOSURE

Ms I.C. Rangel has no disclosures. Dr A. Vanood has no disclosures. Dr A.J. Starling has received consulting fees from AbbVie, Allergan, Amgen, Axsome Therapeutics, Everyday Health, Lundbeck, Med-IQ, Medscape, Neurolief, Satsuma, and WebMD.

REFERENCES

1. Burch RC, Buse DC, Lipton RB. Migraine: Epidemiology, Burden, and Comorbidity. Neurol Clin 2019;37(4):631–49.
2. Headache disorders. World Health Organization; 2016. Available at: https://www.ajmc.com/view/migraine-overview-and-summary–of-current-and-emerging-treatment-options. Accessed April 12, 2022.
3. Buse DC, Loder EW, Gorman JA, et al. Sex differences in the prevalence, symptoms, and associated features of migraine, probable migraine and other severe headache: results of the American Migraine Prevalence and Prevention (AMPP) Study. Headache 2013;53(8):1278–99.
4. Schroeder RA, Brandes J, Buse DC, et al. Sex and Gender Differences in Migraine-Evaluating Knowledge Gaps. J Womens Health (Larchmt) 2018; 27(8):965–73.
5. Lyngberg AC, Rasmussen BK, Jørgensen T, et al. Incidence of primary headache: a Danish epidemiologic follow-up study. Am J Epidemiol 2005;161(11): 1066–73.
6. Ashina M, Katsarava Z, Do TP, et al. Migraine: epidemiology and systems of care. Lancet 2021;397(10283):1485–95.
7. Allais G, Chiarle G, Sinigaglia S, et al. Gender-related differences in migraine. Neurol Sci 2020;41(Suppl 2):429–36.
8. Baykan B, Ertas M, Karlı N, et al. Migraine incidence in 5 years: a population-based prospective longitudinal study in Turkey. J Headache Pain 2015;16:103.
9. Vetvik KG, MacGregor EA. Sex differences in the epidemiology, clinical features, and pathophysiology of migraine. Lancet Neurol 2017;16(1):76–87.
10. Burch R, Rizzoli P, Loder E. The prevalence and impact of migraine and severe headache in the United States: Updated age, sex, and socioeconomic-specific estimates from government health surveys. Headache 2021;61(1):60–8.
11. Burch R, Rizzoli P, Loder E. The Prevalence and Impact of Migraine and Severe Headache in the United States: Figures and Trends From Government Health Studies. Headache 2018;58(4):496–505.
12. Stovner LJ, Hagen K, Linde M, et al. The global prevalence of headache: an update, with analysis of the influences of methodological factors on prevalence estimates. J Headache Pain 2022;23(1):34.
13. Safiri S, Pourfathi H, Eagan A, et al. Global, regional, and national burden of migraine in 204 countries and territories, 1990 to 2019. Pain 2022;163(2): e293–309.
14. Chai NC, Rosenberg JD, Lee Peterlin B. The epidemiology and comorbidities of migraine and tension-type headache. Tech Reg Anesth Pain Manag 2012; 16(1):4–13.
15. MacGregor EA, Frith A, Ellis J, et al. Incidence of migraine relative to menstrual cycle phases of rising and falling estrogen. Neurology 2006;67(12):2154–8.
16. Burch R. Epidemiology and Treatment of Menstrual Migraine and Migraine During Pregnancy and Lactation: A Narrative Review. Headache 2020;60(1): 200–16.
17. Goadsby PJ, Holland PR, Martins-Oliveira M, et al. Pathophysiology of Migraine: A Disorder of Sensory Processing. Physiol Rev 2017;97(2):553–622.
18. Ferrari MD, Goadsby PJ, Burstein R, et al. Migraine. Nat Rev Dis Primers 2022; 8(1):2.
19. Cui Y, Kataoka Y, Watanabe Y. Role of cortical spreading depression in the pathophysiology of migraine. Neurosci Bull 2014;30(5):812–22.

20. Noseda R, Burstein R. Migraine pathophysiology: anatomy of the trigeminovascular pathway and associated neurological symptoms, cortical spreading depression, sensitization, and modulation of pain. Pain 2013;154(Suppl 1):S44–53.
21. de Vries Lentsch S, Rubio-Beltran E, MaassenVanDenBrink A. Changing levels of sex hormones and calcitonin gene-related peptide (CGRP) during a woman's life: Implications for the efficacy and safety of novel antimigraine medications. Maturitas 2021;145:73–7.
22. Eikermann-Haerter K, Kudo C, Moskowitz MA. Cortical spreading depression and estrogen. Headache 2007;47(Suppl 2):S79–85.
23. Bolay H, Berman NE, Akcali D. Sex-related differences in animal models of migraine headache. Headache 2011;51(6):891–904.
24. Aegidius K, Zwart JA, Hagen K, et al. The effect of pregnancy and parity on headache prevalence: the Head-HUNT study. Headache 2009;49(6):851–9.
25. van Oosterhout WPJ, Schoonman GG, van Zwet EW, et al. Female sex hormones in men with migraine. Neurology 2018;91(4):e374–81.
26. Aloisi AM, Bachiocco V, Costantino A, et al. Cross-sex hormone administration changes pain in transsexual women and men. Pain 2007;132(Suppl 1):S60–7.
27. Pringsheim T, Gooren L. Migraine prevalence in male to female transsexuals on hormone therapy. Neurology 2004;63(3):593–4.
28. Martin VT, Wernke S, Mandell K, et al. Defining the relationship between ovarian hormones and migraine headache. Headache 2005;45(9):1190–201.
29. Allais G, Chiarle G, Bergandi F, et al. The use of progestogen-only pill in migraine patients. Expert Rev Neurother 2016;16(1):71–82.
30. Headache Classification Committee of the International Headache S. The International Classification of Headache Disorders, 3rd edition (beta version). Cephalalgia 2013;33(9):629–808.
31. Martin VT. Ovarian hormones and pain response: a review of clinical and basic science studies. Gend Med 2009;6(Suppl 2):168–92.
32. Granella F, Sances G, Allais G, et al. Characteristics of menstrual and nonmenstrual attacks in women with menstrually related migraine referred to headache centres. Cephalalgia 2004;24(9):707–16.
33. Finocchi C, Strada L. Sex-related differences in migraine. Neurol Sci 2014;35(Suppl 1):207–13.
34. Pavlovic JM, Allshouse AA, Santoro NF, et al. Sex hormones in women with and without migraine: Evidence of migraine-specific hormone profiles. Neurology 2016;87(1):49–56.
35. Somerville BW. The role of estradiol withdrawal in the etiology of menstrual migraine. Neurology 1972;22(4):355–65.
36. Nyholt DR, van den Maagdenberg AM. Genome-wide association studies in migraine: current state and route to follow. Curr Opin Neurol 2016;29(3):302–8.
37. Gormley P, Anttila V, Winsvold BS, et al. Meta-analysis of 375,000 individuals identifies 38 susceptibility loci for migraine. Nat Genet 2016;48(8):856–66.
38. Sutherland HG, Griffiths LR. Genetics of Migraine: Insights into the Molecular Basis of Migraine Disorders. Headache 2017;57(4):537–69.
39. Abanoz Y, Gulen Abanoz Y, Gunduz A, et al. Migraine as a risk factor for young patients with ischemic stroke: a case-control study. Neurol Sci 2017;38(4):611–7.
40. Kurth T, Winter AC, Eliassen AH, et al. Migraine and risk of cardiovascular disease in women: prospective cohort study. BMJ 2016;353:i2610.

41. Adelborg K, Szepligeti SK, Holland-Bill L, et al. Migraine and risk of cardiovascular diseases: Danish population based matched cohort study. BMJ 2018; 360:k96.
42. Kurth T, Gaziano JM, Cook NR, et al. Migraine and risk of cardiovascular disease in women. JAMA 2006;296(3):283–91.
43. Kurth T, Schurks M, Logroscino G, et al. Migraine, vascular risk, and cardiovascular events in women: prospective cohort study. BMJ 2008;337:a636.
44. MacClellan LR, Giles W, Cole J, et al. Probable migraine with visual aura and risk of ischemic stroke: the stroke prevention in young women study. Stroke 2007; 38(9):2438–45.
45. Schurks M, Rist PM, Bigal ME, et al. Migraine and cardiovascular disease: systematic review and meta-analysis. BMJ 2009;339:b3914.
46. Champaloux SW, Tepper NK, Monsour M, et al. Use of combined hormonal contraceptives among women with migraines and risk of ischemic stroke. Am J Obstet Gynecol 2017;216(5):489 e481–7.
47. Fazio G, Ferrara F, Barbaro G, et al. Protrhombotic effects of contraceptives. Curr Pharm Des 2010;16(31):3490–6.
48. ACOG Practice Bulletin No. 206. Use of Hormonal Contraception in Women With Coexisting Medical Conditions. Obstet Gynecol 2019;133(2):e128–50.
49. Jamieson DG, Skliut M. Gender considerations in stroke management. Neurol 2009;15(3):132–41.
50. Scher AI, Gudmundsson LS, Sigurdsson S, et al. Migraine headache in middle age and late-life brain infarcts. JAMA 2009;301(24):2563–70.
51. Palm-Meinders IH, Koppen H, Terwindt GM, et al. Structural brain changes in migraine. JAMA 2012;308(18):1889–97.
52. Craig AD. How do you feel–now? The anterior insula and human awareness. Nat Rev Neurosci 2009;10(1):59–70.
53. Robblee J, Starling AJ. SEEDS for success: Lifestyle management in migraine. Cleve Clin J Med 2019;86(11):741–9.
54. Wells RE, O'Connell N, Pierce CR, et al. Effectiveness of Mindfulness Meditation vs Headache Education for Adults With Migraine: A Randomized Clinical Trial. JAMA Intern Med 2021;181(3):317–28.
55. Nestoriuc Y, Martin A. Efficacy of biofeedback for migraine: a meta-analysis. Pain 2007;128(1–2):111–27.
56. Bae JY, Sung HK, Kwon NY, et al. Cognitive Behavioral Therapy for Migraine Headache: A Systematic Review and Meta-Analysis. Medicina (Kaunas) 2021; 58(1):44.
57. Mallick-Searle T, Moriarty M. Unmet needs in the acute treatment of migraine attacks and the emerging role of calcitonin gene-related peptide receptor antagonists: An integrative review. J Am Assoc Nurse Pract 2020;33(6):419–28.
58. Agostoni EC, Barbanti P, Calabresi P, et al. Current and emerging evidence-based treatment options in chronic migraine: a narrative review. J Headache Pain 2019;20(1):92.
59. VanderPluym JH, Halker Singh RB, Urtecho M, et al. Acute Treatments for Episodic Migraine in Adults: A Systematic Review and Meta-analysis. JAMA 2021;325(23):2357–69.
60. Thorlund K, Toor K, Wu P, et al. Comparative tolerability of treatments for acute migraine: A network meta-analysis. Cephalalgia 2017;37(10):965–78.
61. Lipton RB, Buse DC, Serrano D, et al. Examination of unmet treatment needs among persons with episodic migraine: results of the American Migraine Prevalence and Prevention (AMPP) Study. Headache 2013;53(8):1300–11.

62. Holland PR, Goadsby PJ. Targeted CGRP Small Molecule Antagonists for Acute Migraine Therapy. Neurotherapeutics 2018;15(2):304–12.
63. Parikh S. Lasmiditan for acute treatment of migraine. Drugs Today 2021;57(2): 89–100.
64. Tepper SJ. Acute Treatment of Migraine. Neurol Clin 2019;37(4):727–42.
65. Moisset X, Pereira B, Ciampi de Andrade D, et al. Neuromodulation techniques for acute and preventive migraine treatment: a systematic review and meta-analysis of randomized controlled trials. J Headache Pain 2020;21(1):142.
66. Schwedt TJ, Hentz JG, Sahai-Srivastava S, et al. Patient-Centered Treatment of Chronic Migraine With Medication Overuse: A Prospective, Randomized, Pragmatic Clinical Trial. Neurology 2022;98(14):e1409–21.
67. Ailani J, Burch RC, Robbins MS. Board of Directors of the American Headache S. The American Headache Society Consensus Statement: Update on integrating new migraine treatments into clinical practice. Headache 2021;61(7): 1021–39.
68. Dolati S, Rikhtegar R, Mehdizadeh A, et al. The Role of Magnesium in Pathophysiology and Migraine Treatment. Biol Trace Elem Res 2020;196(2):375–83.
69. D'Onofrio F, Raimo S, Spitaleri D, et al. Usefulness of nutraceuticals in migraine prophylaxis. Neurol Sci 2017;38(Suppl 1):117–20.
70. Hepp Z, Dodick DW, Varon SF, et al. Persistence and switching patterns of oral migraine prophylactic medications among patients with chronic migraine: A retrospective claims analysis. Cephalalgia 2017;37(5):470–85.
71. Argyriou AA, Dermitzakis EV, Vlachos GS, et al. Long-term adherence, safety, and efficacy of repeated onabotulinumtoxinA over five years in chronic migraine prophylaxis. Acta Neurol Scand 2022;145(6):676–83.
72. Croop R, Lipton RB, Kudrow D, et al. Oral rimegepant for preventive treatment of migraine: a phase 2/3, randomised, double-blind, placebo-controlled trial. Lancet 2021;397(10268):51–60.
73. Ailani J, Lipton RB, Goadsby PJ, et al. Atogepant for the Preventive Treatment of Migraine. N Engl J Med 2021;385(8):695–706.
74. Deng H, Li GG, Nie H, et al. Efficacy and safety of calcitonin-gene-related peptide binding monoclonal antibodies for the preventive treatment of episodic migraine - an updated systematic review and meta-analysis. BMC Neurol 2020;20(1):57.
75. Varnado OJ, Manjelievskaia J, Ye W, et al. Treatment Patterns for Calcitonin Gene-Related Peptide Monoclonal Antibodies Including Galcanezumab versus Conventional Preventive Treatments for Migraine: A Retrospective US Claims Study. Patient Prefer Adherence 2022;16:821–39.
76. Negro A, Sciattella P, Rossi D, et al. Cost of chronic and episodic migraine patients in continuous treatment for two years in a tertiary level headache Centre. J Headache Pain 2019;20(1):120.
77. Lipton RB, Munjal S, Alam A, et al. Migraine in America Symptoms and Treatment (MAST) Study: Baseline Study Methods, Treatment Patterns, and Gender Differences. Headache 2018;58(9):1408–26.
78. Rhee TG, Harris IM. Gender Differences in the Use of Complementary and Alternative Medicine and Their Association With Moderate Mental Distress in U.S. Adults With Migraines/Severe Headaches. Headache 2017;57(1):97–108.
79. Korolainen MA, Kurki S, Lassenius MI, et al. Burden of migraine in Finland: health care resource use, sick-leaves and comorbidities in occupational health care. J Headache Pain 2019;20(1):13.

80. Humphries KH, Pu A, Gao M, et al. Angina with "normal" coronary arteries: sex differences in outcomes. Am Heart J 2008;155(2):375–81.
81. MaassenVanDenBrink A, Meijer J, Villalon CM, et al. Wiping Out CGRP: Potential Cardiovascular Risks. Trends Pharmacol Sci 2016;37(9):779–88.
82. Petersen KA, Birk S, Lassen LH, et al. The CGRP-antagonist, BIBN4096BS does not affect cerebral or systemic haemodynamics in healthy volunteers. Cephalalgia 2005;25(2):139–47.
83. Depre C, Antalik L, Starling A, et al. A Randomized, Double-Blind, Placebo-Controlled Study to Evaluate the Effect of Erenumab on Exercise Time During a Treadmill Test in Patients With Stable Angina. Headache 2018;58(5):715–23.
84. Allais G, Chiarle G, Sinigaglia S, et al. Menstrual migraine: a review of current and developing pharmacotherapies for women. Expert Opin Pharmacother 2018;19(2):123–36.
85. Maasumi K, Tepper SJ, Kriegler JS, et al. Menstrual Migraine, Review. Headache 2017;57(2):194–208.
86. Mannix LK, Martin VT, Cady RK, et al. Combination treatment for menstrual migraine and dysmenorrhea using sumatriptan-naproxen: two randomized controlled trials. Obstet Gynecol 2009;114(1):106–13.
87. Bigal M, Sheftell F, Tepper S, et al. A randomized double-blind study comparing rizatriptan, dexamethasone, and the combination of both in the acute treatment of menstrually related migraine. Headache 2008;48(9):1286–93.
88. Allais G, Bussone G, Tullo V, et al. Frovatriptan 2.5 mg plus dexketoprofen (25 mg or 37.5 mg) in menstrually related migraine. Subanalysis from a double-blind, randomized trial. Cephalalgia 2015;35(1):45–50.
89. Brandes JL, Poole A, Kallela M, et al. Short-term frovatriptan for the prevention of difficult-to-treat menstrual migraine attacks. Cephalalgia 2009;29(11):1133–48.
90. MacGregor EA, Brandes JL, Silberstein S, et al. Safety and tolerability of short-term preventive frovatriptan: a combined analysis. Headache 2009;49(9):1298–314.
91. Newman LC, Lipton RB, Lay CL, et al. A pilot study of oral sumatriptan as intermittent prophylaxis of menstruation-related migraine. Neurology 1998;51(1):307–9.
92. Tuchman MM, Hee A, Emeribe U, et al. Oral zolmitriptan in the short-term prevention of menstrual migraine: a randomized, placebo-controlled study. CNS Drugs 2008;22(10):877–86.
93. Mannix LK, Savani N, Landy S, et al. Efficacy and tolerability of naratriptan for short-term prevention of menstrually related migraine: data from two randomized, double-blind, placebo-controlled studies. Headache 2007;47(7):1037–49.
94. Marcus DA, Bernstein CD, Sullivan EA, et al. Perimenstrual eletriptan prevents menstrual migraine: an open-label study. Headache 2010;50(4):551–62.
95. Sances G, Martignoni E, Fioroni L, et al. Naproxen sodium in menstrual migraine prophylaxis: a double-blind placebo controlled study. Headache 1990;30(11):705–9.
96. Allais G, Bussone G, De Lorenzo C, et al. Naproxen sodium in short-term prophylaxis of pure menstrual migraine: pathophysiological and clinical considerations. Neurol Sci 2007;28(Suppl 2):S225–8.
97. Facchinetti F, Sances G, Borella P, et al. Magnesium prophylaxis of menstrual migraine: effects on intracellular magnesium. Headache 1991;31(5):298–301.
98. de Lignieres B, Vincens M, Mauvais-Jarvis P, et al. Prevention of menstrual migraine by percutaneous oestradiol. Br Med J 1986;293(6561):1540.

99. MacGregor EA, Frith A, Ellis J, et al. Prevention of menstrual attacks of migraine: a double-blind placebo-controlled crossover study. Neurology 2006;67(12): 2159–63.
100. Coffee AL, Sulak PJ, Hill AJ, et al. Extended cycle combined oral contraceptives and prophylactic frovatriptan during the hormone-free interval in women with menstrual-related migraines. J Womens Health (Larchmt) 2014;23(4):310–7.
101. Sulak P, Willis S, Kuehl T, et al. Headaches and oral contraceptives: impact of eliminating the standard 7-day placebo interval. Headache 2007;47(1):27–37.
102. Robbins MS, Farmakidis C, Dayal AK, et al. Acute headache diagnosis in pregnant women: a hospital-based study. Neurology 2015;85(12):1024–30.
103. LaHue SC, Gelfand AA, Bove RM. Navigating monoclonal antibody use in breastfeeding women: Do no harm or do little good? Neurology 2019;93(15): 668–72.
104. Parikh SK, Delbono MV, Silberstein SD. Managing migraine in pregnancy and breastfeeding. Prog Brain Res 2020;255:275–309.
105. Childress KMS, Dothager C, Gavard JA, et al. Metoclopramide and Diphenhydramine: A Randomized Controlled Trial of a Treatment for Headache in Pregnancy when Acetaminophen Alone Is Ineffective (MAD Headache Study). Am J Perinatol 2018;35(13):1281–6.
106. Dudman DC, Tauqeer F, Kaur M, et al. A systematic review and meta-analyses on the prevalence of pregnancy outcomes in migraine treated patients: a contribution from the IMI2 ConcePTION project. J Neurol 2022;269(2):742–9.
107. Magro I, Nurimba M, Doherty JK. Headache in Pregnancy. Otolaryngol Clin North Am 2022;55(3):681–96.
108. Blech B, Starling AJ. Noninvasive Neuromodulation in Migraine. Curr Pain Headache Rep 2020;24(12):78.
109. Wells RE, Turner DP, Lee M, et al. Managing Migraine During Pregnancy and Lactation. Curr Neurol Neurosci Rep 2016;16(4):40.
110. MacGregor EA. Migraine in pregnancy and lactation. Neurol Sci 2014;35(Suppl 1):61–4.
111. Brin MF, Kirby RS, Slavotinek A, et al. Pregnancy outcomes following exposure to onabotulinumtoxinA. Pharmacoepidemiol Drug Saf 2016;25(2):179–87.
112. Sader E, Rayhill M. Headache in Pregnancy, the Puerperium, and menopause. Semin Neurol 2018;38(6):627–33.
113. Dodick DW. CGRP ligand and receptor monoclonal antibodies for migraine prevention: Evidence review and clinical implications. Cephalalgia 2019;39(3): 445–58.
114. Datta P, Rewers-Felkins K, Kallem RR, et al. Transfer of Low Dose Aspirin Into Human Milk. J Hum Lact 2017;33(2):296–9.
115. Hutchinson S, Marmura MJ, Calhoun A, et al. Use of common migraine treatments in breast-feeding women: a summary of recommendations. Headache 2013;53(4):614–27.
116. Pancheri C, Maraone A, Roselli V, et al. The role of stress and psychiatric comorbidities as targets of non-pharmacological therapeutic approaches for migraine. Riv Psichiatr 2020;55(5):262–8.
117. Klenofsky B, Pace A, Natbony LR, et al. Curr Pain Headache Rep 2019;23(1):1.
118. Suh S, Cho N, Zhang J. Sex Differences in Insomnia: from Epidemiology and Etiology to Intervention. Curr Psychiatry Rep 2018;20(9):69.
119. Seeman MV. Why Are Women Prone to Restless Legs Syndrome? Int J Environ Res Public Health 2020;17(1):368.

120. Tiseo C, Vacca A, Felbush A, et al. Migraine and sleep disorders: a systematic review. J Headache Pain 2020;21(1):126.
121. Fang X, Patel C, Gudesblatt M. Multiple Sclerosis: Clinical Updates in Women's Health Care Primary and Preventive Care Review. Obstet Gynecol 2020;135(3): 757–8.
122. Gerosa M, De Angelis V, Riboldi P, et al. Rheumatoid arthritis: a female challenge. Womens Health (Lond) 2008;4(2):195–201.
123. Zucchi D, Elefante E, Calabresi E, et al. One year in review 2019: systemic lupus erythematosus. Clin Exp Rheumatol 2019;37(5):715–22.
124. Breen ID, Brumfiel CM, Patel MH, et al. Evaluation of the Safety of Calcitonin Gene-Related Peptide Antagonists for Migraine Treatment Among Adults With Raynaud Phenomenon. JAMA Netw Open 2021;4(4):e217934.
125. Gerard AO, Merino D, Van Obberghen EK, et al. Calcitonin gene-related peptide-targeting drugs and Raynaud's phenomenon: a real-world potential safety signal from the WHO pharmacovigilance database. J Headache Pain 2022; 23(1):53.
126. Yunus MB. The role of gender in fibromyalgia syndrome. Curr Rheumatol Rep 2001;3(2):128–34.
127. Fichera G, Polizzi A, Scapellato S, et al. Craniomandibular Disorders in Pregnant Women: An Epidemiological Survey. J Funct Morphol Kinesiol 2020;5(2):36.
128. Kim YS, Kim N. Sex-Gender Differences in Irritable Bowel Syndrome. J Neurogastroenterol Motil 2018;24(4):544–58.
129. Goncalves DA, Camparis CM, Speciali JG, et al. Treatment of comorbid migraine and temporomandibular disorders: a factorial, double-blind, randomized, placebo-controlled study. J Orofac Pain 2013;27(4):325–35.
130. Marcus DA, Bernstein C, Rudy TE. Fibromyalgia and headache: an epidemiological study supporting migraine as part of the fibromyalgia syndrome. Clin Rheumatol 2005;24(6):595–601.
131. Kang JH. Effects on migraine, neck pain, and head and neck posture, of temporomandibular disorder treatment: Study of a retrospective cohort. Arch Oral Biol 2020;114:104718.
132. Xie Y, Zhou G, Xu Y, et al. Effects of Diet Based on IgG Elimination Combined with Probiotics on Migraine Plus Irritable Bowel Syndrome. Pain Res Manag 2019;2019:7890461.
133. Parikh SK, Young WB. Migraine: Stigma in Society. Curr Pain Headache Rep 2019;23(1):8.
134. Young WB, Park JE, Tian IX, et al. The stigma of migraine. PLoS One 2013;8(1): e54074.
135. Parikh SK, Kempner J, Young WB, et al. Stigma, Effective Interventions. Curr Pain Headache Rep 2021;25(11):75.
136. Estave PM, Beeghly S, Anderson R, et al. Learning the full impact of migraine through patient voices: A qualitative study. Headache 2021;61(7):1004–20.
137. Korkmaz S, Kazgan A, Korucu T, et al. Psychiatric symptoms in migraine patients and their attitudes towards psychological support on stigmatization. J Clin Neurosci 2019;62:180–3.
138. Gvantseladze K, Do TP, Hansen JM, et al. The Stereotypical Image of a Person With Migraine According to Mass Media. Headache 2020;60(7):1465–71.

Gender Issues in Epileptic Patients

Maggie L. McNulty, MD

KEYWORDS

• Epilepsy • Women • Contraception • Catamenial seizures • Pregnancy
• Teratogenic

KEY POINTS

- There are unique hormonal considerations to recognize when treating women with epilepsy including how fluctuations in estrogen and progesterone may alter a woman's susceptibility to seizures.
- Adequate contraceptive counseling for women of childbearing age should review the potential bidirectional effect that certain anti-seizure medications can have on contraceptives and how certain contraceptives can affect certain antiseizure medication levels.
- Pregnancy planning can be used to transition to an antiseizure medication with favorable teratogenic and neurocognitive profiles, minimize dose and polytherapy, and identify a baseline target drug level to aim throughout pregnancy.
- With aging, there is a consideration for changes as it relates to menopause and bone health for women with epilepsy.

INTRODUCTION

Epilepsy is a very common neurological condition that worldwide affects people of all ages, races, and socioeconomic statuses. The World Health Organization estimates that currently approximately 50 million people live with epilepsy. In the United States (US) of America, the Centers for Disease Control and Prevention estimates that 3.4 million people live with active epilepsy which is defined as having doctor-diagnosed epilepsy as well as being on medication to treat seizures and/or having one or more seizure within the last year. The incidence and prevalence of epilepsy have been reported to be slightly higher in men than women.[1] These differences have been postulated to be because of the common risk factors for the development of epilepsy as well as the potential concealment of the disease in certain regions or countries by women due to sociocultural reasons. Although the treatment approaches for both women and men are similar, there are special aspects that must be considered when caring for women with epilepsy (WWE).

Department of Neurology, Rush University Medical Center, 1725 West Harrison Street Suite 885, Chicago, IL 60612, USA
E-mail address: maggie_mcnulty@rush.edu

Neurol Clin 41 (2023) 249–263
https://doi.org/10.1016/j.ncl.2022.10.003
neurologic.theclinics.com
0733-8619/23/

DISCUSSION

Hormonal Considerations

There is a bidirectional relationship between hormones and epilepsy whereby hormones influence epilepsy, and additionally, whereby epilepsy affects hormones. Neuro-steroids are steroid molecules that can alter the brain's excitability, and thus, have an effect on the occurrence of seizures. The two main sex steroid hormones that impact WWE are estrogen and progesterone with estradiol and allopregnanolone serving as the active forms. Estrogen is neuroexcitatory or "pro-convulsant" via enhancement of glutamate excitation by potentiating *N*-methyl-D-aspartate receptor activity.[2] This was shown to be clinically relevant in 1959 when intravenous injections of the conjugated estrogenic substance, Premarin®, were administered to 16 female patients with epilepsy of whom 11 patients showed an increase in epileptogenic activity and 4 experienced clinical seizures.[3] This is in contrast to progesterone which promotes neuro-inhibition via its bioactive metabolite allopregnanolone and works as a positive modulator of γ-aminobutyric acid conductance.[4] Both estrogen and progesterone are tertiary products of the hypothalamic-pituitary-gonadal system with direct, reciprocal connections to the temporo-limbic pathways, particularly the amygdala, which may explain how epilepsy can affect and disrupt hormonal cycles. Cells of the hypothalamus that produce gonadotropin-releasing hormone are at risk for injury by seizures and can lead to the abnormal release of follicle-stimulating hormone and luteinizing hormone.

Menarche and Seizure Onset

The age of seizure onset in WWE as it relates to the age of menarche has been a topic of research. For women, menarche serves as an easily identifiable time point that represents reproductive maturation. At menarche, the levels of neuroactive steroids in the blood increase 10-fold. In a retrospective study using data from the Epilepsy Birth Control Registry (EBCR), a web-based survey of 1144 WWE between the ages of 18 and 47 years in a community setting, it was found that more WWE had seizure onset during the year of menarche than during any other year constituting a risk ratio of 3.96 (**Fig. 1**). Additionally, 49% of seizure onset occurred between 2 years before menarche and 6 years after menarche.[5] These findings may have implications for potential neuroendocrine treatments to prevent the development of epilepsy in WWE.

Catamenial Epilepsy

Dating back to 1881, Sir William Gowers observed that most of the women in his clinic reported a worsening of seizures perimenstrually.[6] The term "catamenial epilepsy" has varying definitions but generally refers to cyclic seizure exacerbation in relation to the menstrual cycle. An average menstrual cycle lasts 28 days with day 1 being the first day of menstruation and day 14 representing the day of ovulation. There are hormonal fluctuations that occur during these periods where estrogen peaks at mid-ovulation and progesterone rapidly declines immediately before menstruation. The reported prevalence of catamenial epilepsy varies from 33% to 70% largely dependent on the definition used.[7] There are three distinct patterns of seizure exacerbation identified. During menstruation (C1 pattern) and ovulation (C2 pattern), the estrogen-to-progesterone ratio is at its highest, leading to a favorable proconvulsant state.[8] The C3 pattern occurs with those that experience inadequate luteal phase cycles where there is low progesterone production with unopposed estrogen production.

The National Institute of Health Progesterone Trial Treatment was a randomized, placebo-controlled, double-blind study of women with intractable epilepsy with and

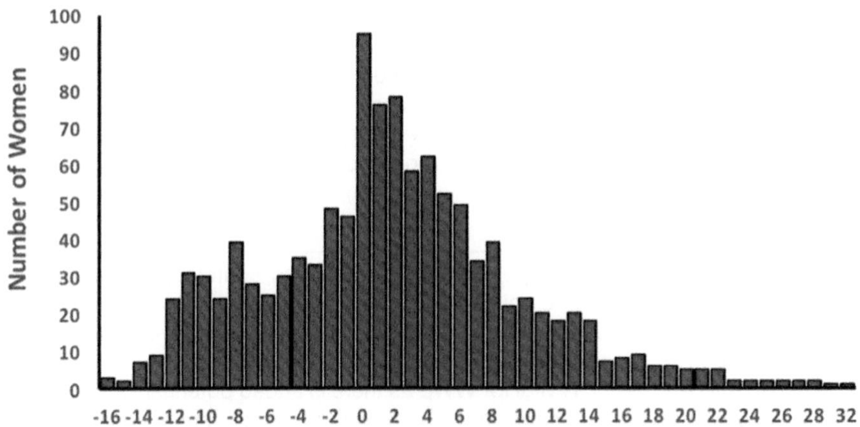

Fig. 1. The analysis of the relationship between the age of seizure onset and the age of menarche finds that more women with epilepsy had their age of seizure onset during the year of menarche than at any other year concerning menarche and significantly more so than expected (95/1144, 8.3% v 24/1144, 2.1%, $P<.0001$). ANOVA analysis, however, finds that the model (R^2 value) explains only 1% of the variance. (*From* Herzog AG, Mandle HB, MacEachern DB. Does the age of seizure onset relate to menarche and does it matter? Seizure. 2019;69:1-6; with permission.)

without a catamenial pattern who were randomized 2:1 to be treated with natural progesterone lozenges to be taken on days 14 to 28 of treatment cycle or placebo.[9] In this study, the prevalence of catamenial epilepsy by pattern was found to be 39.8% for C1, 33.9% for C2, and 47.1% for C3. The findings of this study found that cyclic progesterone is comparable to placebo in the treatment of intractable focal seizures in WWE, however, a secondary analysis, identified a subset of women with C1 or the perimenstrual pattern of $\geq$ three-fold seizure exacerbation to be responsive (defined as $\geq$ 50% seizure reduction) to progesterone treatment. Other potential treatments of catamenial epilepsy that have been considered include medroxyprogesterone acetate, acetazolamide, clobazam, and temporary increases in the dose of a patient's usual anti-seizure medications (ASM) at specific times during the menstrual cycle.[10–12] However, currently, there is no US Food and Drug Administration-approved medication for the treatment of catamenial epilepsy.

Reproductive Alterations

There have been conflicting results with regard to fertility being altered for WWE. Several observations have found a higher prevalence of amenorrhea, menstrual irregularities, premature menopause, and polycystic ovarian syndrome (PCOS) in WWE.[13] PCOS occurs in 5% to 6% of women in the general population but 10% to 20% of WWE and is notably increased in those exposed to valproate via its induction of androgen synthesis within the ovaries. Additionally, women treated with enzyme-inducing ASMs such as phenobarbital, phenytoin, and carbamazepine have been noted to less likely achieve pregnancy which is likely related to alterations in the levels of various sex hormones by the enzyme-inducing medication.[14] Most studies have noted birth rates in WWE to be 37% to 88% of other groups whereas other studies have noted the number of children born to WWE did not differ overall from the reference group.[15–17]

The Women With Epilepsy: Pregnancy Outcomes and Deliveries study was a multicenter, prospective, observational cohort study comparing fertility in WWE with fertility in control women without epilepsy in those without prior known infertility.[18] This study showed no difference in median time to pregnancy, live births, or miscarriage rates between the two groups suggesting that WWE without prior known infertility can successfully achieve pregnancy at similar rates as those women without epilepsy.

Contraception

In any woman of reproductive age, discussion regarding contraception and family planning is important given that unintended pregnancies have been associated with higher rates of unfavorable fetal and maternal outcomes including congenital anomalies, spontaneous abortions, premature delivery, low birth weight, and infant mortality. In particular, this discussion is vital for WWE as there is added potential for ASM teratogenicity as well as the possibility for bidirectional drug–drug interactions between hormonal contraception and ASMs.[19]

The definition of a highly effective form of contraception is a less than 10% failure rate. In the general population, hormonal birth control is considered highly effective, however, in WWE, there is potential for interaction of the enzyme-inducing ASMs with hormonal contraception leading to an increased elimination rate of the hormonal contraception causing a potential unintended pregnancy[20] (**Fig. 2**). Additionally, for some medications, hormonal contraception can increase the metabolism of the ASM leading to lower levels and increased risk of seizures.

The EBCR survey study found that 30.3% of WWE do not use highly effective contraception and that 46.6% use a systemic hormonal form of contraception that may be considered less effective in WWE.[21] In this same survey, 78.9% of WWE reported having at least one unintended pregnancy compared to the general US

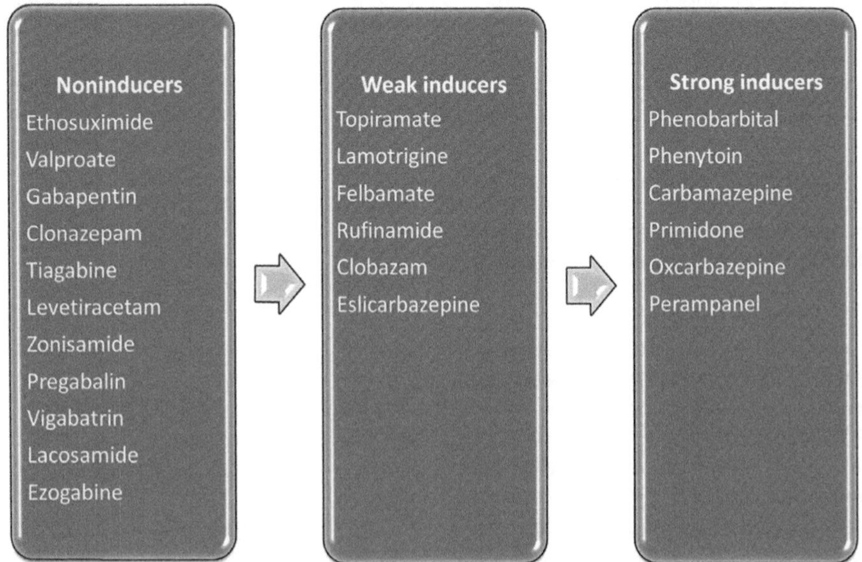

Fig. 2. Degree of induction of sex steroid hormones metabolism. (*From* Vélez-Ruiz NJ, Pennell PB. Issues for Women with Epilepsy. Neurol Clin. 2016;34(2):411-425, ix; with permission.)

population which reports 45% to 51% of pregnancies as unintended.[20] The intrauterine device (IUD) had the lowest failure rate in the EBCR survey study. The hormonal contraception that was used in those on enzyme-inducing ASMs had a significantly greater failure rate than the unintended pregnancy rate using a barrier method. This finding contrasts with what is seen in the general population where hormonal contraceptive has a higher efficacy protecting against pregnancy in comparison with a barrier method. In general, for those treated with enzyme-inducing ASMs, IUD is a preferable option for contraception given its safety profile and high efficacy. Even the levonorgestrel IUD is an option as it is unlikely to be impacted by enzyme-inducing ASM due to localized hormonally mediated changes that work to prevent pregnancy. Another reversible contraceptive option is intramuscular medroxyprogesterone acetate, however, due to its side effect profile that includes weight gain, depression, and hirsutism, it is not always considered as a first-line option.[7]

Estrogen-containing hormonal contraception can also increase the elimination of ASMs that are metabolized via glucuronidation which is of particular significance for WWE treated with lamotrigine. For those on combined oral contraception treatment, the metabolism of lamotrigine is accelerated by approximately 50%.[22] Therefore, counseling WWE regarding the importance of discussing with their physician any plans to start estrogen-containing hormonal contraception is of utmost importance as monitoring of lamotrigine levels would be recommended due to the potential of hormonal contraception to lower certain anti-seizure medication levels leading to breakthrough seizures.

Pregnancy

Globally, it is estimated that 15 million WWE are of childbearing age.[23] Commonly, many questions arise regarding pregnancy including but not limited to the potential teratogenicity of anti-seizure medication exposure, adverse neurocognitive and behavioral outcomes, changes in seizure control during pregnancy, general complications during pregnancy and/or delivery as well as questions as it relates to the postpartum period including the safety of breastfeeding. For WWE who would like to conceive, the encouraging news is that most of them can have normal pregnancies and deliver healthy children; preconception counseling can help to address concerns and inform WWE and their partners of strategies to potentially mitigate risks so that the best-informed decisions can be made.

TERATOGENICITY AND NEUROCOGNITIVE OUTCOMES

A balance must be struck between the potential teratogenic effects and adverse neurodevelopmental effects of anti-seizure medication exposure and the maintenance of maternal seizure control during pregnancy. ASM can be associated with major congenital malformations (MCMs), restricted intrauterine growth, and adverse neurocognitive and behavioral development. Uncontrolled seizures during pregnancy though can cause harm to not only the mother but also the fetus.

Major Congenital Malformations and Other Fetal Outcomes

MCMs are birth defects that are life-threatening, have a major impact on the person, and/or require surgical treatment. In the general population, MCM rates vary between 1.6% and 3.2% and WWE not on ASM have similar rates.[24] The main driver of MCMs in those fetuses exposed to ASM relates to first trimester exposures and is approximately 2 to 3x higher than the general population, however, there is more and more evidence to support that type of anti-seizure medication, the dose of the anti-seizure medication, and certain polytherapy combinations that impact the level of risk.[25]

Much of the data regarding MCMs in WWE come from the information obtained from the various international prospective pregnancy registries that track fetal exposures to ASMs. The three ASMs taken in monotherapy shown to have the greatest prevalence of MCMs are valproate (6.7–10.3%), phenobarbital (5.5–6.5%), and topiramate (3.9–4.3%) whereas no increased risk was noted with lamotrigine or levetiracetam[23] (**Table 1** from reference[23]). The type of MCM varies depending on which ASM is used with a high prevalence of cardiac malformations with barbiturates, neural tube defects, and hypospadias with valproate, and increased risk of cleft lip/palate with topiramate.[26–28] Studies have also demonstrated that a dose-dependent effect is seen where higher doses of phenobarbital and valproate as well as phenytoin, carbamazepine, and even lamotrigine lead to higher rates of MCMs.[29,30] Pregnancy registry data and various publications have altered physician prescription trends. Data from the North American Antiepileptic Drug Pregnancy Registry and the Maternal Outcomes and Neurodevelopmental Effects of Antiepileptic Drugs (MONEAD) study—which is a prospective, multicenter, observational study that enrolled healthy control pregnant women as well as pregnant WWE and performed formal neuropsychological assessments in their children at ages 2 years old, 3 years old, and 6 years old—have demonstrated that prescribing trends have changed over time with less frequent use of valproate, phenytoin, and carbamazepine and increasing use of lamotrigine and levetiracetam.[31,32]

Polytherapy has also been associated with an increased risk of MCMs, however, more recent studies suggest that the specific combination of certain ASMs is more impactful than the number of ASMs. The Kerala Registry of Epilepsy and Pregnancy in which 415 of the pregnancies were noted to occur whereas on polytherapy found that the risk of MCMs was mostly driven by combinations of dual therapy that included the use of valproate or topiramate.[33]

In addition to MCMs, the North American Antiepileptic Drug Pregnancy Registry has also studied other fetal outcomes for those exposed in utero to ASM compared to an unexposed control group and has found an associated increased risk of having a small gestational age (SGA) baby and preterm delivery for those exposed to ASMs in utero. SGA is defined as a birth weight below the 10th percentile for the gestational age or optimal birth weight. SGA is associated with worse health outcomes in both the perinatal period as well as later in life. About 11% of babies born in the ASM-exposed group compared to 5% in the unexposed control group were noted to be SGA at birth, and it was found that topiramate, phenobarbital, and zonisamide monotherapies presented the highest risks of having an SGA baby.[34] These conditions include gastric reflux, delayed gastric emptying, feeding/sensory issues, cardiovascular disease, diabetes, and learning difficulties. However, the data currently available are insufficient to determine if the long-term consequences of ASM-related SGA are the same or similar to other known causes of SGA. Preterm delivery, defined as delivering before 37 weeks of gestation was also found to be to have a statistically significant difference and noted in 9.3% of the exposed group compared to 6.2% of the unexposed control group.[34] However, more recent studies have shown no significant difference between preterm birth, 5-minute APGAR score of less than 6, MCMs, neonatal intensive care admissions, or SGA status in pregnant WWE compared to healthy pregnant women without epilepsy.[35] These findings may be related to the shifting trends in ASM prescriptions given to pregnant women to preferentially include levetiracetam and/or lamotrigine.

Neurocognitive and Behavioral Outcomes

Several studies have explored the possibility of adverse neurocognitive and behavioral outcomes in the children born to WWE specifically as it relates to ASM. The

Table 1
Prevalence (%) of major congenital malformations (malformed/exposed) for different monotherapies

Drug	International Registry of Antiepileptic Drugs and Pregnancy (EURAP)		North American AED Pregnancy Registry		UK Epilepsy and Pregnancy Register	
	Prevalence	(95%CIs)	Prevalence	(95%CIs)	Prevalence	(95%CIs)
Carbamazepine	55% (107/1,957)	(4.5–6.6)	3.0% (31/1,033)	(2.1–4.2)	2.6% (43/1,657)	(1.9–3.5)
Lamotrigine	2.9% (74/2,514)	(2.3–3.7)	1.9% (31/1,562)	(1.4–2.8)	2.3% (49/2,098)	(1.8–3.1)
Levetiracetam	2.8% (17/599)	(1.7–4.5)	2.4% (11/450)	(1.4–4.3)	0.7% (2/304)	(0.2–2.4)
Oxcarbazepine	3.0% (10/333)	(1.4–5.4)	2.2% (4/182)	(0.9–5.5)		
Phenobarbital	6.5% (19/294)	(4.2–9.9)	5.5% (11/199)	(3.1–9.6)		
Phenytoin	6.4% (8/125)	(2.8–12.2)	2.9% (12/416)	(1.7–5.0)	3.7% (3/82)	(1.2–10.2)
Topiramate	3.9% (6/152)	(1.5–8.4)	4.2% (15/349)	(2.5–6.8)	4.3% (3/70)	(1.5–11.9)
Valproate	10.3% (142/1,381)	(8.8–12.0)	9.3% (30/323)	(6.6–12.9)	6.7% (82/1,220)	(5.4–8.3)

Data from three prospective registries.

From Tomson T, Battino D, Bromley R, et al. Management of epilepsy in pregnancy: a report from the International League Against Epilepsy Task Force on Women and Pregnancy. Epileptic Disord Int Epilepsy J Videotape. 2019;21(6):497-517; with permission.

Neurodevelopmental Effects of Antiepileptic Drugs (NEAD) study is a prospective, observational multicenter study conducted at 25 epilepsy centers across the US and United Kingdom. The NEAD study found that fetal exposure to valproate was associated with a lower age—6 intelligent quotient (IQ) score in comparison to fetal exposure to lamotrigine, phenytoin, or carbamazepine with a mean IQ score of 98 in those exposed to valproate compared to mean IQ scores ranging from 106 to 109 in the other three ASMs.[36] This finding was seen even after adjusting for maternal IQ scores, ASM dose, gestational age, and use of preconceptual folate. A dose-dependent effect was notable for valproate, however, even in doses less than 800 mg per day, adverse cognitive effects were seen. Similarly, a study from Denmark found that children exposed prenatally to valproate performed worse on academic tests throughout their primary and lower secondary schooling compared with children unexposed to ASMs and that those exposed prenatally to valproate in comparison to lamotrigine still showed significant impairment.[37] This study adds support that the impact of prenatal exposure to neurodevelopmental teratogens is long-term and is not necessarily mitigated over time. In addition to cognitive concerns, population-based studies have shown that in utero valproate exposure has been associated with an increased risk of autistic spectrum disorders (ASDs) with an absolute risk of 4.42% in those exposed to valproate compared with 1.53% in those unexposed.[38] Other studies have found an association between prenatal exposure to valproate with delayed childhood milestones and attention-deficit hyperactivity disorder.[39,40] A cohort study based on a Nordic register reviewed findings from 16,000 children born to mothers with epilepsy on ASM and noted that those exposed to topiramate and valproate monotherapy had a two- to four-fold increased risk of ASDs and intellectual disability.[41]

Additional information on cognitive outcomes of children born to pregnant WWE has been reported by the MONEAD study. Data published with regard to 2-year-old cognitive outcomes revealed no difference in language domain on the Bayley Scales of Infant and Toddler Development between children born to pregnant WWE compared to those children born to women without epilepsy.[42] These findings are encouraging though are most applicable to women taking levetiracetam and/or lamotrigine as these were the medications most used by the pregnant WWE in this study.

Folic Acid Supplementation

Several studies have explored if folic acid helps to mitigate adverse outcomes as it relates to MCMs or neurocognitive outcomes. Folic acid supplementation in the first trimester in the general population has been associated with a risk reduction of MCMs, specifically neural tube defects. The Centers for Disease Control and Prevention recommends that all women of childbearing age take 400 mcg of folate daily, however, generally, the recommendation for WWE is higher doses of folate. There is no clear consensus though on what that dose of folate should be for WWE. The NEAD study found that WWE who used periconceptual folate had children with a higher mean IQ score of 108 compared to 101, and a dose-dependent effect was observed.[36] Additionally, for WWE on ASMs who did not take periconceptual folate, one in three children exhibited autistic traits.[43]

Seizure frequency changes during pregnancy

Seizures, particularly convulsive seizures, during pregnancy have the potential for adverse outcomes to both the mother and the baby including fetal hypoxia, lactic acidosis, and injury related to falls, and therefore, seizure control during pregnancy is of utmost importance.[8] Multiple studies have reported a varying range of increased frequency of seizures during pregnancy ranging from 14% to 62%. Several factors have been found to help predict seizure frequency changes during pregnancy. Baseline seizure frequency before pregnancy can help predict seizure freedom during pregnancy; 79% of women remain seizure free during pregnancy if they were free of seizures in the 12 months before pregnancy.[44] Factors found to be associated more often with increases in seizure frequency during pregnancy include focal onset epilepsy, polytherapy (acting as a surrogate for more intractable epilepsy), poorer preconception control, a >35% drop in levels of ASMs compared with preconceptional levels and spoor medication adherence.[44] However, previously, there has been insufficient evidence to determine if changes in seizure frequency are related to pregnancy itself or other factors.

The MONEAD study attempted to help answer this question by evaluating changes in seizure frequency between two different periods for pregnant WWE compared with nonpregnant WWE over similar periods.[45] Epoch 1 consisted of the time period of pregnancy and 6 weeks postpartum for the pregnant women and the same time was evaluated prospectively for the control group of nonpregnant WWE. Epoch 2 evaluated the period for pregnant WWE from 6 weeks to 9 months postpartum as well as the same time for the control group. The study showed no meaningful difference between pregnant and nonpregnant women in increased seizure frequency during epoch 1 as compared to epoch 2, therefore, concluding that the state of pregnancy itself is not necessarily the driver behind the increase in seizure frequency. The study not surprisingly found that pregnant women were much more likely to have changes in their ASM dose during pregnancy likely related to the changes in ASM drug levels that occur during pregnancy particularly as it pertains to lamotrigine and levetiracetam. The secondary outcomes showed that women who had no seizures during the 9 months prior to pregnancy or enrollment were more likely to remain seizure free during pregnancy than those who experienced seizures, lending support to the results of previous studies showing seizure freedom in the months before pregnancy can be a good predictor for seizure freedom during pregnancy.

Antiseizure medication concentration changes in pregnancy

During pregnancy, it is vital to aim to target preconceptual levels of ASMs where a woman achieved "good seizure control" and to check levels on at least a monthly basis. An increased risk of seizures has been associated with a decrease in medication concentration levels to 65% or less than the individual's target medication concentration.[44] Lamotrigine and levetiracetam, two of the preferred ASMs in pregnancy, have the most notable pharmacokinetic changes in pregnancy with up to 60% to 70% decrease in serum concentration by the end of pregnancy[23] (**Table 2** from reference[23]). The ASM levels can decrease in pregnancy related to physiological changes of pregnancy including increased volume of distribution, increased renal blood flow and glomerular filtration rate (of notable importance for levetiracetam), reduced serum albumin, and increases in estrogen levels leading to accelerated drug glucuronidation with particular significance for lamotrigine. For women of childbearing age, establishing baseline ASM levels and providing adequate counseling explaining these expected level changes during pregnancy as well as the need for frequent blood level monitoring during pregnancy should be discussed at regular clinic visits.

Maternal risks during pregnancy

Maternal mortality as well as obstetric complications have been observed to be higher for WWE compared to women without epilepsy. One study found that the death rate during pregnancy or the postpartum period was 10 times higher in WWE with 79% of

Table 2
Summary of individual antiseizure drug-projected decreases in serum concentrations (if no dose changes are made)

AED	Decrease in Serum Concentration	Decrease in Serum Free (Unbound) Concentration	Recommendations to Perform Therapeutic Drug Monitoring if Available
Phenobarbital	Up to 55%	Up to 50%	Yes
Phenytoin	60–70%	20–40%	Yes, free concentration
Carbamazepine	0–12%	None	Optional
Valproate	Up to 23%	None	Optional, free concentration if done
Oxcarbazepine monohydroxy-derivative (MHD)	36–62%	N/A	Yes
Lamotrigine	0.77 of population: 69% decrease 0.23 of population: 17% decrease	N/A	Yes
Gabapentin	Insufficient data	N/A	Yes
Topiramate	Up to 30%	N/A	Yes
Levetiracetam	40–60%, with maximal decrease reached in first trimester	N/A	Yes
Zonisamide	Up to 35% but little data	N/A	Yes

Abbreviation: N/A, not applicable.

From Tomson T, Battino D, Bromley R, et al. Management of epilepsy in pregnancy: a report from the International League Against Epilepsy Task Force on Women and Pregnancy. Epileptic Disord Int Epilepsy J Videotape. 2019;21(6):497-517; with permission.

the deaths attributed to sudden, unexpected death in epilepsy or SUDEP.[46] Additionally, mortality during delivery hospitalization was noted to be higher in WWE at 80 deaths per 100,000 compared with women without epilepsy at 6 deaths per 100,000.[47] WWE have also been noted to have an increased risk of pre-eclampsia, increased rate of cesarean delivery, and increased risk of hospitalization of greater than 6 days.

Postpartum period and breastfeeding

During the postpartum period, there is a return to pre-pregnancy physiology and metabolism oftentimes necessitating ASM dose re-adjustments back toward pre-pregnancy levels. Because of the potential for an increase in seizure risk in the postpartum period related to sleep deprivation, at times it is reasonable to recommend slightly higher doses of ASMs than the pre-pregnancy dose. Lamotrigine and other drugs metabolized via glucuronidation may increase precipitously in the postpartum period and lowering of the dose should begin as early as postpartum day 3 and scheduled to return to near pre-pregnancy doses by 3 weeks postpartum.[48] For levetiracetam, which is metabolized through renal clearance, these pathways may normalize 2 to 3 weeks postpartum. Other safety considerations that should be discussed include changing the baby on a padded surface on the ground, avoiding bathing the baby alone, establishing multiple areas in the home where the baby can be safely placed, and avoiding co-sleeping in the event of nocturnal seizures.[49,50]

Breastfeeding offers many potential benefits to both mother and baby. Potential benefits to infants include better neurodevelopmental outcomes and decreased rates of obesity, allergies, and sudden infant death syndrome. However, there have been concerns that such benefits may not be translatable to WWE due to the concern for ASM transmission via breast milk. Transmission through the breast milk has been noted with primidone, levetiracetam, gabapentin, lamotrigine, and topiramate.[51] The NEAD study did not find any adverse effects in breastfed children of WWE on ASMs in IQ, verbal/nonverbal memory, or in executive functioning and found positive outcomes at age 6 with adjusted IQ scores 4 points higher in those children who were breastfed.[52] Additionally, the MONEAD study measured the serum of nursing infants and found that 49% of all ASM concentrations were below the lower limit of quantification and found that overall when breastfed infants had measurable levels these levels were low compared with maternal serum drug concentrations.[53] Taken together, the data is reassuring and supportive of the relative safety of breastfeeding while on ASMs.

Menopause and Bone Health

There are limited data available with regard to how menopause may affect WWE differently than those women without epilepsy and how it may affect seizure frequency. A study by Harden and colleagues[54] noted that WWE have increased rates of premature menopause with the median age of menopause being 47 years compared to 51.4 years in the general population. This study also found that women with a higher seizure burden had a statistically significant younger age of onset of menopause. There have been additional reports of women with catamenial epilepsy experiencing an increase in seizure frequency in the perimenopausal period and a decrease after menopause.[55] Some women in the general population may choose to start hormone replacement therapy to minimize symptoms of menopause, however, in a small randomized, double-blind controlled study worsening in seizures in women on hormone replacement therapy was observed when compared to placebo.[56]

Women in comparison with men are at a four times increased risk of osteoporosis.[57] Many ASMs are known to have long-term adverse outcomes of decreased bone mineral density, and therefore, this topic should be considered whenever prescribing ASMs but even more so when treating WWE. The bone loss is seen most notably because of P450 enzyme induction with a resultant acceleration of vitamin D metabolism when using enzyme-inducing ASMs such as phenytoin, phenobarbital, oxcarbazepine, and carbamazepine.[58] Providing counseling to WWE on preventive measures to preserve bone density including exercise, nutrition, and calcium and vitamin D supplementation can offer strategies to help prevent this from occurring as well as the need for monitoring with bone mineral density scans.[59]

SUMMARY

Across a WWE lifespan, many special considerations need to be taken into account including factors as they relate to hormonal fluctuations, medication interactions as they relate to contraception, pregnancy—with a special focus on any potential negative adverse neurodevelopmental outcomes as well as MCMs concerning ASM, and menopause. WWE need adequate counseling on these areas so that they can make better-informed decisions as well as potentially identify the possibility that their seizure patterns are related to hormonal fluctuations, and therefore, offer different avenues of treatment.

CLINICS CARE POINTS

- Up to 70% of women with epilepsy (WWE) may have seizures triggered by hormonal fluctuations in estrogen or progesterone.
- Folic acid supplementation is recommended to all WWE of child bearing potential to reduce risk of MCMs and adverse neurocognitive and behavioral outcomes.
- The precise dosing though is still not known. Levetiracetam and lamotrigine are ASMs that are preferred in pregnancy but levels throughout pregnancy need to be checked regularly to target pre-conception levels where best seizure control was achieved.

REFERENCES

1. Beghi E. The Epidemiology of Epilepsy. Neuroepidemiology 2020;54(2):185–91.
2. Interactions between hormones and epilepsy | Elsevier Enhanced Reader. doi:10.1016/j.seizure.2015.02.012
3. Logothetis J, Harner R, Morrell F, et al. The role of estrogens in catamenial exacerbation of epilepsy. Neurology 1959;9(5):352.
4. Harden CL, Pennell PB. Neuroendocrine considerations in the treatment of men and women with epilepsy. Lancet Neurol 2013;12(1):72–83.
5. Herzog AG, Mandle HB, MacEachern DB. Does the age of seizure onset relate to menarche and does it matter? Seizure 2019;69:1–6.
6. Gowers WR. Epilepsy and other chronic convulsive diseases: their causes, symptoms, and treatment. London, UK: Forgotten Books; 1901.
7. Vélez-Ruiz NJ, Pennell PB. Issues for Women with Epilepsy. Neurol Clin 2016; 34(2):411–25, ix.
8. Bui E. Women's Issues in Epilepsy. Contin Minneap Minn 2022;28(2):399–427.

9. Herzog AG, Fowler KM, Smithson SD, et al. Progesterone vs placebo therapy for women with epilepsy: A randomized clinical trial. Neurology 2012;78(24): 1959–66.
10. Mattson RH, Cramer JA, Caldwell BV, et al. Treatment of seizures with medroxyprogesterone acetate: preliminary report. Neurology 1984;34(9):1255–8.
11. Ansell B, Clarke E. Acetazolamide in Treatment of Epilepsy. Br Med J 1956; 1(4968):650–4.
12. Feely M, Calvert R, Gibson J. Clobazam in catamenial epilepsy. A model for evaluating anticonvulsants. Lancet Lond Engl 1982;2(8289):71–3.
13. Verrotti A, D'Egidio C, Coppola G, et al. Epilepsy, sex hormones and antiepileptic drugs in female patients. Expert Rev Neurother 2009;9(12):1803–14.
14. Svalheim S, Sveberg L, Mochol M, et al. Interactions between antiepileptic drugs and hormones. Seizure 2015;28:12–7.
15. Artama M, Isojärvi JIT, Raitanen J, et al. Birth rate among patients with epilepsy: a nationwide population-based cohort study in Finland. Am J Epidemiol 2004; 159(11):1057–63.
16. Schupf N, Ottman R. Likelihood of pregnancy in individuals with idiopathic/cryptogenic epilepsy: social and biologic influences. Epilepsia 1994;35(4):750–6.
17. Löfgren E, Pouta A, von Wendt L, et al. Epilepsy in the northern Finland birth cohort 1966 with special reference to fertility. Epilepsy Behav EB 2009;14(1): 102–7.
18. Pennell PB, French JA, Harden CL, et al. Fertility and Birth Outcomes in Women With Epilepsy Seeking Pregnancy. JAMA Neurol 2018;75(8):962–9.
19. Stephen LJ, Harden C, Tomson T, et al. Management of epilepsy in women. Lancet Neurol 2019;18(5):481–91.
20. Herzog AG, Mandle HB, Cahill KE, et al. Predictors of unintended pregnancy in women with epilepsy. Neurology 2017;88(8):728–33.
21. Herzog AG, Mandle HB, Cahill KE, et al. Contraceptive practices of women with epilepsy: Findings of the epilepsy birth control registry. Epilepsia 2016;57(4): 630–7.
22. Herzog AG, Blum AS, Farina EL, et al. Valproate and lamotrigine level variation with menstrual cycle phase and oral contraceptive use. Neurology 2009;72(10): 911–4.
23. Tomson T, Battino D, Bromley R, et al. Management of epilepsy in pregnancy: a report from the International League Against Epilepsy Task Force on Women and Pregnancy. Epileptic Disord Int Epilepsy J Videotape 2019;21(6):497–517.
24. Holmes LB, Khoshbin S. The Teratogenicity of Anticonvulsant Drugs. N Engl J Med 2001;344(15):1132–8.
25. Pennell PB. Antiepileptic drugs during pregnancy: what is known and which AEDs seem to be safest? Epilepsia 2008;49(Suppl 9):43–55.
26. de Jong J, Garne E, de Jong-van den Berg LTW, et al. The Risk of Specific Congenital Anomalies in Relation to Newer Antiepileptic Drugs: A Literature Review. Drugs - Real World Outcomes 2016;3(2):131–43.
27. Veroniki AA, Cogo E, Rios P, et al. Comparative safety of anti-epileptic drugs during pregnancy: a systematic review and network meta-analysis of congenital malformations and prenatal outcomes. BMC Med 2017;15(1):95.
28. Weston J, Bromley R, Jackson CF, et al. Monotherapy treatment of epilepsy in pregnancy: congenital malformation outcomes in the child. Cochrane Database Syst Rev 2016;11:CD010224.
29. Tomson T, Battino D, Perucca E. Teratogenicity of antiepileptic drugs. Curr Opin Neurol 2019;32(2):246–52.

30. Hernandez-Diaz S, Huybrechts KF, Desai RJ, et al. Topiramate use early in pregnancy and the risk of oral clefts: A pregnancy cohort study. Neurology 2018; 90(4):e342–51.
31. Annual Update for 2022 – AED. Available at: https://www.aedpregnancyregistry.org/annual-update-for-2022/. Accessed July 12, 2022.
32. Meador KJ, Pennell PB, May RC, et al. Changes in antiepileptic drug-prescribing patterns in pregnant women with epilepsy. Epilepsy Behav EB 2018;84:10–4.
33. Keni RR, Jose M, Sarma PS, et al, Kerala Registry of Epilepsy and Pregnancy Study Group. Teratogenicity of antiepileptic dual therapy: Dose-dependent, drug-specific, or both? Neurology 2018;90(9):e790–6.
34. Hernández-Díaz S, McElrath TF, Pennell PB, et al. Fetal growth and premature delivery in pregnant women on antiepileptic drugs. Ann Neurol 2017;82(3):457–65.
35. Van Marter LJ, Pennell PB, Brown C, et al. Neonatal Outcomes in the MONEAD Study of Pregnant Women with Epilepsy. J Pediatr X 2021;7:100073.
36. Meador KJ, Baker GA, Browning N, et al. Fetal antiepileptic drug exposure and cognitive outcomes at age 6 years (NEAD study): a prospective observational study. Lancet Neurol 2013;12(3):244–52.
37. Elkjær LS, Bech BH, Sun Y, et al. Association Between Prenatal Valproate Exposure and Performance on Standardized Language and Mathematics Tests in School-aged Children. JAMA Neurol 2018;75(6):663–71.
38. Christensen J, Grønborg TK, Sørensen MJ, et al. Prenatal valproate exposure and risk of autism spectrum disorders and childhood autism. JAMA 2013;309(16): 1696–703.
39. Daugaard CA, Pedersen L, Sun Y, et al. Association of Prenatal Exposure to Valproate and Other Antiepileptic Drugs With Intellectual Disability and Delayed Childhood Milestones. JAMA Netw Open 2020;3(11):e2025570.
40. Christensen J, Pedersen L, Sun Y, et al. Association of Prenatal Exposure to Valproate and Other Antiepileptic Drugs With Risk for Attention-Deficit/Hyperactivity Disorder in Offspring. JAMA Netw Open 2019;2(1):e186606.
41. Bjørk MH, Zoega H, Leinonen MK, et al. Association of Prenatal Exposure to Antiseizure Medication With Risk of Autism and Intellectual Disability. JAMA Neurol 2022. https://doi.org/10.1001/jamaneurol.2022.1269.
42. Meador KJ, Cohen MJ, Loring DW, et al. Two-Year-Old Cognitive Outcomes in Children of Pregnant Women With Epilepsy in the Maternal Outcomes and Neurodevelopmental Effects of Antiepileptic Drugs Study. JAMA Neurol 2021;78(8): 927–36.
43. Bjørk M, Riedel B, Spigset O, et al. Association of Folic Acid Supplementation During Pregnancy With the Risk of Autistic Traits in Children Exposed to Antiepileptic Drugs In Utero. JAMA Neurol 2018;75(2):160–8.
44. Reisinger TL, Newman M, Loring DW, et al. Antiepileptic drug clearance and seizure frequency during pregnancy in women with epilepsy. Epilepsy Behav EB 2013;29(1):13–8.
45. Pennell PB, French JA, May RC, et al. Changes in Seizure Frequency and Antiepileptic Therapy during Pregnancy. N Engl J Med 2020;383(26):2547–56.
46. Edey S, Moran N, Nashef L. SUDEP and epilepsy-related mortality in pregnancy. Epilepsia 2014;55(7):e72–4.
47. MacDonald SC, Bateman BT, McElrath TF, et al. Mortality and Morbidity During Delivery Hospitalization Among Pregnant Women With Epilepsy in the United States. JAMA Neurol 2015;72(9):981–8.

48. Polepally AR, Pennell PB, Brundage RC, et al. MODEL-BASED LAMOTRIGINE CLEARANCE CHANGES DURING PREGNANCY: CLINICAL IMPLICATION. Ann Clin Transl Neurol 2014;1(2):99–106.
49. Rousseau JB. Meeting the needs of the postpartum woman with epilepsy. MCN Am J Matern Child Nurs 2008;33(2):84–9.
50. Bui E, Klein AM. Women with epilepsy: a practical management handbook. Cambridge University Press; 2014. https://doi.org/10.1017/CBO9781139178020.
51. Harden CL, Pennell PB, Koppel BS, et al. Practice parameter update: management issues for women with epilepsy–focus on pregnancy (an evidence-based review): vitamin K, folic acid, blood levels, and breastfeeding: report of the Quality Standards Subcommittee and Therapeutics and Technology Assessment Subcommittee of the American Academy of Neurology and American Epilepsy Society. Neurology 2009;73(2):142–9.
52. Meador KJ, Baker GA, Browning N, et al. Breastfeeding in children of women taking antiepileptic drugs: cognitive outcomes at age 6 years. JAMA Pediatr 2014; 168(8):729–36.
53. Birnbaum AK, Meador KJ, Karanam A, et al. Antiepileptic Drug Exposure in Infants of Breastfeeding Mothers With Epilepsy. JAMA Neurol 2020;77(4):441–50.
54. Harden CL, Koppel BS, Herzog AG, et al. Seizure frequency is associated with age at menopause in women with epilepsy. Neurology 2003;61(4):451–5.
55. Harden CL, Pulver MC, Ravdin L, et al. The effect of menopause and perimenopause on the course of epilepsy. Epilepsia 1999;40(10):1402–7.
56. Harden CL, Herzog AG, Nikolov BG, et al. Hormone replacement therapy in women with epilepsy: a randomized, double-blind, placebo-controlled study. Epilepsia 2006;47(9):1447–51.
57. Alswat KA. Gender Disparities in Osteoporosis. J Clin Med Res 2017;9(5):382–7.
58. Pack AM, Walczak TS. Bone health in women with epilepsy: clinical features and potential mechanisms. Int Rev Neurobiol 2008;83:305–28.
59. Carlson C, Anderson CT. Special Issues in Epilepsy: The Elderly, the Immunocompromised, and Bone Health. Contin Minneap Minn 2016;22(1 Epilepsy): 246–61.

Women and Ischemic Stroke

Disparities and Outcomes

Laurel Cherian, MD, MS

KEYWORDS

• Ischemic stroke • Women • Outcome • Disparities

KEY POINTS

- Most strokes in women are due to traditional vascular risk factors, and the importance of controlling these risks cannot be underestimated.
- Several less common stroke etiologies have a female pre-ponderance, including migrainous infarcts, FMD, MoyaMoya disease and syndrome, and reversible cerebral vasoconstriction syndrome.
- Women also experience a variety of sex-specific risk factors, and these risks evolve over the lifespan through menache, pregnancy, peri-partum, and menopause.
- Women may be less likely to recieve acute stroke therapies, such as thrombolytics or endovascular therapy.

GENERAL CONSIDERATIONS

Although men are at higher risk of stroke throughout most of their lifespan, the incidence of stroke in women climbs with age, increasing after menopause and rising sharply after 85 years. This, combined with women's longer life expectancy, results in most of the stroke deaths occurring in women.[1] Disparity in stroke outcomes in women may be related to age, pre-stroke functional status, and comorbidities.[2] Regardless of the cause, the increased disability and post-stroke care requirements of women, particularly in our aging population, highlight the importance of determining successful strategies for stroke prevention, acute stroke treatments, rehabilitation, and effective secondary prevention measures in women.

Traditional vascular risk factors account for most of the strokes in women, but there are sex-specific risk factors, including age at menarche, use of hormonal contraception, pregnancy, post-partum, menopause, and hormonal replacement that require additional expertise to effectively care for the patient. Transgendered individuals may present management challenges when attempting to balance the need to align the patient's sex with their gender with a potential increased risk of neurovascular complications.[3]

Department of Neurological Sciences, Division of Cerebrovascular Diseases, Rush University Medical Center, 1725 West Harrison Street, Suite 1121, Chicago, IL 60612, USA
E-mail address: Laurel_j_cherian@rush.edu

Neurol Clin 41 (2023) 265–281
https://doi.org/10.1016/j.ncl.2022.10.001
0733-8619/23/

Finally, although significant advances have been won in recent years combating stroke, the declines in stroke incidence seem to primarily be driven by fewer strokes in men.[2] The discrepancy in these trends deserves close examination to determine the barriers that may be preventing similar achievements in stroke reduction in women.

TRADITIONAL VASCULAR RISK FACTORS IN WOMEN

The lifetime risk of stroke in women between the ages of 55 and 75 in the United States is one in five.[4] Stroke is the leading cause of disability in women and the third leading cause of death. Traditional vascular risk factors, including hypertension, diabetes, hyperlipidemia, and atrial fibrillation, are the most common causes of stroke in women, with clear racial disparities seen between white versus minority populations[5] with the African–American population being most affected. Thus, although it is important to be cognizant of sex-specific stroke risk factors in women, the importance of aggressive control of traditional vascular risk factors cannot be underestimated.

Hypertension

Hypertension remains the most important modifiable stroke risk factor in both men and women,[6] and may account for as much as 50% of strokes globally.[7] The relationship between hypertension and stroke risk is direct and linear, with an estimated doubling of stroke risk for every 20 mm Hg of systolic and 10 mm Hg of diastolic increase in blood pressure.[8] Hypertension is more common in elderly women than in men, but premenopausal women have a lower incidence of hypertension compared with men, possibly because of the effects of estrogen receptor regulation on the sympathetic nervous system.[9] However, a variety of other sex-specific processes can contribute to the development of hypertension in women, including the use of oral contraceptives, pregnancy complications such as pre-eclampsia, and higher likelihood of fibromuscular dysplasia, which can result in renal artery stenosis.[10] Obesity is more prevalent in women, and in addition to being an independent risk factor for stroke, it contributes to the development of hypertension, carrying a 2 to 6-fold increased risk.[10]

There are hormone-specific changes that may also contribute to the development of hypertension in peri and postmenopausal women. The reduction in the estradiol and the estrogen/testosterone ratio may contribute to endothelial dysfunction that ultimately results in decreased bioavailable nitric oxide and increased endothelin leading to increased salt sensitivity, and increased renal vascular tone.[11]

Most of the individuals over the age of 80 are hypertensive with women representing the larger percentage of individuals in this age group. The number of women with blood pressure that is well controlled in this oldest cohort is lower than in younger cohorts, for unclear reasons, but may include the inability to tolerate titration of antihypertensives to effective doses, a lack of financial security to afford medications, or a failure of the treating physician to treat aggressively enough to achieve appropriate goals.

Racial and ethnic disparities are profound, with African–American women having the highest hypertension prevalence (>40%) of any minority group. Given that hypertension predisposes individuals to coronary artery disease, stroke, and chronic kidney disease, there is subsequently a lowered life expectancy for African–American women compared with their non-Hispanic white and white peers.[10] The likelihood of achieving blood pressure goals in African–American women is also lower, possibly because of access to affordable care and other social determinants of health.

Women may be more prone to experience some side effects from antihypertensives. The development of edema with calcium channel blockers and cough with ACEIs have been noted in some studies. The rate of cough with ACEIs is up to three times higher in African–American women than in other groups.[12] Hyponatremia and hypokalemia are seen more frequently in women with diuretic therapy. The interaction of sex hormones with metabolizing enzymes may lead to differences in both the effect of a given dose as well as its subsequent elimination and adverse effects.[9]

Diabetes

All diabetics have nearly double the risk of stroke compared with non-diabetics, but women carry an excess risk of stroke associated with diabetes that is independent of other sex differences in cardiovascular risk factors, with an increased risk of stroke by 27% in diabetic women compared with men.[13,14] Abdominal adiposity and/or metabolic syndrome also have a higher stroke risk in women compared with men.[15] Not only is the overall risk of stroke increased in female patients with diabetes, but the likelihood of suffering a fatal stroke is also doubled compared with male patients with diabetes who suffer a stroke.[14,16]

Interestingly, diabetic women without a prior history of stroke may have the same risk of suffering a fatal stroke as non-diabetic women with a prior stroke, suggesting that the presence of diabetes may effectively be a stroke equivalent.[14] As previously noted, the progress that has been seen in reducing the incidence of stroke has largely been driven by stroke reduction in men, and it is hypothesized that the lack of a commensurate stroke reduction in women may be driven by the increasing rates of obesity and diabetes across the population, but with a sex-specific increase in stroke risk in women.[14]

Dyslipidemia

Available data suggest that elevated low-density lipoprotein cholesterol and non-high-density lipoprotein cholesterol increase the risk of stroke, but there do not seem to be clear sex differences about stroke risk or treatment recommendations. Some data suggest that women are less likely to be treated with high-intensity statins. Women were underrepresented in the available studies with only about of quarter of participants being women.[17–19]

Concerning primary stroke prevention, it is worth noting that a variety of changes occur during pregnancy with regard to the lipid profile.[20] Cholesterol is essential for the synthesis of steroid hormones and is vital for the healthy development of the fetal organs. The cholesterol levels increase naturally during the second trimester, peak in the third trimester, and typically return to normal around 4 weeks after delivery. The total cholesterol may elevate 25% to 50%, with even larger increases in HDL.[19] Although some studies suggest that elevation of triglycerides during pregnancy may be a risk for future cardiovascular disease,[21–23] treatment of dyslipidemia in pregnancy is generally not recommended as a primary prevention measure because of increased risk of materno-fetal complications.

However, in July 2021, the FDA removed the Pregnancy Category X label against the use of statins in all pregnant patients, noting that the risk/benefit profile may be favorable in some individuals with significant cardiovascular disease risks, such as those with homozygous familial hypercholesterolemia, which affects 1 in 250 women, or those with a prior history of atherosclerotic cardiovascular disease events, such as heart attack or stroke, which include 1.4% of women between the ages of 20 and 39 years.[24] Concerns over statin use in pregnancy centered on the potential for fetal anomalies, but it should be noted that this was observed in animal studies at statin doses higher than those used in humans. Although high-quality data is lacking, the largest observational cohort of statin use in pregnant women showed no increased risk of fetal anomalies after adjusting for confounding factors.[24] However, recommendations against statin use while breastfeeding remain. As such, the decision to treat a woman with a prenatal or peripartum stroke with statins or other lipid-lowering medications should be carefully weighed as atypical stroke etiologies may be more likely. In patients with significant cardiovascular risk factors and peripartum stroke, treatment of dyslipidemia may be reasonable, with careful consideration regarding the decision to hold or continue statins during future pregnancies.

Atrial Fibrillation

Although men have a higher risk of developing atrial fibrillation (Afib), the risk of Afib increases with age, and women have a longer life expectancy. Therefore, the absolute number of women with Afib is higher than men.[25,26] Even after adjustment for hypertension and prior stroke, women have a higher risk of stroke because of Afib as well as higher stroke mortality. In the practice innovation and clinical excellence (PINNACLE) registry, women were significantly less likely to be treated with anticoagulation than men, regardless of the CHA_2DS_2-VASc score.[27] Other studies suggest that women are less likely to undergo ablation and may be under-dosed with anticoagulants.[28] This is despite the fact that there are no known sex-specific differences in the efficacy of anticoagulation for stroke prevention in Afib. The reasons for this are unclear, perhaps because of a fear of greater fall risk in elderly, frail women that may deter physicians from appropriately anticoagulating some women, despite evidence that the benefit of stroke reduction with anticoagulation outweighs the risk of hemorrhage related to falls.[29]

STROKE ETIOLOGIES WITH A FEMALE PREDOMINANCE

Migraine with Aura

Up to 14% of the United States population suffers from migraine with nearly 30% of these individuals experiencing migraine with aura (MwA). The majority are women (3:1 female to male prevalence).[30] MwA increases the risk of stroke by two- to three-fold in both men and women,[14] but possibly more in women, and may also increase the risk of cardiovascular diseases, including myocardial infarction, perioperative stroke, hypertension, venous thromboembolism, and Afib.[31] The risk of stroke in MwA is higher in women under 45 years of age, those who use oral contraceptives, and those who smoke.[30] The mechanism by which migraine increases the risk of stroke is not entirely clear but may be related to endothelial dysfunction, vasospasm, patent foramen ovale, repeated inflammation, or a higher risk of cervical artery dissection (CAD). The aura is central for the association between migraine and stroke, especially during intense cortical spreading depression with prolonged or severe hypoperfusion leading to migrainous infarction.[14] Individuals presenting with reversible cerebral vasocontriction syndrome (RCVS), which also has a female preponderance, often have a history of migraine, suggesting a continuum of vascular irritability.[30] Caution should be used when treating women with MwA who also have other vascular risk factors, particularly those who smoke. Triptans and ergot alkaloids have the potential to induce vasoconstriction, and the decision to offer or continue therapy in high-risk individuals must be carefully considered, recognizing that undertreated migraine can be a severely disabling condition, causing significant disruption to an individual's ability to function. Data on the newer calcitonin gene-related peptide receptor antagonists are somewhat limited at this point with some studies claiming little to no vascular side effects.[32] However, there is the pathophysiologic potential for the induction of vasospasm with these agents and long-term outcome data should be monitored closely as the use of these medications becomes more common.

Fibromuscular Dysplasia

Fibromuscular dysplasia (FMD) is a non-inflammatory disease of medium-sized arteries that can result in stenosis, occlusion, dissection, and/or aneurysm. Although any artery may be affected, there is a predilection for the renal, extracranial carotid, and extracranial vertebral arteries (65% of cases). Up to 90% of individuals with FMD are women.[33] The cause for the female preponderance of FMD is unclear. Hormonal factors have been speculated to play a role, but there is a lack of epidemiologic evidence to support this. FMD has not been associated with the number of pregnancies or the use of oral contraceptives or other hormones.[34] Spontaneous CAD is a rare cause of stroke that is associated with FMD.

Moyamoya Disease and Syndrome

Moyamoya disease (MMD) causes stenosis and occlusion of the internal carotid arteries leading to transient ischemic attacks, seizures, cerebral infarction, and intracranial hemorrhage. Over time, small, compensatory collateral vessels form at the distal carotid arteries leading to the disease's classic angiographic appearance. Although the cause of MMD is not entirely clear, there may be a genetic component as up to 11% of cases are familial.[35] Sex-specific factors may also play a role as the incidence of MMD in women is nearly 2:1 compared with men.[4] Clinical presentation is bimodal, with pediatric cases more commonly presenting with seizure or ischemic events, and adult cases more commonly presenting with hemorrhagic events.[36] Pediatric cases were noted to be more likely to be females and to also have an associated family history of MMD.[36]

MMD is up to 4.6 times more common in populations of East Asian descent, particularly Japanese and Korean individuals as compared with Caucasians. The natural history of the disease seems to be similar in different populations. In addition to being more common in women, there may be sex-specific differences in the disease course. A study examining preoperative symptoms and long-term outcomes after revascularization found that women were at higher risk for preoperative transient ischemic attacks and had a higher 5-year cumulative risk of post-operative adverse events despite successful revascularization.[37] Authors emphasized, however, that both men and women benefited from revascularization and that there was no sex-specific difference in functional neurologic outcomes between sexes.

Reversible Cerebral Vasoconstriction Syndrome

RCVS classically presents with recurrent thunderclap headaches, transient ischemic attack, cerebral infarction, seizures, and/or cortical subarachnoid hemorrhage, with an associated appearance of segmental constriction of the intracranial vessels, which resolves within 3 months.[38] An association with posterior reversible encephalopathy syndrome (PRES) has also been noted leading to a conclusion that both may represent varying degrees of volatility in cerebrovascular tone. An extensive list of triggers exists, including the use of serotonin and norepinephrine reuptake inhibitors, tacrolimus, marijuana use, and nasal decongestants.[38] Other environmental triggers have been reported, such as rapid temperature changes, and even consumption of extremely spicy foods. However, one of the most widely recognized triggers is hormonal fluctuations, such as those experienced in pregnancy and the peripartum time frame. Up to two-thirds of post-partum RCVS occurs within the first week post-partum.[38] Although many patients are exposed to vasoconstrictive agents during labor and delivery, RCVS has also been reported in women with no identifiable trigger other than the physiologic changes surrounding birth, suggesting that hormonal fluctuations alone may be enough to incite onset.

Compared with men, non-pregnant women with RCVS were more likely to have migraine, have a history of depression, and use serotonergic antidepressants.[39] Women were more likely than men to suffer clinical deterioration, have more infarcts, and have worse angiographic severity scores. However, clinical outcomes at the time of discharge from the hospital were similar.

Treatment of RCVS includes management of elevated blood pressure, if present, control of seizures, work-up for potential alternate etiologies, and removal of potential triggers. It is worth noting that some studies have advocated for use of a conventional cerebral angiogram to confirm the diagnosis, whereas others have reported that this procedure itself, particularly the injection of contrast agent, may exacerbate the condition and should be avoided. It is also important to be aware that the characteristic imaging appearance of segmental vascular constriction may lag behind the clinical presentation by a week or more. In individuals with a high level of clinical suspicion for RCVS, repeat imaging in 1 week may help confirm the diagnosis.

SEX-SPECIFIC STROKE RISK FACTORS

Age at Menarche

The Women's Ischemia Syndrome Evaluation study found that women with early (before age 12) or late (after age 15) menarche were at increased risk of having adverse cardiovascular events, and this effect was still present after controlling for traditional vascular risk factors, suggesting that age at menarche may be an independent risk factor.[40] The analysis revealed a J-shaped relationship, with a higher risk for early menarche. Interestingly, exposure to estrogen was not thought to be the causative factor in these findings, and the authors hypothesized that other factors associated with early menarche, including psychosocial stressors, over-nutrition, and metabolic syndrome may be responsible, whereas factors associated with late menarche, such as polycystic ovary syndrome, excessive exercise, and undernutrition, may play a role.

Hormonal Contraception

Estrogen-containing systemic contraceptives are generally recommended against in women with a history of stroke and should also be avoided in women with MwA, particularly if they also smoke or have other vascular risk factors. The use of long-acting reversible contraception, such as intrauterine devices, allows for substantially lower systemic hormonal exposure and may be the most sensible option for women of childbearing age with a history of stroke or cerebrovascular risk factors. The risk of stroke does not seem to increase with transdermal or vaginal estrogen.[41] Progesterone-only hormonal contraception is also an option but carries the additional burden of strict timing of administration to avoid pregnancy as well as more potential for side effects, such as breast tenderness, acne, alteration in sex drive, headaches, and nausea/vomiting. It should be noted, however, that the risk of stroke is higher during and after pregnancy than it is with any form of hormonal contraception, so finding an effective and well-tolerated birth control method, even if it may be higher risk than other methods, is very important for high-risk women of childbearing age.[42]

Pregnancy/Post-Partum

Pregnancy/post-partum is a prothrombotic state, with an increase in a variety of procoagulant factors, including increases in fibrinogen and prothrombin fragments and a decrease in protein C and S. As such, pregnancy/post-partum carries an elevated risk of stroke for women, with nearly a three-fold increase in the incidence of stroke, evenly divided between ischemic stroke (IS), intracerebral hemorrhage (ICH), and cerebral dural venous sinus thrombosis (CDVST), compared with non-pregnant/post-partum individuals of the same age.[43] The stroke risk is roughly equal between pregnancy (18.3/100k) and post-partum (14.7/100k), but the post-partum rate has been climbing in recent years in conjunction with increases in CAD and HTN.[44]

The risk in the post-partum time frame was traditionally thought to persist for up to 6 weeks post-partum, but more recent studies have suggested that post-partum stroke risk may persist longer, at least 12 weeks post-partum.[45] This would better align with laboratory data showing that although some coagulation markers normalized within the 6-week time frame post-partum, others remain abnormal 8 to 12 weeks after delivery.

Hypertension, in particular, has a profound effect on stroke risk in pregnancy/post-partum, with a more than five-fold increase in the risk of stroke associated with hypertensive disorders of pregnancy, and this risk is exacerbated when hypertension is combined with other cardiac risks, such as congenital heart disease (OR 13.1), Afib (OR 8.1), primary thrombocytopenia (OR 5.5), or migraine (OR 4.5).[46] Other stroke etiologies are specific to pregnancy,[2] including amniotic fluid embolism, cardio-embolism related to dilated peripartum cardiomyopathy, choriocarcinoma, HELLP (hemolysis, elevated liver enzymes, and low platelet count) syndrome, posterior reversible encephalopathy syndrome, peripartum infection, and CAD secondary to hyperemesis gravidarum, which may be incited by repetitive, forceful Valsalva with vomiting.

As noted earlier, elevated blood pressure during pregnancy may inform more than just the cerebrovascular risk during pregnancy itself. Individuals diagnosed with hypertensive disorders of pregnancy have a 3.7x higher risk of later developing hypertension[47] and women with hypertensive disorders of pregnancy also have a 1.8x higher lifetime risk of stroke than women without it.[48]

Angiotensin-converting enzyme inhibitors (ACEIs), angiotensin receptor blockers, and direct renin inhibitors are contraindicated in the second and third trimesters of pregnancy. Pregnant patients should be transitioned to α-methyldopa, nifedipine, and/or labetalol (**Table 1**). Severe pre-eclampsia or eclampsia should be treated with intravenous magnesium sulfate. Additionally, close monitoring of patients with chronic hypertension is important as blood pressure may decline in the first and second trimesters with some women needing to decrease or hold their chronic hypertension medications if they become hypotensive during this time frame. The American College of Gynecology recommends against very low sodium diets in pregnant patients as this may cause low intravascular volume.[49]

Low-dose prophylaxis with aspirin is beneficial during pregnancy in high-risk individuals, such as those at risk of developing pre-eclampsia, and is typically started at the end of the first trimester and continued through delivery.[50] Women with an indication for antiplatelet therapy for stroke prevention may continue aspirin 81mg pre-conception, during the first trimester, and beyond.[51] Data on other antiplatelets in pregnancy are more limited resulting in low-dose aspirin remaining the agent of choice during pregnancy. For patients requiring anticoagulation during pregnancy, heparin products such as enoxaparin, are preferred to warfarin or direct oral anticoagulants as they do not cross the placenta and are not teratogenic.[52–54] In individuals who are unable to tolerate heparin because of heparin-induced thrombocytopenia or other allergies, fondaparinux may be a reasonable alternative.[55–60]

Age at Menopause

It should first be noted that there is a distinction between surgical versus natural menopause and stroke risk. With surgical menopause, there is an abrupt decline in

Table 1
Safety of antihypertensives in pregnancy

Agent	Mechanism of Action	Potential Side Effects	FDA Class	Breastfeeding
α-methyldopa	Alpha2 agonist	Drug of choice according to NHBEP; safety after first trimester well documented, including 7 y follow-up of offspring	B	Compatible
Labetalol	Alpha and beta blocker	May be associated with fetal growth restriction	C	Usually compatible
Nifedipine	Calcium channel blocker Dihydropyridine	May inhibit labor and have synergistic action with magnesium sulfate in BP lowering; little experience with other calcium entry blockers	C	Usually compatible
Hydralazine	Selectively relaxes arteriolar smooth muscle by an unknown mechanism	Few controlled trials, long experience with few adverse events documented; useful in combination with sympatholytic agent; may cause neonatal thrombocytopenia	D	Usually compatible
β-Receptor blockers	Competitive antagonists that block the receptor sites for endogenous catecholamines epinephrine and norepinephrine	May decrease uteroplacental blood flow; may impair fetal response to hypoxic stress; risk of growth restriction when started in first or second trimester (atenolol); may be associated with neonatal hypoglycemia at higher doses	D	

Hydrochlorothiazide	Acts on distal convoluted tubules and inhibits the sodium chloride co-transporter system	Majority of controlled studies in normotensive pregnant women rather than hypertensive patients; can cause volume contraction and electrolyte disorders; may be useful in combination with methyldopa and vasodilator to mitigate compensatory fluid retention	B
Contraindicated ACEIs and angiotensin type 1 receptor antagonists	Decrease formation of angiotensin II, a vasoconstrictor, and increase the level of bradykinin, a vasodilator	Leads to fetal loss in animals; human use associated with cardiac defects, fetopathy, oligohydramnios, growth restriction, renal agenesis and neonatal anuric renal failure, which may be fatal	D

Data from Refs.[80–82]

the loss of ovarian hormones, whereas with natural menopause, the decline occurs more gradually.[61] This distinction may complicate the interpretation of studies on menopause and stroke risk, which have often failed to distinguish between the two. Additional factors, such as age at menarche, use of hormonal contraceptives, and use of hormonal replacement therapy, may also complicate the interpretation of data on menopause and stroke risk. A study that assessed these items as potential confounders, as well as the presence of traditional risk factors, found that later menopause has been associated with a lower risk of total stroke and IS, consistent with a 2% relative risk reduction for each year that menopause is later.[61] In particular, the youngest age cohort of menopause (before age 40) was associated with a 1.62x higher risk of IS compared with the reference (age 50–54 years). Further analysis of surgical versus non-surgical menopause found that the surgical menopause group had non-significant associations with total stroke risk. It should be noted that individuals who underwent hysterectomy or unilateral oophorectomy were categorized as part of the surgical menopause group, which may have affected results. Menopause was not associated with ICH, possibly because of the low number of hemorrhagic events.

The authors hypothesized that early menopause may impart increased risk of total and IS risk by declines in estradiol, but note that, paradoxically, postmenopausal hormone therapy has been associated with increased stroke risk. This suggests that the mechanism of the protective effect of later menopause on reduced stroke risk is likely more complex than simple hormone levels. The timing of menopause may be driven by a variety of physiologic processes and may be reflective of an individual's vascular risk profile, such as hypertension, hyperlipidemia, and diabetes.[62] A study from the Women's Health Initiative found that women with older age at childbirth were more likely to survive till 90 years[63] also suggesting that fertility in older age may be a marker for overall health and a lower risk profile. Further studies examining associations between the timing of menopause and cause of stroke would be informative in determining if and how hormonal changes may predispose women to stroke.

Transgender Hormone Supplementation: Male to Female

For the over 1.4 million individuals in the US whose gender is not congruent with their sex assigned at birth,[64] gender-affirming hormone supplementation may provide a highly valued medical intervention that increases the individual's health and well-being. The effects of these therapies on stroke risk is an evolving area of research, and the combination of gender-affirming hormones with other risk factors may increase the risk of stroke in transgender individuals.[3] It is worth noting that in addition to traditional vascular risk factors, transgender individuals may have additional risks that include barriers to accessing medical care, higher rates of victimization and stigmatization, chronic stress, and higher rates of mental illness, substance use disorders, and sexually transmitted infections. The rates of depression and anxiety in transgender individuals may be over double that of the general population.[65] The rates of traditional vascular risk factors are also higher in the transgender population. The reasons for this are unclear but may be related to a wide array of psychosocial stressors and barriers to care.[65] In a small case series of trans-women (male to female), subjects were younger and had higher rates of tobacco and stimulant use, hepatitis C and HIV.[3] The majority presented with current use of estrogen though only a third were continued on therapy at the time of discharge after stroke.[3]

Cross-sex hormonal therapy (CSHT) may consist of estrogens, androgen antagonists, and/or gonadotropin-releasing hormone agonists. Our current understanding of the risks of these therapies is extrapolated from use in non-transgender populations, such as hormone replacement therapy for postmenopausal women, which has shown an increased risk of stroke with estrogen-containing therapy. Although data are currently limited, with most available data focusing on the risk of venous thromboembolism, the use of low-dose, transdermal estrogen and use of oral bio-identical estrogens over high-dose oral ethinylestradiol may be safer.[3]

Despite the possible increased risk of stroke, the positive impact of gender-affirming hormone therapy on mental health should not be underestimated. Efforts should be made to establish a strong therapeutic relationship with transgender stroke patients ideally as part of a care team experienced with CSHT and transgender care.

TREATMENT CONSIDERATIONS FOR WOMEN WITH STROKE

Acute Stroke Treatment in Pregnancy

IS, ICH, and CDVST occur at roughly equal rates during pregnancy. The incidence of IS in pregnancy is 30/100,000 pregnancies, with most strokes occurring in the peripartum period.[49] Pregnancy itself is a relatively prothrombotic state, and there are associated conditions of pregnancy, such as peripartum cardiomyopathy, that may increase the risk of IS. Conversely, stroke mimics, such as migraine, which may change in character, severity, and frequency during pregnancy, or hypertensive disorders of pregnancy, such as pre-eclampsia and eclampsia, may have associated focal neurologic deficits.

Additionally, atypical stroke etiologies, such as amniotic fluid embolism, are mechanistically unlikely to respond to thrombolytic therapy. Pregnant women were excluded from clinical trials on thrombolytics because of a concern for potential harm, predominantly the possibility of intrauterine bleeding. Other pregnancy-specific concerns with thrombolytic therapy include premature labor, placental abruption, and fetal demise. As such, existing data on the use of thrombolytics in pregnancy is of low quality, limited to case reports and case series. One case series reviewing 18 pregnant patients who received alteplase reported no maternal deaths attributed to thrombolytics, no major bleeding events, four minor bleeding events, one preterm delivery with a good outcome, and three fetal deaths (no fetal deaths were related to thrombolytics).[66] Most available cases have occurred earlier in pregnancy, although there are case reports as late as 39+ weeks,[67] leaving even more uncertainty in the time frame where stroke is most common in pregnancy.

Alteplase is not known to be teratogenic and at 32 kDa is too large a molecule to cross the placenta.[66] Thrombotic events in general, and IS in particular, are among the leading causes of maternal morbidity and mortality worldwide and are the most common cause of maternal mortality in the developed world. As such, the administration of alteplase in pregnancy may be reasonable in many situations, whereby the benefit is likely to outweigh the risk.[66,68] The risks and benefits of tenecteplase (TNK, which is rapidly being adopted as the thrombolytic of choice for acute stroke treatment at many centers, has even less available data than alteplase). TNK, like alteplase, is assigned Pregnancy Category C by the FDA. With a molecular size of 65 kDa and higher fibrin specificity,[69] TNK likely has a similar, or possibly more favorable, risk profile to alteplase. As the adoption of TNK becomes more widespread, data needs to be collected on its use in pregnant patients.

Endovascular therapy (EVT) is also a treatment option in pregnant patients, either in conjunction with thrombolytics or alone, for patients with large vessel occlusion (LVO). Although forgoing thrombolytics in favor of EVT in pregnant patients would decrease the risk of hemorrhagic complications, the thrombus location and the potential for transfer delays to a comprehensive stroke center should be considered in decision-making for thrombolytic therapy. Although EVT likely presents little risk to the pregnancy itself, vessel wall changes during pregnancy could increase risks of vascular wall injury with endovascular devices,[70] which may be more pronounced when trying to access more distal vessels.

The decision to treat with thrombolytics and/or EVT should include a detailed discussion of the risks and benefits of each, with a focus on pregnancy-specific concerns, including gestational age and the presence of any pregnancy-related conditions, such as thrombocytopenia.

Sex-Specific Outcomes for Acute Stroke Therapies

Thrombolytic therapy is a mainstay of acute stroke treatment, typically available at the first hospital of presentation and sometimes even in the pre-hospital setting, such as on a mobile stroke unit. Multiple studies have found no difference in outcomes between men and women among those treated with thrombolytics,[71–73] an improvement compared with the typical sex difference in outcomes seen among the stroke population at large, whereby women are less likely than men to have a good functional outcome.[74]

Unfortunately, women are less likely to be treated with thrombolytics than men. Sex-specific reasons for ineligibility for thrombolytic therapy could include higher rates of Afib in women with associated use of anticoagulants, a higher percentage of women who live alone and may not be discovered in time after stroke onset, or atypical stroke symptoms delaying diagnosis.[75]

Nonetheless, even among groups of eligible patients, the sex disparity for women persists. According to a meta-analysis of studies with sex-specific data on thrombolytic treatment of acute stroke, women may be as much as 30% less likely to be treated with thrombolytics when presenting with acute stroke.[75] This sex disparity persisted after taking into account patient eligibility, geographic/regional location, and after controlling for age, stroke severity, and comorbidities.[75] Given that thrombolytic treatment may be a powerful equalizer against sex disparities in stroke outcomes, it is critically important to better understand how this treatment gap can be overcome.

EVT has revolutionized the treatment of large vessel IS, transforming what was once an almost universally catastrophic event into a treatable medical condition with a reasonable likelihood of good functional outcome. Both men and women benefit from EVT to treat LVO[76] with some studies finding similar outcomes for men and women,[77] whereas others have found that women have may inferior 90-day clinical outcomes compared with men[78] and are less likely to return to work post-stroke.[79] With current studies examining the possibility of moving entirely away from a time-based clock to a tissue-based clock and exploring the treatment of individuals with large core infarcts, it will be important to study sex disparities.

SUMMARY

Sex-specific differences in the prevalence, etiology, treatment, and outcomes of stroke in women highlight a need for a comprehensive understanding of the existing literature to effectively care for patients. Additionally, there is a need for future research focusing on these differences. Women experience a unique set of stroke risk factors during their reproductive years, and then, often outlive their male counterparts to experience a time of elevated risk of stroke in senescence. Systemic bias and barriers to stroke care need to be examined, particularly the lower rates of treatment with thrombolytics for acute IS, and appropriate preventive measures, such as anticoagulation for Afib. Given that most strokes in women occur because of traditional vascular risk factors, aggressive control of these factors should be pursued, particularly given the array of effective treatment options available. Finally, cultural factors need to be examined to determine how to better support women stroke survivors to combat the disparities seen in post-stroke outcomes such as the likelihood of returning to work or living independently. A comprehensive approach to understanding and addressing stroke in women is needed to combat existing disparities and optimize stroke care.

CLINICS CARE POINTS

- Woman have worse post-stroke outcomes than men, with minority women suffering disproportionately.
- Most strokes in women are due to traditional vascular risk factors and aggressive treatment is critical. For example, the risk of stroke doubles for every 20mmHg of systolic and 10mmHg of diastolic increase in BP.
- Intra-uterine devices are an excellent contraceptive choice in stroke survivors, given the high level of efficacy and low systemic hormone exposure.
- In a woman with a history of stroke, sspirin can be continued pre-conception and throughout pregnancy.
- Women respond equallly well to thrombolytics for acute stroke treatment, but are less likely to be treated.

REFERENCES

1. Persky RW, Turtzo LC, McCullough LD. Stroke in women: disparities and outcomes. Curr Cardiol Rep 2010;12(1):6–13.
2. Christensen H, Bushnell C. Stroke in Women. Continuum (Minneap Minn) 2020; 26(2):363–85.
3. LaHue SC, Torres D, Rosendale N, et al. Stroke Characteristics, Risk Factors, and Outcomes in Transgender Adults: A Case Series. Neurologist 2019;24(2):66–70.
4. Benjamin EJ, Muntner P, Alonso A, et al. Heart Disease and Stroke Statistics-2019 Update: A Report From the American Heart Association. Circulation 2019; 139(10):e56–528.
5. Wassertheil-Smoller S. Stroke in women. Nutr Metab Cardiovasc Dis 2010;20(6): 419–25.
6. O'Donnell MJ, Xavier D, Liu L, et al. Risk factors for ischaemic and intracerebral haemorrhagic stroke in 22 countries (the INTERSTROKE study): a case-control study. Lancet 2010;376(9735):112–23.
7. Boehme AK, Esenwa C, Elkind MS. Stroke Risk Factors, Genetics, and Prevention. Circ Res 2017;120(3):472–95.
8. Gaciong Z, Sinski M, Lewandowski J. Blood pressure control and primary prevention of stroke: summary of the recent clinical trial data and meta-analyses. Curr Hypertens Rep 2013;15(6):559–74.
9. Psaltopoulou T, Sergentanis TN, Panagiotakos DB, et al. Mediterranean diet, stroke, cognitive impairment, and depression: A meta-analysis. Ann Neurol 2013;74(4):580–91.
10. Wenger NK, Arnold A, Bairey Merz CN, et al. Hypertension Across a Woman's Life Cycle. J Am Coll Cardiol 2018;71(16):1797–813.

11. Bushnell C, Chireau M. Preeclampsia and Stroke: Risks during and after Pregnancy. Stroke Res Treat 2011;2011:858134.
12. Seely EW, Ecker J. Chronic hypertension in pregnancy. Circulation 2014;129(11): 1254–61.
13. Chambers JC, Fusi L, Malik IS, et al. Association of maternal endothelial dysfunction with preeclampsia. JAMA 2001;285(12):1607–12.
14. Rossi R, Chiurlia E, Nuzzo A, et al. Flow-mediated vasodilation and the risk of developing hypertension in healthy postmenopausal women. J Am Coll Cardiol 2004;44(8):1636–40.
15. Hypertension in pregnancy. Report of the American College of Obstetricians and Gynecologists' Task Force on Hypertension in Pregnancy. Obstet Gynecol 2013; 122(5):1122–31.
16. Os I, Oparil S, Gerdts E, et al. Essential hypertension in women. Blood Press 2004;13(5):272–8.
17. Peters SA, Huxley RR, Woodward M. Diabetes as a risk factor for stroke in women compared with men: a systematic review and meta-analysis of 64 cohorts, including 775,385 individuals and 12,539 strokes. Lancet 2014;383(9933): 1973–80.
18. Madsen TE, Howard VJ, Jimenez M, et al. Impact of Conventional Stroke Risk Factors on Stroke in Women: An Update. Stroke 2018;49(3):536–42.
19. Rodriguez-Campello A, Jimenez-Conde J, Ois A, et al. Sex-related differences in abdominal obesity impact on ischemic stroke risk. Eur J Neurol 2017;24(2): 397–403.
20. Stevens RJ, Coleman RL, Adler AI, et al. Risk factors for myocardial infarction case fatality and stroke case fatality in type 2 diabetes: UKPDS 66. Diabetes Care 2004;27(1):201–7.
21. Mansi IA. Statins in Primary Prevention: Uncertainties and Gaps in Randomized Trial Data. Am J Cardiovasc Drugs *: Drugs devices, other interventions* 2016; 16(6):407–18.
22. Yao X, Gersh BJ, Lopez-Jimenez F, et al. Generalizability of the FOURIER trial to routine clinical care: Do trial participants represent patients in everyday practice? Am Heart J 2019;209:54–62.
23. Aggarwal NR, Patel HN, Mehta LS, et al. Sex Differences in Ischemic Heart Disease: Advances, Obstacles, and Next Steps. Circ Cardiovasc Qual Outcomes 2018;11(2):e004437.
24. Vondra S, Kunihs V, Eberhart T, et al. Metabolism of cholesterol and progesterone is differentially regulated in primary trophoblastic subtypes and might be disturbed in recurrent miscarriages. J Lipid Res 2019;60(11):1922–34.
25. Wang J, Moore D, Subramanian A, et al. Gestational dyslipidaemia and adverse birthweight outcomes: a systematic review and meta-analysis. Obes Rev : official J Int Assoc Study Obes 2018;19(9):1256–68.
26. Jin WY, Lin SL, Hou RL, et al. Associations between maternal lipid profile and pregnancy complications and perinatal outcomes: a population-based study from China. BMC pregnancy and childbirth 2016;16:60.
27. Wiznitzer A, Mayer A, Novack V, et al. Association of lipid levels during gestation with preeclampsia and gestational diabetes mellitus: a population-based study. Am J Obstet Gynecol 2009;201(5):482 e481–488.
28. Bateman BT, Hernandez-Diaz S, Fischer MA, et al. Statins and congenital malformations: cohort study. BMJ 2015;350:h1035.

29. Ko D, Rahman F, Schnabel RB, et al. Atrial fibrillation in women: epidemiology, pathophysiology, presentation, and prognosis. Nat Rev Cardiol 2016;13(6): 321–32.
30. Piccini JP, Hammill BG, Sinner MF, et al. Incidence and prevalence of atrial fibrillation and associated mortality among Medicare beneficiaries, 1993-2007. Circ Cardiovasc Qual Outcomes 2012;5(1):85–93.
31. Thompson LE, Maddox TM, Lei L, et al. Sex Differences in the Use of Oral Anticoagulants for Atrial Fibrillation: A Report From the National Cardiovascular Data Registry (NCDR((R))) PINNACLE Registry. J Am Heart Assoc 2017;6(7).
32. Avgil Tsadok M, Gagnon J, Joza J, et al. Temporal trends and sex differences in pulmonary vein isolation for patients with atrial fibrillation. Heart Rhythm 2015; 12(9):1979–86.
33. Man-Son-Hing M, Nichol G, Lau A, et al. Choosing antithrombotic therapy for elderly patients with atrial fibrillation who are at risk for falls. Arch Intern Med 1999;159(7):677–85.
34. Oie LR, Kurth T, Gulati S, et al. Migraine and risk of stroke. J Neurol Neurosurg Psychiatry 2020;91(6):593–604.
35. Dodick DW, Shewale AS, Lipton RB, et al. Migraine Patients With Cardiovascular Disease and Contraindications: An Analysis of Real-World Claims Data. J Prim Care Community Health 2020;11:2150132720963680.
36. Kudrow D, Pascual J, Winner PK, et al. Vascular safety of erenumab for migraine prevention. Neurology 2020;94(5):e497–510.
37. Singh AK, Tantiwongkosi B, Moise AM, et al. Stroke-like migraine attacks after radiation therapy syndrome: Case report and review of the literature. Neuroradiol J 2017;30(6):568–73.
38. Goldfinch AI, Kleinig TJ. Stroke-like migraine attacks after radiation therapy syndrome: a case report and literature review. Radiol Case Rep 2017;12(3):610–4.
39. Olin JW, Froehlich J, Gu X, et al. The United States Registry for Fibromuscular Dysplasia: results in the first 447 patients. Circulation 2012;125(25):3182–90.
40. Olin JW, Gornik HL, Bacharach JM, et al. Fibromuscular dysplasia: state of the science and critical unanswered questions: a scientific statement from the American Heart Association. Circulation 2014;129(9):1048–78.
41. Sato Y, Kazumata K, Nakatani E, et al. Characteristics of Moyamoya Disease Based on National Registry Data in Japan. Stroke 2019;50(8):1973–80.
42. Kim JS. Moyamoya Disease: Epidemiology, Clinical Features, and Diagnosis. J Stroke 2016;18(1):2–11.
43. Khan N, Achrol AS, Guzman R, et al. Sex differences in clinical presentation and treatment outcomes in Moyamoya disease. Neurosurgery 2012;71(3):587–93 ; discussion 593.
44. Ducros A. Reversible cerebral vasoconstriction syndrome. Lancet Neurol 2012; 11(10):906–17.
45. Topcuoglu MA, McKee KE, Singhal AB. Gender and hormonal influences in reversible cerebral vasoconstriction syndrome. Eur Stroke J 2016;1(3):199–204.
46. Lee JJ, Cook-Wiens G, Johnson BD, et al. Age at Menarche and Risk of Cardiovascular Disease Outcomes: Findings From the National Heart Lung and Blood Institute-Sponsored Women's Ischemia Syndrome Evaluation. J Am Heart Assoc 2019;8(12):e012406.
47. Lokkegaard E, Nielsen LH, Keiding N. Risk of Stroke With Various Types of Menopausal Hormone Therapies: A National Cohort Study. Stroke 2017;48(8):2266–9.
48. Carlton C, Banks M, Sundararajan S. Oral Contraceptives and Ischemic Stroke Risk. Stroke 2018;49(4):e157–9.

49. Swartz RH, Cayley ML, Foley N, et al. The incidence of pregnancy-related stroke: A systematic review and meta-analysis. Int J Stroke 2017;12(7):687–97.
50. Kuklina EV, Tong X, Bansil P, et al. Trends in pregnancy hospitalizations that included a stroke in the United States from 1994 to 2007: reasons for concern? Stroke 2011;42(9):2564–70.
51. Kamel H, Navi BB, Sriram N, et al. Risk of a thrombotic event after the 6-week postpartum period. N Engl J Med 2014;370(14):1307–15.
52. Leffert LR, Clancy CR, Bateman BT, et al. Hypertensive disorders and pregnancy-related stroke: frequency, trends, risk factors, and outcomes. Obstet Gynecol 2015;125(1):124–31.
53. Bellamy L, Casas JP, Hingorani AD, et al. Pre-eclampsia and risk of cardiovascular disease and cancer in later life: systematic review and meta-analysis. BMJ 2007;335(7627):974.
54. Wu P, Haththotuwa R, Kwok CS, et al. Preeclampsia and Future Cardiovascular Health: A Systematic Review and Meta-Analysis. Circ Cardiovasc Qual Outcomes 2017;10(2).
55. ACOG Committee Opinion No. 743. Low-Dose Aspirin Use During Pregnancy. Obstet Gynecol 2018;132(1):e44–52.
56. Swartz RH, Ladhani NNN, Foley N, et al. Canadian stroke best practice consensus statement: Secondary stroke prevention during pregnancy. Int J Stroke 2018;13(4):406–19.
57. Tang AW, Greer I. A systematic review on the use of new anticoagulants in pregnancy. Obstet Med 2013;6(2):64–71.
58. Ginsberg JS, Hirsh J. Use of antithrombotic agents during pregnancy. Chest 1998;114(5 Suppl):524S–30S.
59. Lameijer H, JJJ Aalberts, van Veldhuisen DJ, et al. Efficacy and safety of direct oral anticoagulants during pregnancy; a systematic literature review. Thromb Res 2018;169:123–7.
60. Mazzolai L, Hohlfeld P, Spertini F, et al. Fondaparinux is a safe alternative in case of heparin intolerance during pregnancy. Blood 2006;108(5):1569–70.
61. Welten S, Onland-Moret NC, Boer JMA, et al. Age at Menopause and Risk of Ischemic and Hemorrhagic Stroke. Stroke 2021;52(8):2583–91.
62. Christensen H, Cordonnier C. Age At Menopause: A Female Risk Factor of Stroke? Stroke 2021;52(8):2592–3.
63. Shadyab AH, Gass ML, Stefanick ML, et al. Maternal Age at Childbirth and Parity as Predictors of Longevity Among Women in the United States: The Women's Health Initiative. Am J Public Health 2017;107(1):113–9.
64. Meerwijk EL, Sevelius JM. Transgender Population Size in the United States: a Meta-Regression of Population-Based Probability Samples. Am J Public Health 2017;107(2):e1–8.
65. Denby KJ, Cho L, Toljan K, et al. Assessment of Cardiovascular Risk in Transgender Patients Presenting for Gender-Affirming Care. Am J Med 2021;134(8):1002–8.
66. Gartman EJ. The use of thrombolytic therapy in pregnancy. Obstet Med 2013;6(3):105–11.
67. Aaron S, Mannam PR, Shaikh A, et al. Acute Ischemic Stroke in Term Pregnancy Treated with Recombinant Tissue Plasminogen Activator. Case Rep Neurol 2020;12(Suppl 1):4–8.
68. Demchuk AM. Yes, intravenous thrombolysis should be administered in pregnancy when other clinical and imaging factors are favorable. Stroke 2013;44(3):864–5.

69. Melandri G, Vagnarelli F, Calabrese D, et al. Review of tenecteplase (TNKase) in the treatment of acute myocardial infarction. Vasc Health Risk Manag 2009;5(1): 249–56.
70. Akhter T, Larsson A, Larsson M, et al. Artery wall layer dimensions during normal pregnancy: a longitudinal study using noninvasive high-frequency ultrasound. Am J Physiol Heart Circ Physiol 2013;304(2):H229–34.
71. Lorenzano S, Ahmed N, Falcou A, et al. Does sex influence the response to intravenous thrombolysis in ischemic stroke?: answers from safe implementation of treatments in Stroke-International Stroke Thrombolysis Register. Stroke 2013; 44(12):3401–6.
72. Bushnell CD, Chaturvedi S, Gage KR, et al. Sex differences in stroke: Challenges and opportunities. J Cereb Blood Flow Metab 2018;38(12):2179–91.
73. Kent DM, Buchan AM, Hill MD. The gender effect in stroke thrombolysis: of CASES, controls, and treatment-effect modification. Neurology 2008;71(14): 1080–3.
74. Reeves MJ, Fonarow GC, Zhao X, et al. Quality of care in women with ischemic stroke in the GWTG program. Stroke 2009;40(4):1127–33.
75. Reeves M, Bhatt A, Jajou P, et al. Sex differences in the use of intravenous rt-PA thrombolysis treatment for acute ischemic stroke: a meta-analysis. Stroke 2009; 40(5):1743–9.
76. Goyal M, Menon BK, van Zwam WH, et al. Endovascular thrombectomy after large-vessel ischaemic stroke: a meta-analysis of individual patient data from five randomised trials. Lancet 2016;387(10029):1723–31.
77. Chalos V, de Ridder IR, Lingsma HF, et al. Does Sex Modify the Effect of Endovascular Treatment for Ischemic Stroke? Stroke 2019;50(9):2413–9.
78. Dmytriw AA, Ku JC, Yang VXD, et al. Do Outcomes between Women and Men Differ after Endovascular Thrombectomy? A Meta-analysis. AJNR Am J Neuroradiol 2021;42(5):910–5.
79. Hahn M, Groschel S, Hayani E, et al. Sex Disparities in Re-Employment in Stroke Patients With Large Vessel Occlusion Undergoing Mechanical Thrombectomy. Stroke 2022;53:2528–37.
80. Podymow T, August P. Update on the use of antihypertensive drugs in pregnancy. Hypertension 2008;51(4):960–9.
81. Mustafa R, Ahmed S, Gupta A, et al. A comprehensive review of hypertension in pregnancy. J Pregnancy 2012;2012:105918.
82. Brown CM, Garovic VD. Drug treatment of hypertension in pregnancy. Drugs 2014;74(3):283–96.

Gender Differences in Intracerebral Hemorrhage

Nicholas Dykman Osteraas, MD, MS

KEYWORDS

• Sex differences • Intracerebral hemorrhage • Intraparenchymal hemorrhage

KEY POINTS

- Intracerebral hemorrhage has many potential secondary causes, many of which have gender differences.
- Physiologic differences between men and women play a role, as do differences in risk factors.
- Health care and family bias may influence treatment decisions and outcomes.

INTRODUCTION

Nontraumatic intracerebral hemorrhages (ICHs) are the second most common type of disabling stroke after ischemic stroke (IS), accounting for around 26% of cases globally.[1] In the United States, recent data suggest an annual incidence of 23 to 25 per 100,000,[2,3] with recently increasing rates in the young and middle age,[2] and higher rates in men (25.67 compared with 19.17 per 100,000 in women).[3] Mortality rates in the United States are 13.96 per 100,000 for men, and slightly lower at 11.35 per 100,000 for women.[2] Although commonly studied and reported as a single disease entity, ICH is best understood as a manifestation of different potential pathophysiologic processes, many of which vary in prevalence between men and women and are discussed further.

Globally, there is variation between countries and populations regarding incidence and mortality. Data reporting validity can vary as well, because some IS and subarachnoid hemorrhage (SAH) cases can be grouped in together with ICHs under the umbrella category of "stroke." Naturally this contributes to the challenging nature of the study of ICH.[1,4] The variation between countries regarding incidence and outcome is to be expected, however, because ICH does not occur in an isolated fashion, but rather in a context of risk factors, which vary between both individuals and regions. Treatment and recovery from ICH likewise both occur in the context of a health care system, and these systems of course vary between and within countries.[5]

Department of Neurological Sciences, Division of Cerebrovascular Diseases, Rush University Medical Center, 1725 West Harrison Street Suite 118, Chicago, IL 60612, USA
E-mail address: nicko@gwu.edu

Neurol Clin 41 (2023) 283–296
https://doi.org/10.1016/j.ncl.2022.10.002

Differences between sexes in epidemiology, along with causes, risk factors, interventions, as well as recovery and outcomes are covered. It is important to keep in mind that there are a variety of interacting variables, contributing to disparate findings in the literature. As stated by Gokhale and colleagues,[4] the relationship between gender and ICH is not straightforward given the interaction of gender with other factors such as age and ethnicity. To add to these, we can include any pertinent factor that may significantly vary between genders and influence ICH epidemiology and outcomes, such as substance use,[6] anticoagulant use, and smoking among many other pertinent factors, which are covered in more detail.

Differences in Epidemiology

Gender differences in epidemiology vary widely based on study geography.[1,4] Little variation in incidence between men and women has been found in European and Australian studies, and higher rates in men in North America, Japan, and China.[4] In addition to geographic variations in health care systems, additional factors that vary between geographic settings such as diet, availability and implementation of primary and secondary ICH prevention, age and related demographics, substance use patterns, as well as potential ethnic and/or racial differences can also potentially play a role.[7] All these interacting factors together can be challenging to account for when attempting to isolate gender-specific differences.[4,8]

In many geographic areas and health care systems, women present with ICH at older ages than men[9] (although this is not the case in all cohorts),[6] so it follows that specific causes associated with lobar ICH in the elderly, such as cerebral amyloid angiopathy, may be more common in women as a result of age differences in presentation as opposed to other sex-specific factors that could in theory predispose women to higher rates of lobar ICH. Conversely, ICH in young people may be more likely to be associated with substance use for a similar reason, and so it follows that ICH could potentially be more closely related to cultural and psychological predispositions to substance abuse in specific cohorts than to inherent biologic differences between men and women.[6]

Overall, the relative risk of ICH seems to be higher in men when compared with women,[10] with a robust meta-analysis of more than 11 epidemiologic data sets demonstrating an odds ratio of 1.6 in men.[4]

Differences in Intervention

The cornerstones of acute management for ICH (which ideally should not differ between men and women) include blood pressure (BP) control, reversal of any anticoagulation, investigation into potential secondary causes, admission to a hospital floor able to provide close neurologic monitoring with trained nursing staff, along with evaluation of cases by neurosurgery.[11,12] Regarding BP control, no sex differences in outcomes using "intense" BP reduction with a systolic BP of less than 140 mm Hg have been found in a posthoc analysis of the Antihypertensive Treatment in Intracerebral Hemorrhage-2 (ATACH-2) trial.[13] However, a pooled analysis of the Intensive Blood Pressure Reduction in Acute Cerebral Hemorrhage (INTERACT) trial 1 demonstrated a greater odds of 3-month mortality in men in the intensive arm (odds ratio [OR], 1.22, $P = .022$).[14]

The clinicians who care for patients with ICH and offer medical, surgical, rehabilitative, and palliative services are human, and despite the best of intentions, are subject to possible practice variation based on unconscious bias.[15,16] Although women may have a slightly lower ICH risk when compared with men when using direct oral anticoagulation medications,[17,18] women may be less likely to be prescribed anticoagulants in the setting of atrial fibrillation in the first place.[18] In those who are prescribed anticoagulants and suffer ICH, one retrospective study identified that women on oral anticoagulation were nearly *half* as likely as men to receive reversal agents ($P = .007$).[19] A single-center study demonstrated a nearly 3-fold likelihood of external ventricular drain (EVD) utilization in men when compared with women, despite controlling for differences in bleed location, shift, and clinical decline among other reasons for EVD utilization in the management of patients with ICH.[20] Other work has been unable to find clear evidence of bias leading to differences in treatment.[21]

Differences in Pathophysiology and Presentation

There are multiple different potential causes of ICH, along with multiple risk factors that contribute to ICH risk, many of these related to factors that may vary between genders. A portion of these factors are more closely related to inherent physiologic differences between men and women (for example, risks of ICH associated with pregnancy), and others are more closely related to demographic, social, and psychological factors (such as different rates of cocaine and alcohol use between sexes in certain age ranges, socioeconomic status, and geographic areas).[6,22,23] An excellent example of the interaction between age, gender, and risk factors is the work of Umeano and colleagues,[6] who demonstrated a contradictory finding compared with most literature, with a cohort of women presenting with ICH approximately 4 years younger than men (61.1 + 14.5 vs 65.8 + 17.3 years, $P = .03$). This observation was explained by a much greater extent of substance abuse in the women in this North Carolina cohort (35% vs 8.9%, $P < .0001$).[6]

This discussion of risk factors and ICH risk is not to distract from the biologic effects that gender has on ICH. Simplistically, genetic differences lead to differences in the hormonal environment, which has downstream effects on platelet activation, vasomotor reactivity, and endogenous fibrinolytic systems. As a specific example, slit guidance ligand (SLIT3) protein and G protein-coupled receptor 26 (GPR26) are involved in estrogen and serotonin modulation with potential sex-linked effects on ICH occurrence.[24] These differences in the hormonal environment between men and women likely play a role in ICH risk overall[25] and may play a more prominent role in specific secondary causes of ICH such as ICH associated with reversible cerebral vasoconstriction syndrome (RCVS).

Patients with ICH often present with focal neurologic deficits; seizure, headache, and disturbances of consciousness are also at times present, and most are hypertensive. No difference in headache as a presenting symptom among those with primary ICH was reported in a meta-analysis of 5 studies.[26] Hemorrhage location differences between genders seem to vary by region, with some regions and literature reporting no differences in bleed location, and some with an increase in lobar bleeds in women.[4] Other specific gender differences in presentation in the setting of secondary causes of ICH, such as in the setting of RCVS, are discussed further in more detail in association with these specific causes.

Most ICHs in patients younger than 70 years are related pathophysiologically to uncontrolled hypertension, which over time results in lipohyalinosis and the formation of Charcot-Bouchard aneurysms,[27] setting the stage for ICH. These bleeds are classically located in deep gray matter, although a fair number can be lobar in location.[28] Immediately posthemorrhage, blood-brain barrier breakdown contributes to perihematomal edema, which can result in postbleed neurologic deterioration. There is evidence that this so-called secondary injury may be less extensive in women.[29]

ICH in the setting of pregnancy may, in many cases, have a distinct pathophysiologic process, and different risk factors when compared with the nonpregnant population.[30] Eclampsia, postpartum angiopathy, posterior reversible encephalopathy syndrome (PRES), and RCVS are thought to share a common pathophysiology of increased brain barrier permeability and disordered vasomotor reactivity (likely mediated in part by estrogen) with some common triggering or inciting factors (such as vasoactive medications) along with overlapping clinical and radiographic presentations.[30,31]

Not only RCVS (however, specifically in the setting of tetrahydrocannabinol-mediated RCVS in certain cohorts, males predominate)[32] but also hemorrhagic complications are much more likely in women when compared with men (OR, 2.57; $P = .001$).[33] In the setting of postpartum specifically, the bleed location may be more likely parenchymal as opposed to the subarachnoid space (the opposite pattern is generally found in RCVS outside of pregnancy).[34] Blood in the subarachnoid space or parenchymal hemorrhage may complicate cases of PRES in a minority of cases, and analysis of several data sets suggests this is a risk for poor outcome. Interestingly, analysis of the same data suggested that PRES in the context of pregnancy was more likely to be associated with a favorable outcome.[35] One retrospective study demonstrated that hemorrhagic RCVS was associated with a longer hospital stay but not necessarily worse outcome.[33]

Cerebral Dural Venous Sinus Thrombosis

Cerebral dural venous sinus thrombosis (CDVST) involves occlusion of the dural sinuses and draining veins of the central nervous system (CNS), which can subsequently result in ICH after ensuing venous edema and infarction. CDVST can be incidentally found with no immediate pathophysiologic consequence if the occlusion is not complete and/or other veins are able to compensate. Although clinicians generally think of the large cerebral veins when considering this condition, cortical vein thrombosis can occur as well (either in isolation or as an extension of a larger clot). When ICH complicates CDVST, blood may present radiographically on initial head computed tomography (CT) as lobar ICH and/or convexity SAH. States of increased coagulability, such as those associated with oral contraceptive use or physiologic changes of pregnancy, contribute significantly to an increase risk of CDVST in women, with one cohort publication demonstrating 20% of CDVST cases in women occurring in the setting of pregnancy.[36] Female sex is not a risk for poor prognosis after CDVST, although pregnancy may complicate treatment.[37] Unlike other causes of ICH, anticoagulation is used as treatment along with careful neurologic monitoring; this is not always successful and sometimes surgical intervention is required in the event of neurologic decline despite adequate anticoagulation (**Fig. 1**).

Vascular Malformations

ICH related to vascular malformation, such as arteriovenous malformations, dural arteriovenous fistulas, and cerebral cavernous malformations are a more common cause of ICH in the young, up to nearly 50% of ICH cause in one cohort.[38] One Chinese retrospective series found ICH secondary to vascular malformations occurring more commonly in women,[39] and a separate single-center Japanese study demonstrated a nearly 3-fold risk of rebleed among women with ICH due to vascular malformations.[40] Another study examining outcomes in more than 50 centers in China found a nearly 2.5 times likelihood for poor outcome among women with bleeds occurring in association with a vascular malformation.[41] This gender difference has been hypothesized to be partially related to differences in hormonal receptors, but immunohistochemical analysis has not proved this.[42]

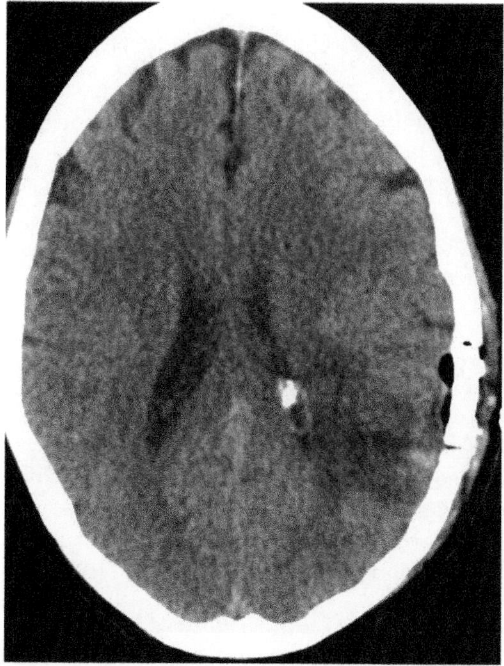

Fig. 1. Axial plain head CT of a 56-year-old woman on estrogen-containing oral contraceptives with headache, aphasia, and extensive CDVST, who declined despite therapeutic anticoagulation, requiring decompressive hemicraniectomy.

Cerebral Amyloid Angiopathy

Cerebral amyloid angiopathy (CAA) is a common cause of lobar ICH in the elderly.[43–45] Amyloid protein deposition in the vasculature leading to weakening of the vessel walls along with an inflammatory reaction is thought be the mechanism underlying the pathophysiologic process. This condition can manifest clinically as sudden persistent neurologic deficits with lobar ICH (**Fig. 2**), potentially along with history of memory impairment, and radiographically on MRI the presence of cortical microbleeds along with cortical superficial siderosis and enlarged perivascular spaces.[44] Patchy or confluent T2-hyperintense lesions in the cortex and subcortical white matter can at times be visualized on MRI in association with microbleeds, which can be associated with subacute cognitive changes, headaches, seizures, and stroke-like symptoms suggesting CAA-related inflammation.[44]

Some mouse models of CAA have demonstrated more severe cognitive impairment and higher rates of microbleeds in females,[43,46] potentially mediated by a more aggressive inflammatory response to the amyloid depositions.[47] However, other models have not demonstrated a clear sex-linked difference in microbleeds and cognitive impairment.[48]

Moyamoya Disease

Moyamoya disease (MMD) refers to a progressive occlusive vasculopathy, traditionally associated with gradual narrowing of the terminal portion of the internal carotid arteries with resulting sprouting of the classic “puff of smoke” lenticulostriates, most visible on conventional angiography. Although IS is the more commonly known

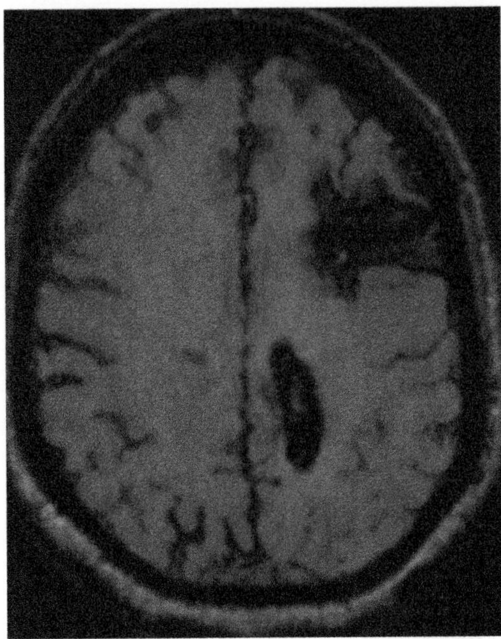

Fig. 2. Axial MRI of the brain—susceptibility weighted imaging—of a 63-year-old woman with multiple lobar hemorrhages, with probable diagnosis of CAA.

complication of the disease, ICH can occur as well,[49–51] at times diagnosed during pregnancy,[51] with the highest bleeding risk between 24 weeks and delivery.[52] MMD is also a more common disease in women, with a 2.9 to 1.1 ratio when compared with men depending on the geographic area of the study.[53–55]

Radiographically, women have a greater likelihood of enlarged perivascular spaces on imaging (OR, 2.67; $P = .34$) and are more likely to receive a diagnosis of bilateral MMD (OR, 0.6, $P = .04$).[56,57] Bleeds in the setting of MMD can occur in similar locations to those associated with hypertension, such as the basal ganglia and thalamus[58]; they are more likely to involve blood in the ventricular system,[59] and can be in atypical locations as well such as the corpus callosum,[58] or in multiple simultaneous locations.[60] Female sex trended closely toward being a significant risk factor for rebleeding in one study ($P = .08$).[61]

The disease needs to be differentiated from a moyamoya radiographic pattern (frequently described as a moyamoya syndrome) that can occur as a result of many other secondary causes, some of which have significant sex differences in the underlying disease causing the syndrome. As an example, a moyamoya radiographic pattern in association with autoimmune thyroiditis has a nearly 10 times higher incidence in women when compared with men.[62]

Hemorrhagic Transformation of Ischemic Stroke

Hemorrhagic transformation of an IS is common, ranging from petechial and clinically insignificant (**Fig. 3**), to transformation of most of the stroke bed with associated neurologic decline. Hemorrhagic transformation is a well-known potential complication of IS and associated thrombolytic therapy (**Fig. 4**), in which case the cause of the ICH is not a mystery. There are cases, however, in which a patient

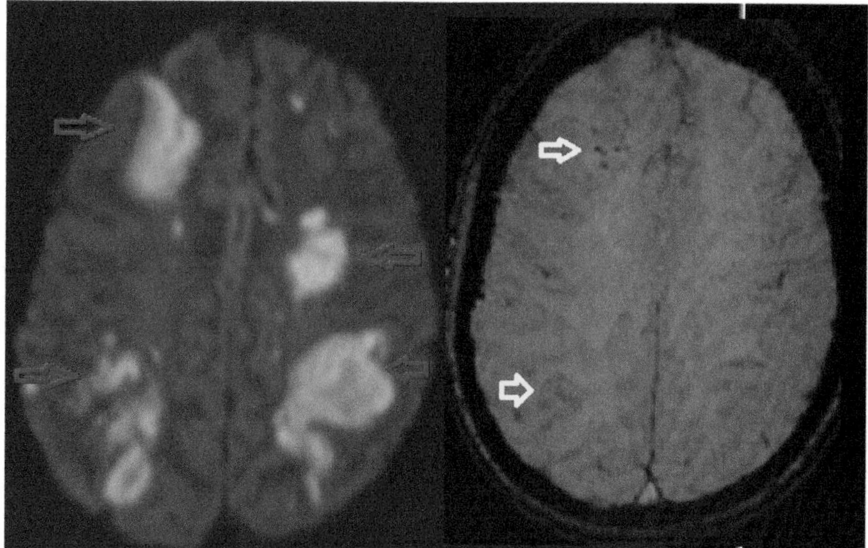

Fig. 3. Axial diffusion-weighted (*A*) and susceptibility-weighted (*B*) MRI of the brain of a 52-year-old woman with multiple infarctions secondary to RCVS (*red arrows*) with petechial hemorrhagic changes (*yellow arrows*) on susceptibility-weighted sequence.

may present to the emergency room with an apparently acute ICH on initial head CT that is the result of a transformed IS. A careful history in combination with MRI can be very useful in ferreting out a transformed IS as the cause in such situations.

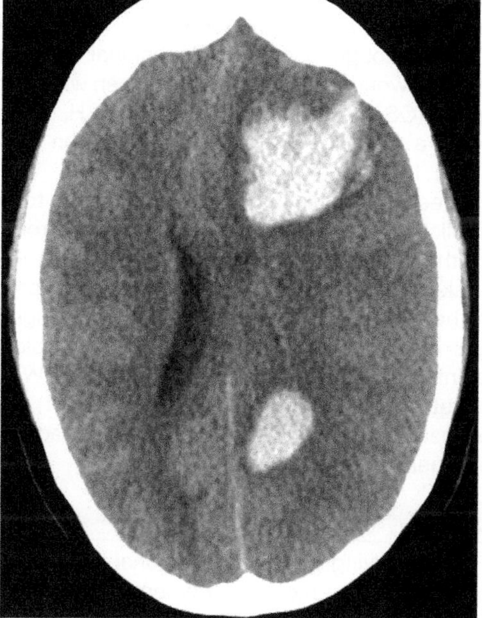

Fig. 4. Axial plain head CT of a 50-year-old woman with hemorrhagic complications after receiving lytic therapy for suspected ischemic stroke.

Infection and Malignancy

ICH can be a complication of infectious CNS encephalitis. Among the most common of viral CNS infections is herpes simplex encephalitis, which has a special predilection for the temporal lobes, resulting in both ischemic and hemorrhagic complications. Cardiac and CNS infections can result in mycotic aneurysms with subsequent rupture and resultant ICH. Meta-analyses have not demonstrated a difference in functional outcome between men and women with infectious encephalitis.[63] Recently, ICH has been reported in association with infection in the setting of coronavirus disease 2019 (COVID-19), more commonly in men (64%–74%).[64–66] Many patients hospitalized with COVID-19 were exposed to treatment doses of anticoagulation, which may have complicated the process of determining the ICH mechanism.[65]

Either primary CNS tumors or solid metastases from systemic malignancy can present initially with ICH. Although hemorrhagic changes within a primary CNS malignancy are easily detected, metastatic hemorrhagic lesions that are most commonly encountered in the gray-white junction may require elaborate workup. Hematologic malignancies and chemotherapy-induced thrombocytopenia are both associated with increased risk of ICH.[67].

Differences in Modifiable Contributing Risk Factors

Hypertension is a well-known risk factor for ICH. In general, men have higher mean arterial pressure readings than women, but this is influenced by both age and race (among other factors as well, such as diet and salt sensitivity).[68] On the other hand, women may be less likely to be adherent to recommended antihypertensive regimens, with a recent large meta-analysis demonstrating lower self-reports of compliance with antihypertensives among women older than 65 years (OR, 0.84; $P = .02$).[69]

Heavy alcohol intake has been associated with an increased risk for ICH.[70] Although in general men have higher rates of harmful alcohol use, this gap has recently been closing.[23–71] In addition, men may have a stronger pathophysiologic association between high BP in response to alcohol than women.[72] Smoking is a risk factor for ICH in both genders, and although there are wide regional variations in smoking rates between men and women, worldwide there are more men who smoke than women.[73] Obstructive sleep apnea (OSA) is also a risk factor for ICH, with one study demonstrating a trend toward a statistically significant interaction between women with OSA and ICH risk (OR, 1.12; $P = .057$).[74]

The association between statin use and ICH risk continues to be an area of active investigation with conflicting data. Recently published data from the Danish Stroke Registry found that both current statin and longer duration of statin use may be associated with reduced risk of ICH in both men and women.[75] It is of note that historically women are less likely than men to receive aggressive lipid management and to be prescribed statins for primary and secondary prevention of cardiovascular conditions including myocardial infarction (67.0% vs 78.4%, $P < .001$). Women are also more likely to discontinue statin therapy (10.9% vs 6.1%; $P < .001$),[76] with similar results found in other studies that also account for the interaction of racial and socioeconomic variables in addition to gender.[77–79]

Differences in Outcome

Although there may be underlying genetic or hormonal factors contributing to differences in outcome in ICH between men and women, it is important to keep in mind that such disparities may potentially vary between sexes given differences in age, associated comorbidities, mediating factors such as treating clinical/hospital practice variations, and family preferences regarding aggressiveness of interventions. It should therefore be no surprise that sex differences in the outcome of patients with ICH has been somewhat conflicting, with some studies demonstrating increased risk of mortality in men,[1,2,9,14,80,81] and some with increased risk in women.[82,83] Part of this discrepancy may be related to challenges associated with accounting for differences in potentially confounding variables listed earlier; after controlling for age, one study found higher rates of death or discharge to hospice in women with ICH (OR, 1.304; $P < .0001$).[83] As an example of the effect that age differences may have in outcome, it can be assumed that conditions associated with increased age such as atrial fibrillation (AF) may be more likely to co-occur in an old cohort of patients, independent of sex.[84] Patients with a lobar bleed along with a diagnosis of AF can be challenging to optimally manage, given the need for anticoagulation, and this could in part explain why females may be more likely to experience poor outcomes caused by a subsequent IS after ICH (OR, 1.3; $P = .004$).[85]

A prognostic marker for worse outcome in the setting of ICH is hemorrhage expansion.[86] Male sex has been associated with higher rates of expansion (OR, 1.7; $P = .007$) in some studies but not in others.[14–87] Assuming patients survive the initial bleed, mortality in ICH survivors is still significantly increased compared with age-matched cohorts without ICH. EVD insertion in ICH-related hydrocephalus was less common in women when compared with men ($P = .016$), raising concerns about sex biases and social factors limitations. Mortality has been largely attributed to superimposed infections, cardiac causes, and recurrent ICH among other less common causes. Regarding specific post-ICH complications, men overall are at higher risk for pneumonia and sepsis (21.9 vs 15.5%, $P < .001$ and 3.4 vs 1.6%, $P = .009$, respectively),[88] whereas women who survive ICH may be less likely to die from infection (OR 0.9, $P = .001$). A Japanese cohort detected nearly seven times higher rates of post-ICH deep vein thrombosis detection in women when compared with men.[89] Very early implementation of "Do not resuscitate" orders have been found to occur at nearly 3 times the rate in women with ICH when compared with men[90]; this has been shown in a separate work to be related to poor outcome, but it is unclear to what extent this may be a causal relationship.[91,92]

Differences between sexes in ICH are in part attributable to physiologic differences and demographic and social/behavioral risk factors, along with patient interface with the health care system as well as the interaction effects between all these factors. Some current work on sex differences in ICH may be limited in examining all potential factors involved in sex differences, which likely contributes to discordant findings in the literature. Further epidemiologic work should continue to incorporate ICH cause, associated contributing risk factors, and detailed demographics to the extent possible. Potential clinician, family, and health care system bias in treatment and interventions can be challenging to study but must continue to be addressed.

CLINICS CARE POINTS

- Blood pressure control and reversal of anticoagulation are cornerstones of acute management.
- Caution needs to be utilized with early DNR orders so that a self fulfiling prophecy does not occur.
- A higher index of suspicion for less common eitiologies of ICH is especailly important in the setting of pregnancy.

REFERENCES

1. Krishnamurthi RV, Ikeda T, Feigin VL. Global, regional and country-specific burden of ischaemic stroke, intracerebral haemorrhage and subarachnoid haemorrhage: a systematic analysis of the global burden of disease study 2017. Neuroepidemiology 2020;54:171–9.
2. Bako AT, Pan A, Potter T, et al. Contemporary Trends in the Nationwide Incidence of Primary Intracerebral Hemorrhage. Stroke 2022;29:e70–4.
3. DeLago AJ Jr, Singh H, Jani C, et al. An observational epidemiological study to analyze intracerebral hemorrhage across the United States: Incidence and mortality trends from 1990 to 2017. J Stroke Cerebrovasc Dis 2022;31:106216.
4. Gokhale S, Caplan LR, James ML. Sex differences in incidence, pathophysiology, and outcome of primary intracerebral hemorrhage. Stroke 2015;46:886–92.
5. Aiken LH, Sermeus W, Van den Heede K, et al. Patient safety, satisfaction, and quality of hospital care: cross sectional surveys of nurses and patients in 12 countries in Europe and the United States. Bmj 2012;344.
6. Umeano O, Phillips-Bute B, Hailey CE, et al. Gender and age interact to affect early outcome after intracerebral hemorrhage. PloS one 2013;8:e81664.
7. Kittner SJ, Sekar P, Comeau ME, et al. Ethnic and racial variation in intracerebral hemorrhage risk factors and risk factor burden. JAMA Netw open 2021;4: e2121921–.
8. Lee KY, So WZ, Ho JS, et al. Prevalence of intracranial hemorrhage amongst patients presenting with out-of-hospital cardiac arrest: A systematic review and meta-analysis. Resuscitation 2022;176:136–49.
9. Xing Y, An Z, Zhang X, et al. Sex differences in the clinical features, risk factors, and outcomes of intracerebral hemorrhage: a large hospital-based stroke registry in China. Scientific Rep 2017;7:1–9.
10. Appelros P, Stegmayr B, Terént A. Sex differences in stroke epidemiology: a systematic review. Stroke 2009;40:1082–90.
11. Greenberg SM, Ziai WC, Cordonnier C, et al. Guideline for the Management of Patients With Spontaneous Intracerebral Hemorrhage: A Guideline From the American Heart Association/American Stroke Association. Stroke 2022. 10.1161/STR. 0000000000000407.
12. Mc Lernon S, Nash PS, Werring D. Acute spontaneous intracerebral haemorrhage: treatment and management. Br J Neurosci Nurs 2022;18:116–24.
13. Fukuda-Doi M, Yamamoto H, Koga M, et al. Sex differences in blood pressure–lowering therapy and outcomes following intracerebral hemorrhage: results from ATACH-2. Stroke 2020;51:2282–6.
14. Sandset EC, Wang X, Carcel C, et al. Sex differences in treatment, radiological features and outcome after intracerebral haemorrhage: pooled analysis of intensive blood pressure reduction in acute cerebral haemorrhage trials 1 and 2. Eur stroke J 2020;5:345–50.
15. Chelimsky G, Simpson P, Feng M, et al. Does Unconscious Bias Affect How Pediatricians Manage Their Patients? WMJ 2022;121:18–25.
16. Capers IVQ. How clinicians and educators can mitigate implicit bias in patient care and candidate selection in medical education. ATS scholar 2020;1:211–7.
17. Law SW, Lau WC, Wong IC, et al. Sex-based differences in outcomes of oral anticoagulation in patients with atrial fibrillation. J Am Coll Cardiol 2018;72:271–82.
18. Yong CM, Tremmel JA, Lansberg MG, et al. Sex differences in oral anticoagulation and outcomes of stroke and intracranial bleeding in newly diagnosed atrial fibrillation. J Am Heart Assoc 2020;9:e015689.

19. Grundtvig J, Ovesen C, Steiner T, et al. Sex-Differences in Oral Anticoagulant-Related Intracerebral Hemorrhage. Front Neurol 2022;13:832903.
20. Wang SS-Y, Bögli SY, Nierobisch N, et al. Sex-Related Differences in Patients' Characteristics, Provided Care, and Outcomes Following Spontaneous Intracerebral Hemorrhage. Neurocrit Care 2022;1–10.
21. Guha R, Boehme A, Demel SL, et al. Aggressiveness of care following intracerebral hemorrhage in women and men. Neurology 2017;89:349–54.
22. McHugh RK, Votaw VR, Sugarman DE, et al. Sex and gender differences in substance use disorders. Clin Psychol Rev 2018;66:12–23.
23. Agabio R, Pisanu C, Luigi Gessa G, et al. Sex differences in alcohol use disorder. Curr Med Chem 2017;24:2661–70.
24. Chung J, Montgomery B, Marini S, et al. Genome-wide interaction study with sex identifies novel loci for intracerebral hemorrhage risk. Arteriosclerosis, Thromb Vasc Biol 2019;39. A571-A.
25. Roy-O'Reilly M, McCullough LD. Sex differences in stroke: the contribution of coagulation. Exp Neurol 2014;259:16–27.
26. Ali M, van Os HJ, van der Weerd N, et al. Sex differences in presentation of stroke: a systematic review and meta-analysis. Stroke 2022;53:345–54.
27. Magid-Bernstein J, Girard R, Polster S, et al. Cerebral hemorrhage: pathophysiology, treatment, and future directions. Circ Res 2022;130:1204–29.
28. Jolink WM, Wiegertjes K, Rinkel GJ, et al. Location-specific risk factors for intracerebral hemorrhage: Systematic review and meta-analysis. Neurology 2020;95: e1807–18.
29. Wagner I, Volbers B, Kloska S, et al. Sex differences in perihemorrhagic edema evolution after spontaneous intracerebral hemorrhage. Eur J Neurol 2012;19: 1477–81.
30. Miller EC, Sundheim KM, Willey JZ, et al. The impact of pregnancy on hemorrhagic stroke in young women. Cerebrovasc Dis 2018;46:10–5.
31. Roth J, Deck G. Neurovascular disorders in pregnancy: A review. Obstet Med 2019;12:164–7.
32. Jensen J, Leonard J, Salottolo K, et al. The epidemiology of reversible cerebral vasoconstriction syndrome in patients at a Colorado comprehensive stroke center. J Vasc Interv Neurol 2018;10:32.
33. Patel SD, Topiwala K, Saini V, et al. Hemorrhagic reversible cerebral vasoconstriction syndrome: A retrospective observational study. J Neurol 2021;268:632–9.
34. Pacheco K, Ortiz JF, Parwani J, et al. Reversible Cerebral Vasoconstriction Syndrome in the Postpartum Period: A Systematic Review and Meta-Analysis. Neurol Int 2022;14:488–96.
35. Chen Z, Zhang G, Lerner A, et al. Risk factors for poor outcome in posterior reversible encephalopathy syndrome: systematic review and meta-analysis. Quantitative Imaging Med Surg 2018;8:421.
36. Pan L, Ding J, Ya J, et al. Risk factors and predictors of outcomes in 243 Chinese patients with cerebral venous sinus thrombosis: A retrospective analysis. Clin Neurol Neurosurg 2019;183:105384.
37. Kalita J, Misra UK, Singh VK, et al. Does gender difference matter in cerebral venous thrombosis? J Clin Neurosci 2022;102:114–9.
38. Ruíz-Sandoval JL, Cantú C, Barinagarrementeria F. Intracerebral hemorrhage in young people: analysis of risk factors, location, causes, and prognosis. Stroke 1999;30:537–41.

39. Tong X, Wu J, Lin F, et al. The effect of age, sex, and lesion location on initial presentation in patients with brain arteriovenous malformations. World Neurosurg 2016;87:598–606.
40. Yamada S, Takagi Y, Nozaki K, et al. Risk factors for subsequent hemorrhage in patients with cerebral arteriovenous malformations. J Neurosurg 2007;107: 965–72.
41. Hao Z, Lei C, Liu J, et al. Sex-specific differences in clinical characteristics and outcomes among patients with vascular abnormality-related intracerebral hemorrhage. World Neurosurg 2019;129:e669–76.
42. Kulungowski AM, Hassanein AH, Nosé V, et al. Expression of androgen, estrogen, progesterone, and growth hormone receptors in vascular malformations. Plast Reconstr Surg 2012;129:919e-24e.
43. Maniskas M, Hudobenko J, Urayama A, et al. Abstract WP397: Longitudinal Sex Differences in Cerebral Amyloid Angiopathy. Stroke 2020;51. AWP397-AWP.
44. Chen S-J, Tsai H-H, Tsai L-K, et al. Advances in cerebral amyloid angiopathy imaging. Ther Adv Neurol Disord 2019;12. 1756286419844113.
45. Charidimou A, Boulouis G, Xiong L, et al. Cortical Superficial Siderosis Evolution: a biomarker of cerebral amyloid angiopathy and intracerebral hemorrhage risk. Stroke 2019;50:954–62.
46. Maniskas ME, Mack AF, Morales-Scheihing D, et al. Sex differences in a murine model of Cerebral Amyloid Angiopathy. Brain Behav Immunity-Health 2021;14: 100260.
47. Finger C, Lee J, Manwani B. Sex differences in cerebral amyloid angiopathy: the role of Monocytes/Macrophages (S2. 008). AAN Enterprises; 2022.
48. Edler MK, Johnson CT, Ahmed HS, et al. Age, sex, and regional differences in scavenger receptor CD36 in the mouse brain: Potential relevance to cerebral amyloid angiopathy and Alzheimer's disease. J Comp Neurol 2021;529:2209–26.
49. Lin Y-H, Huang H, Hwang W-Z. Moyamoya disease with Sjogren disease and autoimmune thyroiditis presenting with left intracranial hemorrhage after messenger RNA-1273 vaccination: A case report. Medicine 2022;101.
50. Chen J-B, Lei D, He M, et al. Clinical features and disease progression in moyamoya disease patients with Graves disease. J Neurosurg 2015;123:848–55.
51. Williams DL, Martin IL, Gully RM. Intracerebral hemorrhage and Moyamoya disease in pregnancy. Can J Anesth 2000;47:996–1000.
52. Inayama Y, Kondoh E, Chigusa Y, et al. Moyamoya disease in pregnancy: a 20-year single-center experience and literature review. World Neurosurg 2019;122: 684–91. e2.
53. Ghaffari-Rafi A, Ghaffari-Rafi S, Leon-Rojas J. Socioeconomic and demographic disparities of moyamoya disease in the United States. Clin Neurol Neurosurg 2020;192:105719.
54. Hoshino H, Izawa Y, Suzuki N. Epidemiological features of moyamoya disease in Japan. Neurologia medico-chirurgica 2012;52:295–8.
55. Kleinloog R, Regli L, Rinkel GJ, et al. Regional differences in incidence and patient characteristics of moyamoya disease: a systematic review. J Neurol Neurosurg Psychiatry 2012;83:531–6.
56. Kuribara T, Mikami T, Komatsu K, et al. Prevalence of and risk factors for enlarged perivascular spaces in adult patients with moyamoya disease. BMC Neurol 2017; 17:1–9.
57. Khan N, Achrol AS, Guzman R, et al. Sex differences in clinical presentation and treatment outcomes in moyamoya disease. Neurosurgery 2012;71:587–93.

58. Abuoliat ZA, AlFarhan BA, Alshahrani AA, et al. Atypical location of intracerebral hemorrhage in moyamoya disease. Cureus 2017;9.
59. Nah H-W, Kwon SU, Kang D-W, et al. Moyamoya disease-related versus primary intracerebral hemorrhage: location and outcomes are different. Stroke 2012;43: 1947–50.
60. Yu J, Yuan Y, Li W, et al. Moyamoya disease manifested as multiple simultaneous intracerebral hemorrhages: A case report and literature review. Exp Ther Med 2016;12:1440–4.
61. Kang S, Liu X, Zhang D, et al. Natural Course of Moyamoya Disease in Patients With Prior Hemorrhagic Stroke: Clinical Outcome and Risk Factors. Stroke 2019; 50:1060–6.
62. Phi JH, Wang K-C, Lee JY, et al. Moyamoya syndrome: a window of moyamoya disease. J Korean Neurosurg Soc 2015;57:408–14.
63. Christie S, Chan V, Mollayeva T, et al. Systematic review of rehabilitation intervention outcomes of adult and paediatric patients with infectious encephalitis. BMJ open 2018;8:e015928.
64. Leasure AC, Khan YM, Iyer R, et al. Intracerebral hemorrhage in patients with COVID-19: an analysis from the COVID-19 cardiovascular disease registry. Stroke 2021;52:e321–3.
65. Margos NP, Meintanopoulos AS, Filioglou D, et al. Intracerebral hemorrhage in COVID-19: A narrative review. J Clin Neurosci 2021;89:271–8.
66. Lin G, Xu X, Luan X, et al. A Longitudinal Research on the Distribution and Prognosis of Intracerebral Hemorrhage During the COVID-19 Pandemic. Front Neurol 2022;690.
67. Raghavan A, Wright CH, Wright JM, et al. Outcomes and clinical characteristics of intracranial hemorrhage in patients with hematologic malignancies: a systematic literature review. World Neurosurg 2020;144:e15–24.
68. Sandberg K, Ji H. Sex differences in primary hypertension. Biol sex differences 2012;3:1–21.
69. Biffi A, Rea F, Iannaccone T, et al. Sex differences in the adherence of antihypertensive drugs: a systematic review with meta-analyses. BMJ open 2020;10: e036418.
70. An SJ, Kim TJ, Yoon B-W. Epidemiology, risk factors, and clinical features of intracerebral hemorrhage: an update. J stroke 2017;19:3.
71. Peltier MR, Verplaetse TL, Mineur YS, et al. Sex differences in stress-related alcohol use. Neurobiol Stress 2019;10:100149.
72. Taylor B, Irving HM, Baliunas D, et al. Alcohol and hypertension: gender differences in dose–response relationships determined through systematic review and meta-analysis. Addiction 2009;104:1981–90.
73. Islami F, Torre LA, Jemal A. Global trends of lung cancer mortality and smoking prevalence. Translational Lung Cancer Res 2015;4:327.
74. Geer JH, Falcone GJ, Vanent KN, et al. Obstructive sleep apnea as a risk factor for intracerebral hemorrhage. Stroke 2021;52:1835–8.
75. Rudolph DA, Hald SM, Rodríguez LAG, et al. Association of Long-term Statin Use With the Risk of Intracerebral Hemorrhage: A Danish Nationwide Case-Control Study. Neurology 2022. https://doi.org/10.1212/WNL.0000000000200713.
76. Peters SA, Colantonio LD, Zhao H, et al. Sex differences in high-intensity statin use following myocardial infarction in the United States. J Am Coll Cardiol 2018;71:1729–37.

77. Nanna MG, Wang TY, Xiang Q, et al. Sex differences in the use of statins in community practice: patient and provider assessment of lipid management registry. Circ Cardiovasc Qual Outcomes 2019;12:e005562.
78. Stocks NP, McElroy H, Ryan P, et al. Statin prescribing in Australia: socioeconomic and sex differences. Med J Aust 2004;180:229–31.
79. Gamboa CM, Colantonio LD, Brown TM, et al. Race-sex differences in statin use and low-density lipoprotein cholesterol control among people with diabetes mellitus in the reasons for geographic and racial differences in stroke study. J Am Heart Assoc 2017;6:e004264.
80. Olié V, Grave C, Tuppin P, et al. Patients Hospitalized for Ischemic Stroke and Intracerebral Hemorrhage in France: Time Trends (2008–2019), In-Hospital Outcomes, Age and Sex Differences. J Clin Med 2022;11:1669.
81. Willers C, Lekander I, Ekstrand E, et al. Sex as predictor for achieved health outcomes and received care in ischemic stroke and intracerebral hemorrhage: a register-based study. Biol sex differences 2018;9:1–9.
82. Ganti L, Jain A, Yerragondu N, et al. Female gender remains an independent risk factor for poor outcome after acute nontraumatic intracerebral hemorrhage. Neurol Res Int 2013;2013.
83. Craen A, Mangal R, Stead TG, et al. Gender differences in outcomes after nontraumatic intracerebral hemorrhage. Cureus 2019;11.
84. Kaiser J, Schebesch K-M, Brawanski A, et al. Long-term follow-up of cerebral amyloid angiopathy-associated intracranial hemorrhage reveals a high prevalence of atrial fibrillation. J Stroke Cerebrovasc Dis 2019;28:104342.
85. Kuohn LR, Leasure AC, Acosta JN, et al. Cause of death in spontaneous intracerebral hemorrhage survivors: multistate longitudinal study. Neurology 2020;95: e2736–45.
86. Lv X-N, Li Q. Imaging predictors for hematoma expansion in patients with intracerebral hemorrhage: a current review. Brain Hemorrhages 2020;1:133–9.
87. Marini S, Morotti A, Ayres AM, et al. Sex differences in intracerebral hemorrhage expansion and mortality. J Neurol Sci 2017;379:112–6.
88. Marini S, Morotti A, Lena UK, et al. Men experience higher risk of pneumonia and death after intracerebral hemorrhage. Neurocrit Care 2018;28:77–82.
89. Kawase K, Okazaki S, Toyoda K, et al. Sex difference in the prevalence of deep-vein thrombosis in Japanese patients with acute intracerebral hemorrhage. Cerebrovasc Dis 2009;27:313–9.
90. Nakagawa K, Vento MA, Seto TB, et al. Sex differences in the use of early do-not-resuscitate orders after intracerebral hemorrhage. Stroke 2013;44:3229–31.
91. Hemphill JC III, Newman J, Zhao S, et al. Hospital usage of early do-not-resuscitate orders and outcome after intracerebral hemorrhage. Stroke 2004; 35:1130–4.
92. Zahuranec D, Morgenstern L, Sanchez B, et al. Do-not-resuscitate orders and predictive models after intracerebral hemorrhage. Neurology 2010;75:626–33.

Neurologic Disorders in Women and Sleep

Fidaa Shaib, MD

KEYWORDS

• Sleep disorder • Neurologic disorder • Sleep-disordered breathing • Sleep quality • Insomnia • Sleepiness • Restless legs • Parasomnia

KEY POINTS

- There are limited data describing sleep disorders in women with neurologic disorders.
- There is a bidirectional relationship between neurologic disorders and sleep.
- Standard tools may not be applicable for screening for sleep disorders in women in general and more specifically in women with neurologic disorders because of overlap of symptoms.
- Evaluation for sleep disorders should be included in the work-up of women with neurologic disorders.
- Management of sleep disorders impacts quality of life in women with neurologic disorders.

Sleep disorders in women remain underrecognized and underdiagnosed mainly because of gender bias in researching and characterizing sleep disorders in women. Symptoms of common sleep disorders are frequently missed in the general female population.[1] Sleep disorders in women with neurologic disorders is further underrecognized and underdiagnosed mainly because of significant overlapping of sleep disorder symptoms with those of the primary neurologic illness. There is also significant lack of data related to sleep disorders in women in general and those with neurologic disorders specifically. Given the bidirectional relationship with sleep and neurologic disorders, it remains critical to be aware of the presentation and impact of sleep disorders in this patient population. **Table 1** provides a summary of common sleep disorders/symptoms that are discussed in this article, including diagnostic criteria,[2] work-up, and therapy.

EPILEPSY

There is a bidirectional relationship between sleep and epilepsy. Sleep stages influence the frequency and subtypes of seizures and sleep deprivation and comorbid

Pulmonary, Critical Care, and Sleep Medicine, Baylor College of Medicine, McNair Campus, 7200 Cambridge Street, Houston, TX 77030, USA
E-mail address: Shaib@bcm.edu

Neurol Clin 41 (2023) 297–314
https://doi.org/10.1016/j.ncl.2023.01.004 **neurologic.theclinics.com**
0733-8619/23/

Table 1
Common sleep disorders and symptoms

Sleep Disorder/Symptom	Definition	Work-up	Therapy
Sleep-disordered breathing	Group of breathing disorders that occur during sleep include obstructive sleep apnea, central sleep apnea, and hypoventilation	• Clinical assessment • Diagnostic sleep study • Home sleep apnea testing (not indicated for patients with advanced neurologic disease)	• Positive airway pressure • Noninvasive positive pressure ventilation • Upper airway surgery • Mandibular advancing device • Hypoglossal nerve stimulation • Behavioral and positional therapy
Sleep quality and insomnia	Difficulty with initiating or maintaining sleep or poor sleep quality that occurs despite adequate sleep opportunity and results in daytime impairment	• Clinical assessment • Tools: Insomnia Severity Index, Sleep Diary, Pittsburgh Sleep Quality Index	• Sleep hygiene (not effective as stand-alone therapy) • Cognitive behavioral therapy for insomnia • Light therapy • Pharmacotherapy
Excessive sleepiness	Symptoms of excessive daytime sleepiness that could be isolated or as a result of an underlying sleep disorder, sleep disruption, circadian misalignment, or insufficient sleep	• Clinical assessment • Work-up for specific suspected sleep disorder • Multiple Sleep Latency Test • Tools: Epworth Sleepiness Score, sleep diary, actigraphy	• Management of underlying sleep disorder • Counseling on dangers of sleepiness and safety • Counseling on importance of obtaining adequate sleep
Restless leg syndrome/Willis-Ekbom disease and periodic limb movement disorder	Movement disorders that affect sleep onset or sleep continuity and result in sleep disruption and daytime impairment	• Clinical assessment • Work up for underlying cause: medication or metabolic (ferritin, iron levels, vitamin D) • Sleep study for periodic limb movement disorder • Tools: International Restless Legs Scale	• Iron and vitamin D replacement as indicated • Medication change if patient condition allows • Pharmacotherapy with alpha-2-delta ligands, dopamine agonists, and narcotics in severe cases

Parasomnia	A group of abnormal sleep behaviors or experiences that can occur during or at end of a sleep period, such as REM behavior disorder and nightmares	• Clinical assessment • Work-up for underlying cause: sleep disorder or medications	• Counseling on safety to self and others • Treatment of underlying sleep disorder • Evaluation for underlying neurodegenerative disease • Pharmacotherapy with clonazepam and melatonin
Circadian disorders	Disorders of sleep timing causing misalignment with the 24-h biologic rhythm	• Clinical assessment • Tools: sleep diary, actigraphy, melatonin measurements	• Melatonin • Light therapy • Chronotherapy

sleep disorders affects seizure control.[3] Sleep disorders are common in patients with epilepsy with an estimated prevalence of 24% to 55%.[4]

Poor sleep quality is common in patients with epilepsy. It is reported in up to 70% of patients with Pittsburgh Sleep Quality Index greater than five.[5] Insomnia prevalence varies among different studies between 36.0% and 74.4% with higher prevalence reported in women compared with men with epilepsy (68% vs 32%; $P = 0.02$).[6] Although insomnia severity indices were independently associated with depression and anxiety in persons with epilepsy, the association between anxiety and insomnia severity was seen in women.[7]

Obstructive sleep apnea (OSA) in patients with epilepsy is more common in men (39.1%) compared with women (9.7%). Although true in men with epilepsy and OSA, depression and not OSA is a risk factor for daytime sleepiness in women with epilepsy making the Epworth Sleepiness Score (ESS) less useful as a screening tool.[7] Continuous positive airway pressure (CPAP) therapy results in five times improvement in seizure control when compared with those untreated.[8] Therapy with vagus nerve stimulator is reported to increase severity of sleep-disordered breathing (SDB) mainly in males.[9]

Excessive daytime sleepiness (EDS) as measured with ESS is higher in patients with epilepsy compared with matched control subjects (42% vs 25%; $P = 0.026$).[10]

Sudden unexpected death in epilepsy has an estimated incidence of 1.4/1000 patient-years[11] and is more common in males[12]; it is suspected that postictal central sleep apnea (CSA), brainstem dysfunction, and associated bradycardia leads to asystole and death.[13]

Restless leg syndrome (RLS) and bruxism are increased in patients with epilepsy compared with control subjects.[14]

Significant overlap in symptoms of epilepsy and parasomnia warrants concomitant sleep and neurologic evaluation and the use of specific scales, particularly with frontal lobe epilepsy and parasomnias.[15]

STROKE

Patients are at increased risk for poor sleep quality and insomnia after stroke with higher prevalence in women up to 41%.[16] Treatment of insomnia in poststroke patients is challenging because of increased risk for cognitive and communication impairment in addition to significant hypnotic side effects.[17] Cognitive behavioral therapy in insomnia remains the best recommended therapy, although data are limited in poststroke patients.

Sleep apnea is a known risk factor for ischemic stroke; women younger than 35 years old with sleep apnea have the highest risk for stroke compared with men or women of older age groups.[18] In postmenopausal women, insomnia, snoring, and risk for SDB predict an increased risk for ischemic stroke.[19] Stroke survivors commonly suffer from sleep apnea immediately and on long-term follow-up after a stroke. Male sex is a risk factor in this population for OSA and CSA[20] with worse severity compared with female sex.[21]

Fatigue is common in stroke patients and is in part related to poor sleep quality.[22]

Stroke-related RLS has been reported as a result of anatomic lesions mainly in the lenticulostriate area and the ventral brainstem.[23] No gender difference has been reported.[24]

Parasomnias including REM behavior disorder (RBD) can occur following a stroke and in up to 46% of those with brainstem infarcts especially with lesions involving the medioventral pons.[25]

HEADACHES

Migraine

Women are three times more likely than men to suffer from headaches, predominantly migraine. The prevalence of migraine tends to increase at menarche and to decline after menopause, with this variation mediated by hormonal changes.[26] The relationship between migraine and sleep is complex: migraine may disrupt sleep, and sleep disruption may lower the threshold for migraine. Compared with episodic migraine (EM), patients with chronic migraine (CM), especially women, are more likely to have sleep disorders[27] and more migraine triggers that may lead to sleep disturbance.[28] Women with migraine tend to nap more, with the naps duration associated with headache severity and nocturnal sleep disturbance.[29]

The bidirectional association between migraine and insomnia is well recognized,[30] with a significantly higher prevalence of insomnia among migraineurs. Digital cognitive therapy for insomnia in women with CM is effective in reducing headache frequency, with 65.7% response rate, with a third of patients completing the therapy in one study converting from CM to EM.[31]

Women with CM are at increased risk for sleep apnea and poor sleep quality.[27] Headaches could also be one of the presenting symptoms of SDB.[32] Although men are more likely to suffer from SDB, studies evaluating the impact of gender difference on OSA symptoms and comorbidities showed that women with OSA reported more morning headaches (50.0% vs 28.4%; $P < 0.001$) when compared with men.[33,34]

The association of RLS with migraine is well described. A recent systematic review reported an RLS prevalence of 13.7% to 25% in migraineurs, with higher prevalence CM compared with EM (34.3% vs 16%).[35] Increased risk and severity of RLS was also observed in patients with family history of migraine,[36] with RLS being five times higher in migraineurs with dopaminergic premonitory symptoms.[37] The comorbid association of RLS and migraine is thought to be related to an overlap of multiple pathophysiologic mechanisms including the shared hypothalamic dopaminergic dysfunction, disturbance in iron metabolism, and the recently reported role of vitamin D. A recent study evaluating the association between migraine complicated with RLS and vitamin D levels, showed a higher prevalence of RLS in patients with migraine compared with control subjects (6.62% vs 22.29%; $P < 0.001$),[37] with the lower vitamin D levels in patients with migraine and RLS compared with those with migraine without RLS.[38] The choice of therapy for migraine should take into consideration the risk of exacerbation of RLS symptoms and vice versa. It is expected that treatment of RLS and resulting improved sleep quality and duration will have a favorable effect on migraine. However, treatment of RLS with dopamine agonists may trigger a migraine attack, whereas dopamine antagonists have a favorable effect as migraine therapy.[39] Restless leg–like syndrome has been reported in several case series as an emergent adverse effect of the migraine-preventive calcitonin gene-related peptide monoclonal antibodies.[40]

The prevalence of EDS, defined as ESS of greater than 10, was found to increase with headache frequency, with no relationship to migraine status.[41] However, 20% of migraine sufferers manifested EDS during a migraine exacerbation; this was associated with the migraine severity and the presence of depression.[42] When it comes to specific disorders of excessive sleepiness, migraine and narcolepsy seem to share common pathophysiology involving the hypothalamic orexinergic system; the evidence for a clear association is still lacking.[35]

In a study where women accounted for 84% of the subjects, bruxism during sleep was shown to be associated with increased risk of CM, EM, and episodic tension-type headache.[43] When evaluating grinding patterns, grinding sites in women with migraine and bruxism were significantly more extensive compared with those without migraine.[44]

Women who are shift workers are more likely to experience migraine when compared with men shift workers and daytime workers.[45] This, however, could be caused by high prevalence of migraine among women, with changes in sleep-wake rhythm being a common migraine trigger. Additionally, shift work seems to be associated with chronification of migraine and higher headache-related disability.[46]

Cluster Headache

Cluster headache (CH) is a rare primary headache disorder more common in men. It has a diurnal and biseasonal rhythm, and often occurs during vulnerable period at end of a sleep cycle.[47]

Patients with CH usually have decreased sleep quality, and have difficulty adjusting sleep rhythm. Common triggers for CH include reduced sleep quality and quantity.[48] Women with CH (although rare) tend to have insufficient sleep and poor sleep quality.[49]

In a study of 186 subjects, predominantly men with CH, Ofte and colleagues[50] reported no difference in the frequency of insomnia among the sexes; worth noting that men with CH reported higher prevalence of insomnia compared with women with migraine in the same geographic area.

There is no clear relationship between CH and SDB; however, evaluation for sleep quality and underlying SDB is warranted in patients with primary headache disorders, predominantly migraine and CH.

A direct association between RLS and CH has not been documented. Theoretically, the decreased melatonin and the increased dopaminergic activity in CH could be protective against RLS.[51,52]

The circadian nature (diurnal and seasonal) of CH suggests a close relationship with the circadian system. This is further supported by multiple alterations in biomarkers of circadian biology, such as melatonin, in addition to the expression of circadian genes in CH.[53] Interesting to note that diurnal attack cycle is delayed by 1 hour in women compared with men, suggesting functional differences in the hypothalamus.[54] Treatment with melatonin has been shown to be successful in preventing CH.[55]

TRAUMATIC BRAIN INJURY

Traumatic brain injury (TBI) is a significant cause of disability worldwide.[56] Sleep disturbances have been reported in 50% of young adults with TBI,[57] and are more common in older patients, specifically OSA, insomnia, and daytime sleepiness (80.0%, 51.2%, and 36.3%, respectively).[58] Although TBI is more common in men, women have worse 6-month outcomes with more mental health and postconcussion symptoms,[59] and women with mild TBI were shown to have more neurobehavioral impairment.[60]

Sleep disruption remains one of the most prevalent outcomes of TBI. Post-TBI sleep disturbances are more common in older women compared with control subjects (21.7% vs 9.6%; $P = 0.024$), and nighttime sleep disturbance, measured using the Nighttime Behavioral Disturbances domain of the Neuropsychiatric Inventory-Questionnaire that evaluates nighttime awakenings, early wake up time, or daytime sleepiness, was more common in men with TBI compared with the men with non-TBI (19.8% vs 14.8%; $P = 0.305$).[61] In a cohort of postconcussion patients (60.8% women), women had higher perception of sleep changes, which was associated with significant increase in severity of sleep disturbances clinically and statistically when compared with men.[62]

Insomnia is the most common sleep disorder post-TBI, occurring in 30% to 60% of patients, with the insomnia prevalence decreasing exponentially with TBI severity.[63,64] Women with TBI, especially caused by domestic violence, often report worse insomnia symptoms.[65] Insomnia remission in TBI may occur in up to 60% of patients at 5 years postinjury; persistent insomnia was less frequently observed in men.[66]

The prevalence of OSA and CSA post-TBI ranges from 25% to 68%, and 36% respectively.[57] No gender difference has been reported.

RLS symptoms were more frequently reported in patients with mild TBI when compared with control subjects (32.4% vs 2.7%; P <0.001),[67] with no noticeable sex differences.

EDS is common after TBI, affecting 40.7% of patients[68]; women are more likely to report more than one symptom of hypersomnia.[69]

Studies showed no statistically significant difference in the occurrence of nightmares following TBI in women compared with men (17.07% vs 21.74%; $P = 0.628$), although women with TBI tend to manifest more negative affect, maladaptive coping, depression, and anxiety compared with men with TBI ($P = 0.005$) irrespective of nightmare status.[70]

Patients with TBI are at increased risk for altered circadian timing, especially delayed sleep phase.[71] The overnight production of melatonin, a hormone closely related to circadian timing, is reduced by 42% in patients post-TBI compared with control subjects with a delay of 1.5 hours.[72] Prolonged-release melatonin (2 mg) was shown to improve sleep quality and efficiency when compared with placebo.[73] Dynamic light therapy may have a favorable impact on sleep disturbance and insomnia with small effect on fatigue.[74]

NEUROMUSCULAR DISORDERS

Amyotrophic Lateral Sclerosis

Amyotrophic lateral sclerosis (ALS) is a progressive neurodegenerative disease affecting the upper and lower motor neurons, resulting in muscle weakness, fasciculations, spasticity, and hyperreflexia. The prevalence of ALS is 5 to 8/100,000, with a lifetime risk of 1:400 in women and 1:300 in men.[75]

Sleep quality impairment measured using the Pittsburgh Sleep Quality Index, including difficulty initiating and maintaining sleep, is reported in 50% to 63% of patients with ALS and is not necessarily associated with EDS.[76]

Insomnia is present in up to 50% of patients with ALS and frequency increased with disease severity. No gender difference has been reported.[77]

Frequency and severity of SDB occurs with disease severity and frequency in males compared with females. Nocturnal hypoventilation is reported in 41.9% of men versus 26.4% in women. Prevalence of OSA is increased in ALS, particularly in men (60%) compared with women (38.9%).[78] CSA is rare (5.4%)[79] and seems to be predominantly in men.[80]

Periodic limb movement disorders (PLMDs) are significantly more common in ALS, compared with healthy control subjects (53.6% vs 15.4%),[81] whereas RLS occurs in 14.6% of patients with ALS compared with 10% of control subjects, with no difference among sexes.[82]

RBD and REM without atonia is scarce with ALS and occurs predominantly in men.[81]

Myasthenia Gravis

Myasthenia gravis (MG) is a rare autoimmune disease of the neuromuscular junction that predominantly affects women between 20 and 40 years of age (3:1 female/

male ratio). A 62% of patients with MG suffer from severe fatigue; however, women with MG tend to report more fatigue[83] with higher fatigue scores.[84]

Insomnia has been reported to occur less frequently in patients with MG compared with the general population; significant attention has to be paid when considering therapeutic options[85] especially risk of disease exacerbation with melatonin use.[86]

SDB caused by weakening of the oropharyngeal muscles strongly affects the quality of life of patients with MG. OSA in patients with MG is associated with male sex and obesity, similar to the general population, with twice as high supine apnea-hypopnea index (AHI) compared with nonsupine AHI.[87] Moreover sleep apnea events were noted to occur mostly in REM sleep in studies that included predominantly female patients.[88]

RLS is more prevalent in MG (47.6%), predominantly in females (57.1%), and is associated with worse quality-of-life scores.[89]

EDS has not been well studied in MG. In a study by Kassardjian and colleagues,[90] seven of eight patients with MG demonstrated hypersomnia on objective testing and not on ESS suggesting that the ESS might not be adequate to evaluate sleepiness in patients with MG.

NEURODEGENERATIVE DISORDERS

Multiple System Atrophy

Multiple system atrophy (MSA) is a group of rare neurologic disorders characterized by autonomic dysfunction, parkinsonism, and ataxia. Women are more likely to receive an early diagnosis, manifest with motor symptoms, and have slightly prolonged disease course, whereas autonomic dysfunction is predominant in men.[91] Faster disease progression has been reported in patients with autonomic dysfunction.[92]

Poor sleep quality with significant sleep fragmentation occurs in 53% of patients, with early awakenings (33%) and insomnia (20%).[93]

Patients with MSA are at increased risk for OSA as a result of upper airway involvement with the disease. Transformation from OSA to CSA has been reported in 13% of patients even before positive airway pressure use and resolution of sleep apnea occurred in 29%.[94] Sleep-related hypoventilation is present in 27% of patients with MSA with no sex difference.[95]

RLS is common in MSA (28%), although the prevalence of PLMD varies among studies and does not correlate with RLS severity or the ESS.[96]

Hypersomnia can occur in 27% to 50% of patients with MSA and is associated with more fatigue, anxiety, cognitive dysfunction, and significant disability.[93,97]

The prevalence of RBD with dream enactment behavior in MSA is up to 88% in with no known sex difference.[91,98]

Parkinson Disease

Parkinson disease (PD) is a neurodegenerative disorder with nonmotor symptoms as the most disabling disease characteristics. Although more prevalent in men, women tend to have a late onset of disease, faster disease progression, inferior quality of life, and higher mortality rate.[99] Disrupted sleep and impaired alertness are most common symptoms of PD. According to the Women's Health Initiative Observational Study among postmenopausal women, sleep disturbance was associated with increased risk of developing PD after 16-year follow-up (10%–30%), especially in those with insomnia (26%), with prolonged sleep duration greater than 9 hours.[100]

Insomnia remains the most common sleep disorder in PD, affecting almost 60% of patients of both sexes, and is thought to be a result of multiple processes including depression and change in circadian rhythm circuits.[101]

The prevalence of OSA in PD ranges from 20% to 60%. Women with PD do not have a higher frequency of OSA[102]; however, they are less likely to receive therapy with CPAP and have lower level of adherence to therapy when compared with men with PD or women without PD.[103]

RLS affects 14% of patients with PD worldwide with higher prevalence in women compared with men (13% vs 11%).[104] Women with PD and RLS have higher incidence of insomnia, constipation, and loss of smell.[105]

EDS affects 21% to 76% of patients with PD[106]; however, data on gender differences in sleepiness in PD are not conclusive. Mahale and colleagues[107] reported increased frequency of daytime sleepiness in females compared with males (45.9% vs 26.9%). A recent meta-analysis reported an association of EDS with male sex in PD, with odds ratio of 1.50 (95% confidence interval, 1.30–1.72).[108]

Probable RBD has been reported in 27% of women with PD, mainly in older patients with high incidence of insomnia and EDS. RBD in women was mostly manifested as vocalization, non–complex motor activity, and without aggressive behavior.[109] Nightmares have also been reported in increased frequency in women (32.4%) compared with men (16.8%) with PD.[107]

Mild Cognitive Impairment and Alzheimer Disease

Mild cognitive impairment predicts an increased risk for developing Alzheimer disease (AD) in addition to other dementias. AD is the most common form of dementia, with women being disproportionally affected by the disease.[110]

Poor sleep quality, difficulty initiating sleep, and less than 5-hour sleep duration are regarded as a modifiable risk factor for cognitive decline that was found to be more common in women.[111] There is a bidirectional link between sleep disturbances and AD, with sleep disturbances and reduced sleep quality occurring in 24.5% of patients with AD.[112] Older women have higher incidence of disrupted sleep and are at increased risk for developing AD and related dementia. This is thought to be mediated through the impact of changes in female sex hormones, mainly estradiol and progesterone, on sleep and memory.[113]

Men with AD have a higher prevalence of OSA and more severe disease compared with women with AD.[114] In women, where AHI may not be the best indicator of sleep apnea severity, the high level of sleep fragmentations resulting from OSA may impair glymphatic system activity and may result in increased risk of neurodegenerative pathology.[115] Treatment with CPAP may improve cognitive function in OSA patients with AD.[116]

Multiple Sclerosis

Multiple sclerosis (MS) is an autoimmune demyelinating disease affecting the central nervous system, with a higher prevalence in women[117] with disease onset between the ages of 20 and 40 years of age.[118]

Females tend to have higher prevalence of poor sleep quality. Impairment of sleep quality in MS is associated with depression and anxiety in women, whereas it is associated with pain in men.[119] In addition, addressing sleep disturbances in MS may result in favorable effect on depression, pain, and physical fatigue.[120] Targeting treatment of insomnia in MS may prove to be a challenging, but is an impactful intervention in the management of MS-related fatigue.[121] Cognitive behavioral therapy for insomnia[122] and hormone-replacement therapy improve sleep quality in women with MS.[123] Menopause may further exacerbate MS symptoms especially with the development of sleep disturbances.[124]

MS may be associated with increased prevalence of OSA (24.7%) especially in men. Severity of SDB does not explain the prevalence of fatigue in patients with MS.[125,126]

Women with MS are at increased risk for developing RLS and associated daytime sleepiness.[127]

Fatigue is a common symptom of MS mainly in women, with increased incidence of EDS, RLS, and poor sleep quality.[128]

OTHER SPECIAL DISORDERS

Rett Syndrome

Rett syndrome a developmental disorder that occurs predominantly in females (1:10,000) and is characterized by regression in psychomotor development resulting in significant impairments in multiple health, behavioral, motor, and cognitive functions.

Sleep disorders are extremely common in Rett syndrome. Those include SDB predominantly in the form of OSA in addition to less frequent CSA.[129] Patients may also exhibit irregular breathing during wakefulness and sleep with alternating periods of hyperventilation and hypoventilation.[130]

In addition, circadian disorders, difficulty initiating and maintaining sleep, daytime naps, nocturnal laughter, and bruxism are highly prevalent in this population.[131]

Craniopharyngioma

Patients with craniopharyngioma are at increased risk for SDB that is worsened by the presence of hypothalamic dysfunction mainly related to significant weight gain. OSA and CSA are common, in addition to central hypersomnia including narcolepsy, and circadian disorders.[132]

Postcraniotomy

Patients recovering from craniotomy for brain tumors suffer from mental and physical fatigue. Mental fatigue scores were higher in women compared with men and were associated with sleep disruption and increased wake after sleep onset time ($r = 0.40$; $P = 0.006$).[133]

SUMMARY

Sleep disorders are common in women with neurologic disorders and have significant impact on health outcomes and quality of life. Special consideration is needed for the assessment, work-up, and management of sleep disorders in this patient population. Further research specific to women with sleep disorder is needed to improve recognition and optimize care.

CLINICS CARE POINTS

- Sleep disorders are underrecognized in women, especially those with neurologic disorders.
- Significant symptom overlap exists between neurologic and sleep disorders making the standard screenign tests for sleep disorders less helpful in the clinical setting.
- Screening for sleep disorders should be part of the intial neurology work up 4, Management of sleep disorders will impact quality of life in patients with neurologic disorders.
- Sleep disorders are common in patients with epilepsy and their management impact the epilepsy control.

- Restless leg syndrome/Willis-Ekbom disease and Periodic Limb Movment Disorder occur with increased frequency in patients with neurologic disorders and pharmacologic therapy should take into consideration risks of exacebation of both conditions.

REFERENCES

1. Basoglu OK, Tasbakan MS. Gender differences in clinical and polysomnographic features of obstructive sleep apnea: a clinical study of 2827 patients. Sleep Breath 2018;22(1):241–9.
2. American Academy of Sleep Medicine. The International Classification of Sleep Disorders. 3rd edition. Darien, IL: M. Sateia; 2014.
3. Moore JL, Carvalho DZ, St Louis EK, et al. Sleep and epilepsy: a focused review of pathophysiology, clinical syndromes, co-morbidities, and therapy. Neurotherapeutics 2021;18(1):170–80.
4. Quigg M, Gharai J, Rulandet S, et al. Insomnia in epilepsy is associated with continuing seizures and worse quality of life. Epilepsy Res 2016;122:91–6.
5. Vendrame M, Yang B, Jackson S, et al. Insomnia and epilepsy: a questionnaire-based study. J Clin Sleep Med 2013;9(2):141–6.
6. Ismayilova V, Demir AU, Tezer FI. Subjective sleep disturbance in epilepsy patients at an outpatient clinic: a questionnaire-based study on prevalence. Epilepsy Res 2015;115:119–25.
7. Jo S, Kim HJ, Kim HW, et al. Sex differences in factors associated with daytime sleepiness and insomnia symptoms in persons with epilepsy. Epilepsy Behav 2020;104(Pt A):106919.
8. Grigg-Damberger M, Foldvary-Schaefer N. Bidirectional relationships of sleep and epilepsy in adults with epilepsy. Epilepsy Behav 2021;116:107735.
9. Kim JS, Lee DE, Bae H, et al. Effects of vagus nerve stimulation on sleep-disordered breathing, daytime sleepiness, and sleep quality in patients with drug-resistant epilepsy. J Clin Neurol 2022;18(3):315–22.
10. Sap-Anan N, Pascoe M, Wang L, et al. The Epworth Sleepiness Scale in epilepsy: internal consistency and disease-related associations. Epilepsy Behav 2021;121(Pt A):108099.
11. Mesraoua B, Tomson T, Brodie M, et al. Sudden unexpected death in epilepsy (SUDEP): definition, epidemiology, and significance of education. Epilepsy Behav 2022;132:108742.
12. Devinsky O, Hesdorffer DC, Thurman DJ, et al. Sudden unexpected death in epilepsy: epidemiology, mechanisms, and prevention. Lancet Neurol 2016;15(10):1075–88.
13. Vilella L, Lacuey N, Hampson JP, et al. Postconvulsive central apnea as a biomarker for sudden unexpected death in epilepsy (SUDEP). Neurology 2019;92(3):e171–82.
14. Happe S. Excessive daytime sleepiness and sleep disturbances in patients with neurological diseases: epidemiology and management. Drugs 2003;63(24):2725–37.
15. Latreille V, St Louis EK, Pavlova M. Co-morbid sleep disorders and epilepsy: a narrative review and case examples. Epilepsy Res 2018;145:185–97.
16. Baylan S, Griffiths S, Grant N, et al. Incidence and prevalence of post-stroke insomnia: a systematic review and meta-analysis. Sleep Med Rev 2020;49:101222.

17. Glass J, Lanctot KL, Herrmann N, et al. Sedative hypnotics in older people with insomnia: meta-analysis of risks and benefits. BMJ 2005;331(7526):1169.
18. Chang CC, Chuang HC, Lin CL, et al. High incidence of stroke in young women with sleep apnea syndrome. Sleep Med 2014;15(4):410–4.
19. Beverly Hery CM, Hale L, Naughton MJ. Contributions of the Women's Health Initiative to understanding associations between sleep duration, insomnia symptoms, and sleep-disordered breathing across a range of health outcomes in postmenopausal women. Sleep Health 2020;6(1):48–59.
20. Baillieul S, Dekkers M, Brill AK, et al. Sleep apnoea and ischaemic stroke: current knowledge and future directions. Lancet Neurol 2022;21(1):78–88.
21. McDermott M, Brown DL, Li C, et al. Sex differences in sleep-disordered breathing after stroke: results from the BASIC project. Sleep Med 2018;43:54–9.
22. Ho LYW, Lai CKY, Ng SSM. Contribution of sleep quality to fatigue following a stroke: a cross-sectional study. BMC Neurol 2021;21(1):151.
23. Ruppert E, Hacquard A, Tatu L, et al. Stroke-related restless legs syndrome: clinical and anatomo-functional characterization of an emerging entity. Eur J Neurol 2022;29(4):1011–6.
24. Wang XX, Feng Y, Tan EK, et al. Stroke-related restless legs syndrome: epidemiology, clinical characteristics, and pathophysiology. Sleep Med 2022;90: 238–48.
25. Tang WK, Hermann DM, Chen YK, et al. Brainstem infarcts predict REM sleep behavior disorder in acute ischemic stroke. BMC Neurol 2014;14:88.
26. Pavlovic JM. Headache in women. Continuum 2021;27(3):686–702.
27. Buse DC, Rains JC, Pavlovic JM, et al. Sleep disorders among people with migraine: results from the Chronic Migraine Epidemiology and Outcomes (CaMEO) study. Headache 2019;59(1):32–45.
28. van Casteren DS, Verhagen IE, Onderwater GL, et al. Sex differences in prevalence of migraine trigger factors: a cross-sectional study. Cephalalgia 2021; 41(6):643–8.
29. Ong JC, Dawson SC, Taylor HL, et al. A micro-longitudinal study of naps, sleep disturbance, and headache severity in women with chronic migraine. Behav Sleep Med 2023;21(2):117–28.
30. Uhlig BL, Engstrøm M, Ødegård SS, et al. Headache and insomnia in population-based epidemiological studies. Cephalalgia 2014;34(10):745–51.
31. Crawford MR, Luik AI, Espie CA, et al. Digital cognitive behavioral therapy for insomnia in women with chronic migraines. Headache 2020;60(5):902–15.
32. Bouloukaki I, Tsiligianni I, Schiza S. Evaluation of obstructive sleep apnea in female patients in primary care: time for improvement? Med Princ Pract 2021; 30(6):508–14.
33. Bostan OC, Akcan B, Saydam CD, et al. Impact of gender on symptoms and comorbidities in obstructive sleep apnea. Eurasian J Med 2021;53(1):34–9.
34. Nigro CA, Dibur E, Borsini E, et al. The influence of gender on symptoms associated with obstructive sleep apnea. Sleep Breath 2018;22(3):683–93.
35. Tiseo C, Vacca A, Felbush A, et al. Migraine and sleep disorders: a systematic review. J Headache Pain 2020;21(1):126.
36. Gozubatik-Celik G, Benbir G, Tan F, et al. The prevalence of migraine in restless legs syndrome. Headache 2014;54(5):872–7.
37. Cologno D, Cicarelli G, Petretta V, et al. High prevalence of dopaminergic premonitory symptoms in migraine patients with restless legs syndrome: a pathogenetic link? Neurol Sci 2008;29(Suppl 1):S166–8.

38. Sun S, Liu C, Jia Y, et al. Association between migraine complicated with restless legs syndrome and vitamin D. Front Neurol 2021;12:777721.
39. Fernandez-Matarrubia M, Cuadrado ML, Sanchez-Barros CM, et al. Prevalence of migraine in patients with restless legs syndrome: a case-control study. Headache 2014;54(8):1337–46.
40. Gonzalez-Quintanilla V, Perez-Pereda S, Gonzalez-Suarez A, et al. Restless legs-like syndrome as an emergent adverse event of CGRP monoclonal antibodies: a report of two cases. Cephalalgia 2021;41(11–12):1272–5.
41. Stavem K, Kristiansen HA, Kristoffersen ES, et al. Association of excessive daytime sleepiness with migraine and headache frequency in the general population. J Headache Pain 2017;18(1):35.
42. Kim J, Cho SJ, Kim WJ, et al. Excessive daytime sleepiness is associated with an exacerbation of migraine: a population-based study. J Headache Pain 2016; 17(1):62.
43. Fernandes G, Franco AL, Goncalves DA, et al. Temporomandibular disorders, sleep bruxism, and primary headaches are mutually associated. J Orofac Pain 2013;27(1):14–20.
44. Kato M, Saruta J, Takeuchi M, et al. Grinding patterns in migraine patients with sleep bruxism: a case-controlled study. Cranio 2016;34(6):371–7.
45. Appel AM, Torok E, Jensen MA, et al. The longitudinal association between shift work and headache: results from the Danish PRISME cohort. Int Arch Occup Environ Health 2020;93(5):601–10.
46. Sandoe CH, Sasikumar S, Lay C, et al. The impact of shift work on migraine: a case series and narrative review. Headache 2019;59(9):1631–40.
47. Barloese M. Current understanding of the chronobiology of cluster headache and the role of sleep in its management. Nat Sci Sleep 2021;13:153–62.
48. de Coo IF, van Oosterhout WPJ, Wilbrink LA, et al. Chronobiology and sleep in cluster headache. Headache 2019;59(7):1032–41.
49. Liaw YC, Wang YF, Chen WT, et al. Sex-related differences in cluster headache: a hospital-based study in Taiwan. Cephalalgia 2022;42(14):1532–42.
50. Ofte HK, Berg DH, Bekkelund SI, et al. Insomnia and periodicity of headache in an arctic cluster headache population. Headache 2013;53(10):1602–12.
51. Florindo D, Daniela C, Giulio C, et al. Cluster headache patients are not affected by restless legs syndrome: an observational study. Clin Neurol Neurosurg 2011; 113(4):308–10.
52. D'Andrea G, Gucciardi A, Perini F, et al. Pathogenesis of cluster headache: from episodic to chronic form, the role of neurotransmitters and neuromodulators. Headache 2019;59(9):1665–70.
53. Burish MJ, Chen Z, Yoo SH. Cluster headache is in part a disorder of the circadian system. JAMA Neurol 2018;75(7):783–4.
54. Lund N, Barloese M, Petersen A, et al. Chronobiology differs between men and women with cluster headache, clinical phenotype does not. Neurology 2017; 88(11):1069–76.
55. Leone M, D'Amico D, Moschiano F, et al. Melatonin versus placebo in the prophylaxis of cluster headache: a double-blind pilot study with parallel groups. Cephalalgia 1996;16(7):494–6.
56. Pervez M, Kitagawa RS, Chang TR. Definition of traumatic brain injury, neurosurgery, trauma orthopedics, neuroimaging, psychology, and psychiatry in mild traumatic brain injury. Neuroimaging Clin N Am 2018;28(1):1–13.

57. Mathias JL, Alvaro PK. Prevalence of sleep disturbances, disorders, and problems following traumatic brain injury: a meta-analysis. Sleep Med 2012;13(7):898–905.
58. Wei L, et al. Sleep disturbances following traumatic brain injury in older adults: a comparison study. J Head Trauma Rehabil 2020;35(4):288–95.
59. Mikolic A, van Klaveren D, Groeniger JO, et al. Differences between men and women in treatment and outcome after traumatic brain injury. J Neurotrauma 2021;38(2):235–51.
60. Villegas E, Hartsock MJ, Aben B, et al. Association between altered cortisol profiles and neurobehavioral impairment after mild traumatic brain injury in college students. J Neurotrauma 2022;39(11–12):809–20.
61. Ledger C, Karameh WK, Munoz DG, et al. Gender role in sleep disturbances among older adults with traumatic brain injury. Int Rev Psychiatry 2020;32(1):39–45.
62. Wiseman-Hakes C, Foster E, Langer L, et al. Characterizing sleep and wakefulness in the acute phase of concussion in the general population: a naturalistic cohort from the Toronto Concussion Study. J Neurotrauma 2022;39(1–2):172–80.
63. Albrecht JS, Wickwire EM. Sleep disturbances among older adults following traumatic brain injury. Int Rev Psychiatry 2020;32(1):31–8.
64. Zhou Y, Greenwald BD. Update on insomnia after mild traumatic brain injury. Brain Sci 2018;8(12).
65. Iverson KM, Dardis CM, Grillo AR, et al. Associations between traumatic brain injury from intimate partner violence and future psychosocial health risks in women. Compr Psychiatry 2019;92:13–21.
66. Lequerica AH, Weber E, Dijkers MP, et al. Factors associated with the remission of insomnia after traumatic brain injury: a traumatic brain injury model systems study. Brain Inj 2020;34(2):187–94.
67. Walker JM, Mulatya C, Hebert D, et al. Sleep assessment in a randomized trial of hyperbaric oxygen in U.S. service members with post concussive mild traumatic brain injury compared to normal controls. Sleep Med 2018;51:66–79.
68. Crichton T, Singh R, Abosi-Appeadu K, et al. Excessive daytime sleepiness after traumatic brain injury. Brain Inj 2020;34(11):1525–31.
69. Wickwire EM, Albrecht JS, Griffin NR, et al. Sleep disturbances precede depressive symptomatology following traumatic brain injury. Curr Neurobiol 2019;10(2):49–55.
70. Nabasny A, Myrga JM, Juengst SB. Neurobehavioral symptoms by gender and experience of nightmares after traumatic brain injury. Rehabil Psychol 2020;65(2):186–91.
71. Castriotta RJ, Murthy JN. Sleep disorders in patients with traumatic brain injury: a review. CNS Drugs 2011;25(3):175–85.
72. Grima NA, Ponsford JL, St Hilaire MA, et al. Circadian melatonin rhythm following traumatic brain injury. Neurorehabil Neural Repair 2016;30(10):972–7.
73. Grima NA, Rajaratnam SMW, Mansfield D, et al. Efficacy of melatonin for sleep disturbance following traumatic brain injury: a randomised controlled trial. BMC Med 2018;16(1):8.
74. Connolly LJ, Rajaratnam SMW, Murray JM, et al. Home-based light therapy for fatigue following acquired brain injury: a pilot randomized controlled trial. BMC Neurol 2021;21(1):262.
75. Boentert M. Sleep and sleep disruption in amyotrophic lateral sclerosis. Curr Neurol Neurosci Rep 2020;20(7):25.

76. Lucia D, McCombe PA, Henderson RD, et al. Disorders of sleep and wakefulness in amyotrophic lateral sclerosis (ALS): a systematic review. Amyotroph Lateral Scler Frontotemporal Degener 2021;22(3–4):161–9.
77. Chowdhury A, Mukherjee A, Sinharoy U, et al. Non-motor features of amyotrophic lateral sclerosis: a clinic-based study. Ann Indian Acad Neurol 2021; 24(5):745–53.
78. Engel M, Glatz C, Helmle C, et al. Respiratory parameters on diagnostic sleep studies predict survival in patients with amyotrophic lateral sclerosis. J Neurol 2021;268(11):4321–31.
79. Reyhani A, Benbir Senel G, Karadeniz D. Effects of sleep-related disorders on the prognosis of amyotrophic lateral sclerosis. Neurodegener Dis 2019; 19(3–4):148–54.
80. Boentert M, Glatz C, Helmle C, et al. Prevalence of sleep apnoea and capnographic detection of nocturnal hypoventilation in amyotrophic lateral sclerosis. J Neurol Neurosurg Psychiatry 2018;89(4):418–24.
81. Lo Coco D, Puligheddu M, Mattaliano P, et al. REM sleep behavior disorder and periodic leg movements during sleep in ALS. Acta Neurol Scand 2017;135(2): 219–24.
82. Liu S, Shen D, Tai H, et al. Restless legs syndrome in Chinese patients with sporadic amyotrophic lateral sclerosis. Front Neurol 2018;9:735.
83. Andersen LK, Aadahl M, Vissing J. Fatigue, physical activity and associated factors in 779 patients with myasthenia gravis. Neuromuscul Disord 2021; 31(8):716–25.
84. Ruiter AM, Verschuuren J, Tannemaat MR. Prevalence and associated factors of fatigue in autoimmune myasthenia gravis. Neuromuscul Disord 2021;31(7): 612–21.
85. Jordan H, Ortiz N. Management of insomnia and anxiety in myasthenia gravis. J Neuropsychiatry Clin Neurosci 2019;31(4):386–91.
86. Nedkova-Hristova V, Velez-Santamaria V, Casasnovas C. Myasthenia gravis exacerbation after melatonin administration: case series from a tertiary referral centre. BMC Neurol 2020;20(1):403.
87. Heo SJ, Jun JS, Park D, et al. Characteristics of obstructive sleep apnea in myasthenia gravis patients: a single center study. Neurol Sci 2019;40(4): 719–24.
88. Fernandes Oliveira E, Nacif SR, Alves Pereira N, et al. Sleep disorders in patients with myasthenia gravis: a systematic review. J Phys Ther Sci 2015; 27(6):2013–8.
89. Ataide MF, da Cunha-Correia C, Petribu KCL. The relationship between restless legs syndrome and quality of life in patients with myasthenia gravis. Eur Neurol 2019;81(3–4):205–8.
90. Kassardjian CD, Kokokyi S, Barnett C, et al. Excessive daytime sleepiness in patients with myasthenia gravis. J Neuromuscul Dis 2015;2(1):93–7.
91. Coon EA, Nelson RM, Sletten DM, et al. Sex and gender influence symptom manifestation and survival in multiple system atrophy. Auton Neurosci 2019; 219:49–52.
92. Foubert-Samier A, Pavy-Le Traon A, Guillet F, et al. Disease progression and prognostic factors in multiple system atrophy: a prospective cohort study. Neurobiol Dis 2020;139:104813.
93. Ghorayeb I, Bioulac B, Tison F. Sleep disorders in multiple system atrophy. J Neural Transm 2005;112(12):1669–75.

94. Ohshima Y, Nakayama H, Matsuyama N, et al. Natural course and potential prognostic factors for sleep-disordered breathing in multiple system atrophy. Sleep Med 2017;34:13–7.
95. Sugiyama A, Terada J, Shionoya Y, et al. Sleep-related hypoventilation and hypercapnia in multiple system atrophy detected by polysomnography with transcutaneous carbon dioxide monitoring. Sleep Breath 2022;26(4):1779–89.
96. Cochen De Cock V. Sleep abnormalities in multiplesystem atrophy. Curr Treat Options Neurol 2018;20(6):16.
97. Wang H, Tang X, Zhou J, et al. Excessive daytime sleepiness is associated with non-motor symptoms of multiple system atrophy: a cross-sectional study in China. Front Neurol 2021;12:798771.
98. Palma JA, Fernandez-Cordon C, Coon EA, et al. Prevalence of REM sleep behavior disorder in multiple system atrophy: a multicenter study and meta-analysis. Clin Auton Res 2015;25(1):69–75.
99. Vaidya B, Dhamija K, Guru P, et al. Parkinson's disease in women: mechanisms underlying sex differences. Eur J Pharmacol 2021;895:173862.
100. Beydoun HA, Naughton MJ, Beydoun MA, et al. Association of sleep disturbance with Parkinson disease: evidence from the Women's Health Initiative. Menopause 2022;29(3):255–63.
101. Mizrahi-Kliger AD, Feldmann LK, Kühn AA, et al. Etiologies of insomnia in Parkinson's disease: lessons from human studies and animal models. Exp Neurol 2022;350:113976.
102. Sun AP, Liu N, Zhang YS, et al. The relationship between obstructive sleep apnea and Parkinson's disease: a systematic review and meta-analysis. Neurol Sci 2020;41(5):1153–62.
103. Dunietz GL, Chervin RD, Burke JF, et al. Obstructive sleep apnea treatment disparities among older adults with neurological disorders. Sleep Health 2020;6(4): 534–40.
104. Yang X, Liu B, Shen H, et al. Prevalence of restless legs syndrome in Parkinson's disease: a systematic review and meta-analysis of observational studies. Sleep Med 2018;43:40–6.
105. Sobreira-Neto MA, Pena-Pereira MA, Sobreira EST, et al. Is restless legs syndrome in Parkinson disease patients associated with any specific factor? Arq Neuropsiquiatr 2021;79(1):38–43.
106. Shen Y, Huang JY, Li J, et al. Excessive daytime sleepiness in Parkinson's disease: clinical implications and management. Chin Med J (Engl) 2018;131(8): 974–81.
107. Mahale R, Yadav R, Pal PK. Does gender differences have a role in determining sleep quality in Parkinson's disease? Acta Neurol Belg 2021;121(4):1001–7.
108. Feng F, Cai Y, Hou Y, et al. Excessive daytime sleepiness in Parkinson's disease: a systematic review and meta-analysis. Parkinsonism Relat Disord 2021;85: 133–40.
109. Mahale RR, Yadav R, Pal PK. Rapid eye movement sleep behaviour disorder in women with Parkinson's disease is an underdiagnosed entity. J Clin Neurosci 2016;28:43–6.
110. Farrer LA, Cupples LA, Haines JL, et al. Effects of age, sex, and ethnicity on the association between apolipoprotein E genotype and Alzheimer disease. A meta-analysis. APOE and Alzheimer Disease Meta Analysis Consortium. JAMA 1997; 278(16):1349–56.

111. Brachem C, Winkler A, Tebrügge S, et al. Associations between self-reported sleep characteristics and incident mild cognitive impairment: the Heinz Nixdorf Recall Cohort Study. Sci Rep 2020;10(1):6542.
112. Moran M, Lynch CA, Walsh C, et al. Sleep disturbance in mild to moderate Alzheimer's disease. Sleep Med 2005;6(4):347–52.
113. Harrington YA, Parisi JM, Duan D, et al. Sex hormones, sleep, and memory: interrelationships across the adult female lifespan. Front Aging Neurosci 2022;14:800278.
114. Gaeta AM, Benítez ID, Jorge C, et al. Prevalence of obstructive sleep apnea in Alzheimer's disease patients. J Neurol 2020;267(4):1012–22.
115. Liguori C, Maestri M, Spanetta M, et al. Sleep-disordered breathing and the risk of Alzheimer's disease. Sleep Med Rev 2021;55:101375.
116. Ancoli-Israel S, Palmer BW, Cooke JR, et al. Cognitive effects of treating obstructive sleep apnea in Alzheimer's disease: a randomized controlled study. J Am Geriatr Soc 2008;56(11):2076–81.
117. Orton SM, Herrera BM, Yee IM, et al. Sex ratio of multiple sclerosis in Canada: a longitudinal study. Lancet Neurol 2006;5(11):932–6.
118. Chitnis T, Glanz B, Jaffin S, et al. Demographics of pediatric-onset multiple sclerosis in an MS center population from the Northeastern United States. Mult Scler 2009;15(5):627–31.
119. Vitkova M, Rosenberger J, Gdovinova Z, et al. Poor sleep quality in patients with multiple sclerosis: gender differences. Brain Behav 2016;6(11):e00553.
120. Vitkova M, Gdovinova Z, Rosenberger J, et al. Is poor sleep quality associated with greater disability in patients with multiple sclerosis? Behav Sleep Med 2018; 16(2):106–16.
121. Johansson K, Wasling P, Axelsson M. Fatigue, insomnia and daytime sleepiness in multiple sclerosis versus narcolepsy. Acta Neurol Scand 2021; 144(5):566–75.
122. Abbasi SM, Alimohammadi NP, Pahlavanzadeh SM. Effectiveness of cognitive behavioral therapy on the quality of sleep in women with multiple sclerosis: a randomized controlled trial study. Int J Community Based Nurs Midwifery 2016;4(4):320–8.
123. Akberzie W, Kataria L. Sleep disorders and aging in women. Clin Geriatr Med 2021;37(4):667–82.
124. Kravitz HM, Joffe H. Sleep during the perimenopause: a SWAN story. Obstet Gynecol Clin North Am 2011;38(3):567–86.
125. Sunter G, Omercikoglu Ozden H, Vural E, et al. Risk assessment of obstructive sleep apnea syndrome and other sleep disorders in multiple sclerosis patients. Clin Neurol Neurosurg 2021;207:106749.
126. Sparasci D, Fanfulla F, Ferri R, et al. Sleep-related breathing disorders in multiple sclerosis: prevalence, features and associated factors. Nat Sci Sleep 2022;14:741–50.
127. Li Y, Munger KL, Batool-Anwar S, et al. Association of multiple sclerosis with restless legs syndrome and other sleep disorders in women. Neurology 2012; 78(19):1500–6.
128. Nociti V, Losavio FA, Gnoni V, et al. Sleep and fatigue in multiple sclerosis: a questionnaire-based, cross-sectional, cohort study. J Neurol Sci 2017;372: 387–92.
129. Leoncini S, Signorini C, Boasiako L, et al. Breathing abnormalities during sleep and wakefulness in Rett syndrome: clinical relevance and paradoxical relationship with circulating pro-oxidant markers. Front Neurol 2022;13:833239.

130. Ramirez JM, Ward CS, Neul JL. Breathing challenges in Rett syndrome: lessons learned from humans and animal models. Respir Physiolo Neurobiol 2013; 189(2):280–7.
131. Tascini G, Dell'Isola GB, Mencaroni E, et al. Sleep disorders in Rett syndrome and Rett-related disorders: a narrative review. Front Neurol 2022;13:817195.
132. Romigi A, Feola T, Cappellano S, et al. Sleep disorders in patients with craniopharyngioma: a physiopathological and practical update. Front Neurol 2021;12: 817257.
133. Kitselaar WM, de Morree HM, Trompenaars MW, et al. Fatigue after neurosurgery in patients with a brain tumor: the role of autonomic dysregulation and disturbed sleep. J Psychosom Res 2022;156:110766.

Neuroimmunological Disorders: The Gender Effect

Edith L. Graham, MD

KEYWORDS

- Multiple sclerosis • Disease-modifying therapy • Pregnancy • Breastfeeding
- Fertility

KEY POINTS

- The use of DMT is not generally recommended during pregnancy in MS patients unless the need outweighs the risks to the fetus.
- Various treatment strategies can reduce both relapse risk and potential harm to baby.
- There is increasing evidence for safety of certain therapies during breastfeeding.
- Neuroimmunologic disorders such as NMOSD, MOGAD, CNS vasculitis and neurosarcoidosis have different therapeutic considerations during pregnancy.

INTRODUCTION

Multiple sclerosis (MS) is a chronic, immune-driven disease characterized by demyelination in the central nervous system (CNS). MS may have a relapsing or progressive course and diagnosis depends on the dissemination of CNS demyelinating lesions in the periventricular, infratentorial, juxta/cortical regions as well as the spinal cord. MS has also been linked to Epstein-Barr virus infection, low vitamin D, obesity, and cigarette smoking.[1–3] MS is three times as common in females and is most often diagnosed between the 20 and 40 years of age and therefore disproportionately affects women of childbearing age.[4–6] The use of disease-modifying therapies (DMTs) for MS and other neuroimmunologic disorders during pregnancy is evolving to maximize therapeutic benefits for the pregnant patient while minimizing harm to the fetus.

SEX AND GENDER DIFFERENCES IN MULTIPLE SCLEROSIS

Being female plays a role in the development of autoimmune diseases given that genes for the immune system are inherited on the X chromosome. Although one X chromosome is inactivated in females, during times of cellular stress, the inactive X

Department of Neurology, Division of Neuroimmunology, Northwestern University, 710 North Lake Shore Drive #1411, Chicago, IL 60611, USA
E-mail address: edith.graham@northwestern.edu

Neurol Clin 41 (2023) 315–330
https://doi.org/10.1016/j.ncl.2022.10.004

chromosome may undergo epigenetic changes contributing to an autoimmune response.[7] Female mice of the XX chromosome are more susceptible to experimental autoimmune encephalomyelitis, the animal model of MS.[8]

The role of hormones in MS is complex. Despite the increased risk of MS in women, estrogen alone is not to blame. In general, the sex hormones estrogen and testosterone tend to be neuroprotective.[9] Estradiol and estriol, two types of estrogen, have been shown to be helpful in mitigating MS symptoms, although their role in the overall disease process is still being elucidated.[10]

In addition to MS affecting more women than men, there are sex differences in the onset and type of MS. Women are more likely to have earlier age of onset and men are more likely to have progressive courses and higher disability.[11]

MENARCHE

Early menarche is associated with earlier onset of disease. For those with younger age at menarche (age 10 to 12), MS onset was around age 29 compared with later menarche (13 to 15), where MS onset was around age 32 ($p = .047$).[10] Another study found association between increased risk of MS with earlier age of menarche, but not earlier age at disease onset.[12] Obesity has been associated with earlier onset of menstruation, and a BMI greater than 30 kg/m^2 at age 18 has also been associated with 2.25 times increased risk of MS.[13]

PREGNANCY AND MULTIPLE SCLEROSIS

Pregnancy is considered protective in MS due to the shift to a more immune-tolerant state as to not attack the growing fetus. This occurs with a shift from cytotoxic Th1 CD4+ T cells to the more tolerant Th2 CD4+ T cells. Th1 cells are also important for cell-mediated immunity, which underlies the pathogenesis of MS and why a decrease in these cells leads to a lower relapse rate. This immune shift is triggered by the extravillous trophoblasts in the developing placenta. During placentation, the extravillous trophoblasts migrate into the maternal uterus and modify its vessels to provide blood flow and nutrients to the developing fetus. The extravillous trophoblasts also play an important role in MS quiescence in pregnancy by secreting soluble HLA-G which induces regulatory type 1 T cells to produce interleukin-10, which in turn increases Th2, promoting maternal tolerance.[14]

Despite the decreased MS relapse rate in pregnancy, there is a disease rebound in the postpartum phase. The Pregnancy in Multiple Sclerosis (PRIMS) study in 1998 was the first large multicenter prospective study of MS in pregnant women.[15] PRIMS assessed 254 women with relapsing-remitting MS during and after 269 pregnancies. Patients were examined at 20-, 28- and 36-week of gestation to determine the relapse rate in each trimester. Relapse rate declined by approximately 70% during the third trimester as compared with the rate in the year before conception. The risk of relapses was increased in the first 3 months postpartum (28%); the relapse rate returned to baseline after month 4 postpartum.

The PRIMS 2-year follow-up study found that women with greater disease activity in the year before pregnancy and during pregnancy had a higher risk of relapse in the 3 months postpartum.[16] Similarly, Hughes and colleagues,[17] followed 900 pregnancies and found use of DMTs in preconception period was associated with a 45% reduction in relapse risk postpartum. Updated postpartum relapse data in 2021 by Anderson and colleagues[18] showed that there is lower annualized relapse rate in the first 3 months postpartum than previously reported; only 17% of patients relapsed postpartum. Most of the patients (>80%) did not experience postpartum relapse.

THERAPEUTIC CONSIDERATIONS BEFORE AND DURING PREGNANCY

As of November 2022, there are 23 different Food and Drug Administration (FDA)-approved DMTs that exist for the treatment of MS, including injectable, oral, and infused medications.[19] One area of practice in MS that has changed over the years is early initiation of early high- or moderate-efficacy treatment, which reduce relapse rate by greater than 50%. Recent research supports that high-efficacy therapy commencement within 2 years of disease-onset is associated with less disability after 6 to 10 years than when such therapies are delayed.[20] In one comparison study of patients who started high efficacy versus moderate efficacy therapy, 68% of patients on high efficacy therapy (vs 36% on moderate efficacy therapy) achieved 'No Evidence of Disease Activity' at 1 year.[21] Moreover, treatment with early high-efficacy therapy delays time to secondary progression.[22]

Pregnancy brings its own set of challenges with DMT planning. Patients with low lesion burden, very few relapses and little to no disability may reasonably be untreated while trying to naturally conceive; however, women with better control of MS in the year before pregnancy have lower relapses during pregnancy. Therefore, most MS specialists will opt for active treatment in the preconception period, with most of the patients now being on DMTs in the year before pregnancy.[18] Timing of medication discontinuation relative to conception often depends on the specific DMT used (**Table 1**).[23]

Glatiramer, Interferons

According to European guidelines, at least 300, and ideally 1000, first-trimester exposed pregnancies to a therapy are needed to ascertain drug safety.[24] Glatiramer acetate and interferon beta (INFβ) both have over 2500 first-trimester exposures reported and are considered safe in pregnancy. In addition, prospective studies for both glatiramer acetate and INFβ have shown reassuring safety data.[25,26]

Glatiramer acetate and interferons are considered mild or low-efficacy therapies. Given trends toward higher efficacy therapies, more recently clinicians and patients opt to use B-cell depleting therapies or monoclonal antibodies peripartum on account of their higher efficacy and the rationale that they do not cross the placenta during the first trimester.[27]

B-Cell Depleting Agents

Ocrelizumab, ofatumumab, and rituximab are IgG1 antibodies. IgG is the predominant means of immunity that is transferred from mother to fetus; however, IgG antibodies do not cross placenta in the first trimester of pregnancy. After the first trimester, these antibodies increase in a linear fashion, with transfer starting minimally at weeks 13 to 18 of gestation and sharply increasing at weeks 22 to 26 and continuing to rise during the third trimester.[27] Since data suggest that most birth defects typically occur during weeks 3 to 8 gestation- and far before the antibody transfer occurs-birth defects should not be associated with the use of these monoclonal antibodies in patients with MS. Many biologics have been in clinical use for more than 5 years now, and despite thousands of cases of use in pregnancy, an increase in birth defects has not to be reported to date beyond the background risk of birth defects of 1 in 33 (3%) in every pregnancy.[28]

Should a patient wish to conceive while receiving B-cell depleting therapy, the time-to-near complete elimination of the antibody, along with the antibody transport across the placenta, can help counsel patient on time of last infusion to trial of conception. The average half-lives (and near complete elimination) of these agents are as follows:

Table 1
Disease-modifying treatments for multiple sclerosis during pregnancy and breastfeeding

	Pregnancy FDA Category	Discontinuation Considerations	Breastfeeding Considerations
Glatiramer acetate (Copaxone)	B	At conception; may continue during pregnancy	May continue[91]
Interferons (Rebif, Avonex, Plegridy)	C	At conception; may continue during pregnancy	May continue[92]
Fumarates (Tecfidera, Vumerity, Bafiertam)	C	Just before or at conception (~1 h half-life)	Not recommended due to small molecule size; 2 patients who breastfed on DMF had low transfer into breastmilk[93]
Teriflunomide (Aubagio)	X	Use rapid cholestyramine elimination protocol	Contraindicated[48]
Sphingosine 1-phosphate receptor inhibitors: fingolimod (Gilenya), ozanimod (Zeposia), ponesimod (Ponvory), siponimod (Mayzent)	C	Stop fingolimod and siponimod 2 mo before conception, ozanimod 3 mo. If switching several months before conception, may need alternate treatment ~2 to 4 wk after discontinuation	No published experience Contraindicated
AntiCD20 agents: ocrelizumab (Ocrevus), ofatumumab (Kesimpta), rituximab (Rituxan)	C	3 mo before conception; Average half-life (near complete elimination): Rituxan 18 d (3 mo) Ocrelizumab 26 d (4.5 mo) Ofatumumab 16 d (2.7 mo)	Rituximab and ocrelizumab are transferred in very low amounts into the breastmilk and considered to be safe.[29] Data limited on ofatumumab
Natalizumab (Tysabri)	C	Switch to B-cell targeted therapy or consider extended-interval dosing during pregnancy with last dose ~34 wk gestation	Transfer into breastmilk low (RID 0.04%), although may have cumulative effects[94]
Alemtuzumab (Lemtrada)	C	4 mo before conception	No published experience; Contraindicated
Cladribine (Mavenclad)	D	6 mo before conception	10 d after last drug administration[94]

rituximab 18 days (3 months), ocrelizumab 26 days (4.5 months), and ofatumumab 16 days (2.7 months). Generally, most patients are recommended to wait 3 months after their last infusion or injection of B-cell depleting agents to conception,[23] given that transmission of antibodies across the placenta usually starts in the second trimester. Exposure to B-cell depleting therapy within 3 months of conception or during pregnancy may transiently decrease newborn blood cell counts, although we have not seen clinical complications related to immune suppression in newborn. This risk may be decreased by using lower doses of rituximab. Off-label use of rituximab in patients planning pregnancy has been effective at doses up to 500 mg every 6 months, with only 2.7% of relapse rare postpartum.[29]

Alemtuzumab

Alemtuzumab is an anti-CD52 monoclonal antibody also used for the treatment of relapsing forms of MS. The FDA label recommends waiting 4 months post-infusion to conceive, although the half-life is 2 weeks with undetectable serum levels within 30 days.[30] There was no observed increased rate of spontaneous abortion in patients treated with alemtuzumab within 4 months of infusion.[30] A single case of neonatal Graves' disease was reported at day 21 in a mother exposed to alemtuzumab within 4 months of pregnancy.[31]

Cladribine

Cladribine—with two oral treatment courses taken approximately 1 year apart—was shown to deplete approximately 40% to 50% of total T- and 80% of total B cells.[32] Patients planning pregnancy should wait at least 6 months after the last dose of cladribine before conception.[33] An analysis of pregnancy outcome in 49 female patients receiving cladribine over 6 months after the last dose, there was no difference in congenital malformation in the exposed patients compared with placebo.[34]

Natalizumab

Natalizumab was approved for MS in 2004 and is an IgG4 monoclonal antibody given through infusion every 4 weeks.[35] Relapse rates increase during pregnancy in women who discontinued use of natalizumab pre-pregnancy, although continuation of natalizumab during pregnancy reduced odds of relapse during gestation.[36] Hellwig and colleagues[37] found that 40% of patients who discontinued natalizumab pre-conception had a relapse during pregnancy, and 10% had clinically meaningful disability postpartum. Given the association with rebound relapse, natalizumab may be continued during pregnancy in high-risk patients.

The Tysabri Pregnancy Exposure Registry looked at 317 pregnancies exposed to natalizumab, and reported a higher birth defect rate than in the Metropolitan Atlanta Congenital Defects Program (5.05% vs 2.67%), although no specific pattern of birth defects emerged. Most patients were last exposed to natalizumab within 3 months before conception or in the first trimester. Of the 4 patients who continued treatment throughout pregnancy, there were no reports of congenital anomalies.[38]

Blockade of α-4 integrins may impact fetal development, in particular fetal hematopoiesis and cardiac development. In most cases, exposure to α-4 integrin blockade in the first or second trimester was not associated with poor outcomes, whereas exposure in the third-trimester was associated with hematological abnormalities.[39] Given risk of transient hematological abnormalities (including anemia and thrombocytopenia) in newborns exposed to natalizumab, the last infusion is often recommended between weeks 28 to 32 of gestation. There have been no cardiac abnormalities in children born to mothers exposed to natalizumab. Extended interval dosing every 6 to 8 weeks has also been considered during pregnancy.

Sphingosine 1-Phosphate Receptor Modulators

Sphingosine 1-phosphate (S1P) modulators such as fingolimod block egress of lymphocytes from the lymph node.[40] Although it is effective at preventing MS relapse, fingolimod withdrawal was associated with high risk of relapse in 52 cases of severe MS rebound.[41] Exposure during pregnancy is associated with a twofold higher risk of major congenital anomalies including congenital heart disease, renal disease, and musculoskeletal abnormalities.[42] Thus, it is recommended to discontinue fingolimod at least 2 months before pregnancy, and to switch to alternate DMT. In cases of accidental pregnancy exposure, fetal organ screening with ultrasound is recommended. Otherwise, sexually active women of child-bearing age should use a method of contraception while on fingolimod and for 2 months afterward.[43] Siponimod, another S1P modulator, should also be discontinued 2 months before pregnancy, whereas ozanimod should be discontinued for at least 3 months before conception due to a long-acting metabolite. For this reason, many practitioners avoid using S1P modulators in patients who may become pregnant.

Fumarates

The fumarates (dimethyl fumarate, diroximel fumarate, monomethyl fumarate) are oral medications taken twice daily, and shown to reduce the number of MS relapses by approximately one-half.[44] Patients planning pregnancy can continue a fumarate treatment until pregnancy test is positive pregnancy test is confirmed given the short half-life of less than 24 hours.[45] An international registry tracking pregnancy outcome in women treated with dimethyl fumarate, showed no increase in risk of spontaneous abortion or birth defect.[46]

Teriflunomide

Teriflunomide is a dihydroorotate dehydrogenase inhibitor and is considered Category X in pregnancy. There is a boxed warning regarding its teratogenicity due to animal studies resulting in embryolethal effects.[47] Despite the warning, there has not been a clear toxic effect in cases of accidental exposure to pregnancy in humans.[48] Given its long half-life and potential risks, it should be discontinued 2 years before pregnancy. In most cases, this is accomplished more quickly with the use of cholestyramine rapid elimination protocol (cholestyramine 8 g by mouth three times daily for 11 days).[48]

RELAPSE DURING PREGNANCY

When MS relapse is suspected during pregnancy, an MRI—which is safe when done without contrast during pregnancy-should be obtained. In a study of over 1.4 million deliveries, fetal exposure to gadolinium contrast showed a higher risk of stillbirth or neonatal death, adjusted RR 1.68, (95% CI, 0.97 to 2.90) compared with control.[49]

Treatment of MS relapse in pregnancy may be considered with balance between disability and teratogenicity. Intravenous (IV) methylprednisolone is considered Category C in pregnancy, with possible increased risk of oral cleft and low birth weight when used during the first trimester. Prednisone, prednisolone or methylprednisolone are metabolized to inactive forms by 11-B-hydroxysteroid dehydrogenase in the placenta allowing less than 10% of maternal dose to reach the fetus. The use of betamethasone or dexamethasone is considered less safe during pregnancy, although dexamethasone may be given to expecting mothers during gestation to promote lung maturation and considered Category A in Australia. In high-risk patients, monthly IV immunoglobulin therapy or monthly IV methylprednisolone may be considered.[50,51] See **Table 2** for a summary of relapse treatments during pregnancy.

OBSTETRIC ANESTHESIA

There still exists misconceptions about the dangers of neuraxial anesthesia in patients with preexisting CNS disorders including MS, and at one time neuraxial anesthesia was considered an absolute contraindication in those patients. Recent data showed no difference in the course of disease progression in MS patients receiving neuraxial compared with epidural anesthesia.[52,53] Further data to better evaluate the safety of these procedures in MS patients is needed.

POSTPARTUM CARE

Postpartum sleep disruption on top of baseline MS fatigue may make caring for one's newborn challenging. Poor sleep also negatively impacts other MS symptoms. Thus, physicians should ensure that patients have adequate support at home to help care for them and their baby. Physicians should also consider offering short-term disability or Family and Medical Leave Act for MS patients who may need extra time recovering from birth. Although screening for postpartum depression is important, recent studies did now show higher depression rate in patients with MS.[54]

BREASTFEEDING

Exclusive breastfeeding is considered protective in MS and has been shown to reduce the relapse rate. In a study Hellwig and colleagues[55] from 2012 which compared women who exclusively breastfed to those who included intermittent formula supplementation or to those who did not breastfeed, the rate of relapse in the first 3 months postpartum was 0.68 in the exclusive breastfeeding group versus 1.5 in the two other groups.

When magnetic resonance imaging is indicated, and according to the American College of Radiology guidelines, gadolinium contrast administration to breastfeeding mother is safe since only a very small amount of gadolinium-based contrast is excreted into the breast milk. In mothers who wish to take extra precautions, breastmilk may be discarded 12 to 24 hours after MRI, but any time beyond that is unnecessary. Specific recommendations regarding individual DMTs can be found in **Table 1**.[56,57]

FERTILITY IN MULTIPLE SCLEROSIS

A 2015 study by Thöne and colleagues[58] showed that patients with relapsing-remitting MS have lower mean levels of anti-Müllerian hormone (AMH) than healthy controls. Most of these women were not on disease-modifying treatment (DMT). In addition, a 2016 study by Sepúlveda and colleagues[59] found that lower AMH levels were associated with higher MS disease activity. This suggests that infertility can lead to higher risk of relapse in MS. It may be that higher disease activity could cause lower AMH levels, or that some third variable might affect both disease activity and AMH level. Conversely, a study by Graves and colleagues[60] in 2018, found that AMH was not significantly different between MS patients and healthy controls.

Women with MS often have a narrow window to become pregnant while receiving treatment. For example, women on B-cell-depleting agents such as ocrelizumab or

Table 2
Pregnancy considerations of therapy for multiple sclerosis relapses[50]

	Pregnancy Category	Possible Fetal Effects	Metabolism
Methylprednisolone (oral or intravenous)	C	Possible increased risk of oral cleft if used in first trimester; low birth weight	Placenta metabolizes to inactive forms via 11b-hydroxysteroid dehydrogenase allowing <10% of maternal dose to reach fetus
Dexamethasone (oral or intravenous)	C	Low birth weight	Crosses placenta with minimal metabolism, leading to likely direct full-dose on the fetus
Intravenous immunoglobulin (IVIG)	C	No known adverse effects	
Therapeutic plasma exchange	Use if relapse is refractory to treatment with steroids		

rituximab are encouraged to conceive between months 3 to 6 after infusion. Women may have difficulty conceiving and may benefit from ART.

An increased risk of MS relapse has been reported with use of ART such as in vitro fertilization and controlled ovarian stimulation with medications such as clomiphene and letrozole. These treatments increase hormonal levels much higher than natural ovulation cycles, which may in turn predispose to MS relapse. A meta-analysis of five studies evaluating the relapse rate of women with MS after ART and all have shown an increase in relapse rate after treatment.[61] These findings have subsequently formed the basis for counseling women with MS contemplating ART. One study of 16 patients found a sevenfold increased relapse rate and ninefold increase in gadolinium-enhancing lesions on MRI brain over the period of treatment with ART. DMT was discontinued for greater than 15 months before ART initiation, thus this could have led to increase in the burden of enhancing lesions.[62]

Gonadotropin-releasing hormone (GnRH) antagonists—with shorte protocols compared with GnRH agonists-are more frequently used to prevent a lutenizing hormone surge during controlled ovarian hyperstimulation (COH). Furthermore, many women choose to freeze all of their oocytes or embryos after COH and consider transvaginal oocyte retrieval (TVOR) rather than proceeding directly to embryo transfer and pregnancy. Most MS patients now-a-day remain on DMT through COH and TVOR as DMT reduces the risk of relapse.[63] Recent and larger cohort studies have failed to show an increased risk of relapse with ART.[61,64]

MENOPAUSE

MS is more likely to enter a progressive phase postmenopause. An observational, multicenter study of 148 perimenopausal women found a decrease in relapse rate and increase in disability as measured by the expanded disability status scale in the 2 years post-menopause.[65] Although we know the MS becomes more degenerative with age, we do not understand the impact of menopause and hormonal effect on disease progression.

In a Swedish survey of women with MS, 40% reported worsening of MS symptoms postmenopause. This, in contrast to 25% of women who reported improvement in symptoms during pregnancy, a time of elevated estrogen.[66] Along those lines, another study found that hormone therapy reduces physical symptoms in post-menopausal MS patients.[67] Estrogen has also been shown to have a protective role in preventing brain atrophy and white matter changes in non-MS patients.[68] The role of estrogen in post-menopausal MS patients requires further research.

NEUROMYELITIS OPTICA SPECTRUM DISORDER

Neuromyelitis optica spectrum disorder (NMOSD) is a demyelinating disorder mediated by antibodies against aquaporin-4 water channels on astrocytes. Unlike MS, NMOSD is associated with a higher risk of pregnancy complications including miscarriage (43%) and preeclampsia (11%).[69]

NMOSD patients accrue increased disease activity and more disability per relapse compared with those with MS, therefore prevention of relapse is extremely important. In general, childbearing patients treated with rituximab typically withhold the medication at least 3 months before conception. In circumstances where patients are at risk for serious neurologic disability from NMO relapse, rituximab can be given closer to conception, or even during pregnancy.[70] Fetuses exposed to rituximab are likely to be born with undetectable CD19 counts, which tend to recover by weeks 6 to 8 of life at which point they can get their 2-month vaccinations.[71,72]

Unlike MS, CD19/CD20 B cell recovery is associated with relapse; thus, patients with NMO require tighter B-cell depletion strategies. Therefore, patients with NMO need early infusion of rituximab in the postpartum period, usually at 2-week postpartum to allow for maternal healing and milk maturation but should not be delayed greater than 4 weeks postpartum to prevent relapse risk.[71]

There is no datum on the use of the recently FDA-approved NMO medications inebilizumab (Uplizna), eculizumab (Soliris), and satralizumab (Enspryng) during pregnancy. Inebilizumab is an IgG1 monoclonal antibody that depletes CD19 B cells; the pharmacodynamics of inebilizumab are expected to be similar to other cell-depleting agents.[73] Eculizumab is an IgG2/4 C5 terminal complement inhibitor. IgG2 does not readily cross the placenta, though IgG4 does. Eculizumab has been used during pregnancy in other conditions such as paroxysmal nocturnal hemoglobinuria, atypical hemolytic uremic syndrome (aHUS), and hemolysis, elevated liver enzymes, and low platelet count (HELLP) syndrome without harm to the fetus.[74] Over 400 cases of eculizumab exposure during pregnancy in paroxysmal nocturnal hemoglobinuria or atypical hemolytic uremic syndrome showed no adverse outcomes.[75] Eculizumab may transfer to the fetus, though effect of the drug typically only lasts a couple weeks postpartum given the shorter half-life.[76,77] Satralizumab, an IL-6 receptor recycling antibody, is similar in mechanism to tocilizumab which has limited safety data in pregnancy. Both satralizumab and tocilizumab are IgG1 antibodies that cross the placenta. In 16 pregnant women exposed to tocilizumab, there were normal fetal outcomes in all except one which had hydrops fetalis.[78]

MYELIN OLIGODENDROCYTE GLYCOPROTEIN ANTIBODY-ASSOCIATED DISORDER

Myelin Oligodendrocyte Glycoprotein Antibody-Associated Disorder (MOGAD) is another rare CNS demyelinating disorder, with less disability with relapses compared with NMO.[78] MOGAD patients with high titer antibodies are at risk for relapsing disease.[79] Monthly maintenance IVIG at a dose of 0.5 g/kg may be one of the most effective treatments at preventing MOGAD relapses and is considered safe during pregnancy.[80] Low-dose prednisone may also be used. Azathioprine is overall less effective in MOGAD, but may be continued during pregnancy as it has not been shown to significantly increase risk of birth defects in other autoimmune disorders.[81]

NEUROSARCOIDOSIS

Neurosarcoidosis is characterized by granulomatous inflammation of the nervous system. Sarcoidosis is associated with higher risk of pre-eclampsia, eclampsia, deep vein thrombosis, pulmonary embolism, premature delivery, cesarean section, and postpartum hemorrhage.[82] As such, thromboprophylaxis may be given to patients with sarcoidosis during pregnancy. Studies on outcomes of pregnancy in patients with neurosarcoidosis are lacking.

Although sarcoidosis is known to be responsive to steroids, it often returns once steroids are withdrawn, necessitating the addition of a steroid-sparing immunosuppressants. Typical agents include infliximab, methotrexate, mycophenolate, and azathioprine. IV infliximab, an IgG1 monoclonal antibody, is increasingly used for neurosarcoidosis.[83] Over 1850 pregnancies have been exposed to infliximab, mostly in patients with inflammatory bowel disease (IBD), with a similar rate of miscarriage, low birth weight, preterm delivery and infant infection compared with the general population.[84] Infliximab can be discontinued 2 months before pregnancy to avoid any fetal exposure, although good infant outcomes have in been reported in women who continued infliximab for IBD throughout pregnancy.[85]

In addition, most patients are on a concomitant oral immunosuppressant to prevent the development of anti-infliximab antibodies. In non-childbearing patients, methotrexate is a common choice given its independent ability to treat sarcoidosis; however, methotrexate is contraindicated in pregnancy given its antineoplastic effects and teratogenicity. Accidental methotrexate exposure was associated with high rate of miscarriage, fetal malformation, and congenital heart defect.[86] Mycophenolate should also not be given during pregnancy as it is associated with an elevated risk of miscarriage and fetal malformation.[87] Concomitant treatment with infliximab and azathioprine or low-dose steroids is safer in child-bearing patients with neurosarcoidosis. Other options include maintenance prednisone throughout pregnancy, with little evidence to support any poor fetal outcomes with its chronic use in pregnancy.[88]

CENTRAL NERVOUS SYSTEM VASCULITIS

CNS vasculitis is an inflammatory disorder of cerebral, and rarely spinal arteries and veins. Cyclophosphamide and pulse steroids are often used as induction therapy, whereas azathioprine, methotrexate, or mycophenolate are used for maintenance.[83] Pregnant patients exposed to cyclophosphamide risk an extremely high chance of in-utero fetal demise.[89] Women must not become pregnant for at least a year after the last dose of cyclophosphamide, and men should not father a child for at least 6 months after receiving such treatment. Breastfeeding is also contraindicated with cyclophosphamide. Considerations for steroid-sparing agents are similar to MOGAD and neurosarcoidosis. Azathioprine or maintenance prednisone can be considered. Rituximab may also be given before pregnancy given some benefit in CNS vasculitis.[90] Mycophenolate and methotrexate must be avoided.

SUMMARY

Several neuroimmunologic disorders tend to affect women of childbearing age. Although relapse risk in patients with MS decreases during pregnancy, patients should still be optimized on DMTs before and after pregnancy to minimize gaps in treatment. Exclusive breastfeeding may reduce the chance of disease relapse postpartum, and many DMTs are considered to be safe while breastfeeding. Treatments of other neuroimmunologic disorders such as NMOSD, MOGAD, neurosarcoidosis, and CNS vasculitis may require rituximab before, and prednisone maintenance or IVIG therapy during pregnancy.

CLINICS CARE POINTS

- Various treatment strategies can reduce both relapse risk and potential harm to baby. B-cell depleting agents including rituximab and ocrelizumab are ideal for MS patients planning pregnancy as they are of high efficacy and their therapeutic effect is longer than their serum concentration.
- Natalizumab and sphingosine 1-phosphate (S1P) inhibitors should be avoided during pregnancy due to rebound risk. If the patient is at high risk for relapse, natalizumab can be continued during pregnancy; however, S1P should be discontinued in all instances.
- Glatiramer acetate and interferon may be either stopped at conception or continued during pregnancy.
- Fumarates should be stopped at conception.
- IgG1 monoclonal antibodies such as rituximab and ocrelizumab have minimal transfer through the breastmilk.

DISCLOSURE

E. Graham has received research funding from Roche Genentech and has participated as a consultant or advisory board member for Atara Biotherapeutics, Genentech, Novartis, Tavistock Life Sciences, Horizon Therapeutics, American College of Physicians.

REFERENCES

1. Bjornevik K, Cortese M, Healy BC, et al. Longitudinal analysis reveals high prevalence of Epstein-Barr virus associated with multiple sclerosis. Science 2022; 375(6578):296–301.
2. Bar-Or A, Pender MP, Khanna R, et al. Epstein-Barr virus in multiple sclerosis: theory and emerging immunotherapies. Trends Mol Med 2020;26(3):296–310 [published correction appears in Trends Mol Med. 2021;27(4):410-411].
3. Thompson AJ, Banwell BL, Barkhof F, et al. Diagnosis of multiple sclerosis: 2017 revisions of the McDonald criteria. Lancet Neurol 2018;17(2):162–73.
4. Wallin MT, Culpepper WJ, Coffman P, et al. The Gulf War era multiple sclerosis cohort: age and incidence rates by race, sex and service. Brain 2012;135(Pt 6):1778–85.
5. Orton SM, Herrera BM, Yee IM, et al. Sex ratio of multiple sclerosis in Canada: a longitudinal study. Lancet Neurol 2006;5(11):932–6.
6. Koch-Henriksen N, Sørensen PS. The changing demographic pattern of multiple sclerosis epidemiology. Lancet Neurol 2010;9(5):520–32.
7. Brooks WH, Renaudineau Y. Epigenetics and autoimmune diseases: the X chromosome-nucleolus nexus. Front Genet 2015;6:22.
8. Smith-Bouvier DL, Divekar AA, Sasidhar M, et al. A role for sex chromosome complement in the female bias in autoimmune disease. J Exp Med 2008;205(5): 1099–108.

9. Kipp M, Amor S, Krauth R, et al. Multiple sclerosis: neuroprotective alliance of estrogen-progesterone and gender. Front Neuroendocrinol 2012;33(1):1–16.
10. Ysrraelit MC, Correale J. Impact of sex hormones on immune function and multiple sclerosis development. Immunology 2019;156(1):9–22.
11. Sloka JS, Pryse-Phillips WE, Stefanelli M. The relation between menarche and the age of first symptoms in a multiple sclerosis cohort. Mult Scler 2006;12(3):333–9.
12. Ramagopalan SV, Valdar W, Criscuoli M, et al. Age of puberty and the risk of multiple sclerosis: a population based study. Eur J Neurol 2009;16(3):342–7.
13. Munger KL, Chitnis T, Ascherio A. Body size and risk of MS in two cohorts of US women. Neurology 2009;73(19):1543–50.
14. Warning JC, McCracken SA, Morris JM. A balancing act: mechanisms by which the fetus avoids rejection by the maternal immune system. Reproduction 2011; 141(6):715–24.
15. Confavreux C, Hutchinson M, Hours MM, et al. Rate of pregnancy-related relapse in multiple sclerosis. pregnancy in multiple sclerosis group. N Engl J Med 1998; 339(5):285–91.
16. Vukusic S, Hutchinson M, Hours M, et al. Pregnancy and multiple sclerosis (the PRIMS study): clinical predictors of postpartum relapse. Brain 2004;127(Pt 6): 1353–60 [published correction appears in Brain. 2004 Aug;127(Pt 8):1912].
17. Hughes SE, Spelman T, Gray OM, et al. Predictors and dynamics of postpartum relapses in women with multiple sclerosis. Mult Scler 2014;20(6):739–46.
18. Anderson A, Krysko KM, Rutatangwa A, et al. Clinical and radiologic disease activity in pregnancy and postpartum in MS. Neurol Neuroimmunol Neuroinflamm 2021;8(2):e959.
19. Disease-Modifying Therapies for MS. Available at: https://www.nationalmssociety.org/Treating-MS/Medications. Accessed August 1, 2022.
20. He A, Merkel B, Brown JWL, et al. Timing of high-efficacy therapy for multiple sclerosis: a retrospective observational cohort study. Lancet Neurol 2020;19(4): 307–16.
21. Simonsen CS, Flemmen HØ, Broch L, et al. Early high efficacy treatment in multiple sclerosis is the best predictor of future disease activity over 1 and 2 years in a norwegian population-based registry. Front Neurol 2021;12:693017.
22. Brown JWL, Coles A, Horakova D, et al. Association of initial disease-modifying therapy with later conversion to secondary progressive multiple sclerosis [published correction appears in JAMA. 2020 Apr 7;323(13):1318]. JAMA 2019; 321(2):175–87.
23. Krysko KM, Bove R, Dobson R, et al. Treatment of women with multiple sclerosis planning pregnancy. Curr Treat Options Neurol 2021;23(4):11.
24. European Medicines Agency (EMA). Evaluation of medicines for human use. Guidelines on risk assessment of medical products on human reproduction and lactation: from data to labeling. 2008. London. Available at: http://www.ema.europa.eu/docs/en_GB/document_library/Scientific_guideline/2009/09/WC500003307.pdf. Accessed August 1, 2022.
25. Herbstritt S, Langer-Gould A, Rockhoff M, et al. Glatiramer acetate during early pregnancy: a prospective cohort study. Mult Scler 2016;22(6):810–6.
26. Thiel S, Langer-Gould A, Rockhoff M, et al. Interferon-beta exposure during first trimester is safe in women with multiple sclerosis-A prospective cohort study from the German Multiple Sclerosis and Pregnancy Registry. Mult Scler 2016;22(6): 801–9.

27. Pentsuk N, van der Laan JW. An interspecies comparison of placental antibody transfer: new insights into developmental toxicity testing of monoclonal antibodies. Birth Defects Res B Dev Reprod Toxicol 2009;86(4):328–44.
28. Centers for Disease Control and Prevention. Update on overall prevalence of major birth defects–Atlanta, Georgia, 1978-2005. MMWR Morb Mortal Wkly Rep 2008;57(1):1–5.
29. Smith JB, Hellwig K, Fink K, et al. Rituximab, MS, and pregnancy. Neurol Neuroimmunol Neuroinflamm 2020;7(4):e734.
30. Lemtrada FDA label (accessdata.fda.gov). Revised 10/2017. Accessed August 1, 2022.
31. Oh J, Achiron A, Celius EG, et al. Pregnancy outcomes and postpartum relapse rates in women with RRMS treated with alemtuzumab in the phase 2 and 3 clinical development program over 16 years. Mult Scler Relat Disord 2020;43:102146.
32. Leist TP, Comi G, Cree BA, et al. Effect of oral cladribine on time to conversion to clinically definite multiple sclerosis in patients with a first demyelinating event (ORACLE MS): a phase 3 randomised trial. Lancet Neurol 2014;13(3):257–67.
33. Hellwig K, Thiel S, Ciplea A, et al. Pregnancy of MS patients treated with cladribine tablets, 2020, AAN. 15 Supplement94. Neurology; 2020.
34. Giovannoni G, Galazka A, Schick R, et al. Pregnancy outcomes during the clinical development program of cladribine in multiple sclerosis: an integrated analysis of safety. Drug Saf 2020;43(7):635–43.
35. Polman CH, O'Connor PW, Havrdova E, et al. A randomized, placebo-controlled trial of natalizumab for relapsing multiple sclerosis. N Engl J Med 2006;354(9): 899–910.
36. Yeh WZ, Widyastuti PA, Van der Walt A, et al. Natalizumab, fingolimod and dimethyl fumarate use and pregnancy-related relapse and disability in women with multiple sclerosis. Neurology 2021;96(24):e2989–3002 [published online ahead of print, 2021 Apr 20].
37. Hellwig K, Tokic M, Thiel S, et al. Multiple sclerosis disease activity and disability following discontinuation of natalizumab for pregnancy. JAMA Netw Open 2022; 5(1):e2144750.
38. Friend S, Richman S, Bloomgren G, et al. Evaluation of pregnancy outcomes from the Tysabri® (natalizumab) pregnancy exposure registry: a global, observational, follow-up study. BMC Neurol 2016;16(1):150.
39. Haghikia A, Langer-Gould A, Rellensmann G, et al. Natalizumab use during the third trimester of pregnancy. JAMA Neurol 2014;71(7):891–5.
40. Kappos L, Radue EW, O'Connor P, et al. A placebo-controlled trial of oral fingolimod in relapsing multiple sclerosis. N Engl J Med 2010;362(5):387–401.
41. Fragoso YD, Adoni T, Gomes S, et al. Severe exacerbation of multiple sclerosis following withdrawal of fingolimod. Clin Drug Investig 2019;39(9):909–13.
42. Hellwig K. Effect of fingolimod on pregnancy outcomes in patients with multiple sclerosis. Stockholm (Sweden): ECTRIMS; 2019.
43. Geissbühler Y, Vile J, Koren G, et al. Evaluation of pregnancy outcomes in patients with multiple sclerosis after fingolimod exposure. Ther Adv Neurol Disord 2018;11. 1756286418804760.
44. Prosperini L, Pontecorvo S. Dimethyl fumarate in the management of multiple sclerosis: appropriate patient selection and special considerations. Ther Clin Risk Manag 2016;12:339–50.
45. Alroughani R, Inshasi J, Al-Asmi A, et al. Disease-modifying drugs and family planning in people with multiple sclerosis: a consensus narrative review from the gulf region. Neurol Ther 2020;9(2):265–80.

46. Hellwig K., An international registry tracking pregnancy outcomes in women treated with dimethyl fumarate. Stockholm, Sweden: ECTRIMS; Neurology, 2020; 94 (15 Supplement).
47. Cada DJ, Demaris K, Levien TL, et al. Teriflunomide. Hosp Pharm 2013;48(3): 231–40.
48. Vukusic S, Coyle PK, Jurgensen S, et al. Pregnancy outcomes in patients with multiple sclerosis treated with teriflunomide: clinical study data and 5 years of post-marketing experience. Mult Scler 2020;26(7):829–36.
49. Ray JG, Vermeulen MJ, Bharatha A, et al. Association between MRI exposure during pregnancy and fetal and childhood outcomes. JAMA 2016;316(9):952–61.
50. Canibaño B, Deleu D, Mesraoua B, et al. Pregnancy-related issues in women with multiple sclerosis: an evidence-based review with practical recommendations. J Drug Assess 2020;9(1):20–36.
51. Achiron A, Kishner I, Dolev M, et al. Effect of intravenous immunoglobulin treatment on pregnancy and postpartum-related relapses in multiple sclerosis. J Neurol 2004;251(9):1133–7.
52. Hebl JR, Horlocker TT, Schroeder DR. Neuraxial anesthesia and analgesia in patients with preexisting central nervous system disorders. Anesth Analg 2006; 103(1). https://doi.org/10.1213/01.ane.0000220896.56427.53.
53. Lu E, Zhao Y, Dahlgren L, et al. Obstetrical epidural and spinal anesthesia in multiple sclerosis. J Neurol 2013;260(10):2620–8.
54. Krysko KM, Anderson A, Singh J, et al. Risk factors for peripartum depression in women with multiple sclerosis. Mult Scler 2022;28(6):970–9.
55. Hellwig K, Haghikia A, Rockhoff M, et al. Multiple sclerosis and pregnancy: experience from a nationwide database in Germany. Ther Adv Neurol Disord 2012; 5(5):247–53.
56. Kubik-Huch RA, Gottstein Alame NM, Frenzel T, et al. Gadopentetate diglumine excretion into human breast milk during lactation. Radiology 2000;216:555–8.
57. Lin SP, Brown JJ. MR contrast agents: physical and pharmocologic basics. JMRI 2007;25:884–99.
58. Thöne J, Kollar S, Nousome D, et al. Serum anti-Müllerian hormone levels in reproductive-age women with relapsing-remitting multiple sclerosis. Mult Scler 2015;21(1):41–7.
59. Sepúlveda M, Ros C, Martínez-Lapiscina EH, et al. Pituitary-ovary axis and ovarian reserve in fertile women with multiple sclerosis: A pilot study. Mult Scler 2016;22(4):564–8.
60. Graves JS, Henry RG, Cree BAC, et al. Ovarian aging is associated with gray matter volume and disability in women with MS. Neurology 2018;90(3):e254–60.
61. Bove R, Rankin K, Lin C, et al. Effect of assisted reproductive technology on multiple sclerosis relapses: Case series and meta-analysis. Mult Scler 2020;26(11): 1410–9.
62. Correale J, Farez MF, Ysrraelit MC. Increase in multiple sclerosis activity after assisted reproduction technology. Ann Neurol 2012;72(5):682–94.
63. Graham E. Assisted reproductive technologies in women with MS: a multicenter analysis of inflammatory activity. West Palm Beach (FL): ACTRIMS; 2022.
64. Mainguy M, Tillaut H, Degremont A, et al. Assessing the risk of relapse requiring corticosteroids after in vitro fertilization in women with multiple sclerosis. Neurology 2022. https://doi.org/10.1212/WNL.0000000000201027.
65. Baroncini D, Annovazzi PO, De Rossi N, et al. Impact of natural menopause on multiple sclerosis: a multicentre study. J Neurol Neurosurg Psychiatry 2019; 90(11):1201–6.

66. Holmqvist P, Wallberg M, Hammar M, et al. Symptoms of multiple sclerosis in women in relation to sex steroid exposure. Maturitas 2006;54(2):149–53.
67. Bove R, White CC, Fitzgerald KC, et al. Hormone therapy use and physical quality of life in postmenopausal women with multiple sclerosis. Neurology 2016; 87(14):1457–63.
68. Kantarci K, Tosakulwong N, Lesnick TG, et al. Brain structure and cognition 3 years after the end of an early menopausal hormone therapy trial. Neurology 2018;90(16):e1404–12.
69. Nour MM, Nakashima I, Coutinho E, et al. Pregnancy outcomes in aquaporin-4-positive neuromyelitis optica spectrum disorder. Neurology 2016;86(1):79–87.
70. Miranda-Acuña J, Rivas-Rodríguez E, Levy M, et al. Rituximab during pregnancy in neuromyelitis optica: a case report. Neurol Neuroimmunol Neuroinflamm 2019; 6(2):e542.
71. Chakravarty EF, Murray ER, Kelman A, et al. Pregnancy outcomes after maternal exposure to rituximab. Blood 2011;117(5):1499–506.
72. Galati A, McElrath T, Bove R. Use of B-Cell-depleting therapy in women of childbearing potential with multiple sclerosis and neuromyelitis optica spectrum disorder. Neurol Clin Pract 2022;12(2):154–63.
73. D'Souza R, Wuebbolt D, Andrejevic K, et al. Pregnancy and neuromyelitis optica spectrum disorder—reciprocal effects and practical recommendations: a systematic review. Front Neurol 2020;11:544434.
74. Hallstensen RF, Bergseth G, Foss S, et al. Eculizumab treatment during pregnancy does not affect the complement system activity of the newborn. Immunobiology 2015;220:452–9.
75. Socié G, Caby-Tosi MP, Marantz JL, et al. Eculizumab in paroxysmal nocturnal haemoglobinuria and atypical haemolytic uraemic syndrome: 10-year pharmacovigilance analysis. Br J Haematol 2019;185(2):297–310.
76. Duineveld C, Wijnsma KL, Volokhina EB, et al. Placental passage of eculizumab and complement blockade in a newborn. Kidney Int 2019;95(4):996.
77. Weber-Schoendorfer C, Schaefer C. Pregnancy outcome after tocilizumab therapy in early pregnancy-a case series from the German Embryotox Pharmacovigilance Center. Reprod Toxicol 2016;60:29–32.
78. Dubey D, Pittock SJ, Krecke KN, et al. Clinical, radiologic, and prognostic features of myelitis associated with myelin oligodendrocyte glycoprotein autoantibody. JAMA Neurol 2019;76(3):301–9.
79. Sechi E, Buciuc M, Pittock SJ, et al. Positive predictive value of myelin oligodendrocyte glycoprotein autoantibody testing. JAMA Neurol 2021;78(6):741–6.
80. Chen JJ, Flanagan EP, Bhatti MT, et al. Steroid-sparing maintenance immunotherapy for MOG-IgG associated disorder. Neurology 2020;95(2):e111–20.
81. Alami Z, Agier MS, Ahid S, et al. Pregnancy outcome following in utero exposure to azathioprine: a French comparative observational study. Therapie 2018;73(3): 199–207.
82. Hadid V, Patenaude V, Oddy L, et al. Sarcoidosis and pregnancy: obstetrical and neonatal outcomes in a population-based cohort of 7 million births. J Perinat Med 2015;43(2):201–7.
83. Gelfand JM, Bradshaw MJ, Stern BJ, et al. Infliximab for the treatment of CNS sarcoidosis: a multi-institutional series. Neurology 2017;89(20):2092–100.
84. Geldhof A, Slater J, Clark M, et al. Exposure to infliximab during pregnancy: post-marketing experience. Drug Saf 2020;43(2):147–61.

85. Dawson AL, Riehle-Colarusso T, Reefhuis J, et al. National birth defects prevention study. maternal exposure to methotrexate and birth defects: a population-based study. Am J Med Genet A 2014;164A(9):2212–6.
86. Coscia LA, Armenti DP, King RW, et al. Update on the teratogenicity of maternal mycophenolate mofetil. J Pediatr Genet 2015;4(2):42–55.
87. Bandoli G, Palmsten K, Forbess Smith CJ, et al. A review of systemic corticosteroid use in pregnancy and the risk of select pregnancy and birth outcomes. Rheum Dis Clin North Am 2017;43(3):489–502.
88. Beuker C, Schmidt A, Strunk D, et al. Primary angiitis of the central nervous system: diagnosis and treatment. Ther Adv Neurol Disord 2018;11. 1756286418785071.
89. Clowse ME, Magder L, Petri M. Cyclophosphamide for lupus during pregnancy. Lupus 2005;14(8):593–7.
90. Salvarani C, Brown RD Jr, Muratore F, et al. Rituximab therapy for primary central nervous system vasculitis: a 6 patient experience and review of the literature. Autoimmun Rev 2019;18(4):399–405.
91. Ciplea AI, Langer-Gould A, Stahl A, et al. Safety of potential breast milk exposure to IFN-β or glatiramer acetate: one-year infant outcomes. Neurol Neuroimmunol Neuroinflamm 2020;7(4):e757.
92. Ciplea AI, Datta P, Rewers-Felkins K, et al. Dimethyl fumarate transfer into human milk. Ther Adv Neurol Disord 2020;13. 1756286420968414.
93. Proschmann U, Haase R, Inojosa H, et al. Drug and neurofilament levels in serum and breastmilk of women with multiple sclerosis exposed to natalizumab during pregnancy and lactation. Front Immunol 2021;12:715195.
94. Yamout BI, Alroughani R. Multiple sclerosis. Semin Neurol 2018;38(2):212–25.

Neuro-Oncology in Women

Clinical Considerations

Lauren Singer, MD*, Ditte Primdahl, MD, Priya Kumthekar, MD

KEYWORDS

• Oncology • Glioma • Meningioma

KEY POINTS

- While gliomas are more common in males than females, females have overall improved survival with treatment with standard of care.
- Sex differences in gliomas are a result of molecular, hormonal, and biologic differences at the cellular level.
- Meningiomas are more commonly found in females and many meningiomas express hormone receptors, including estrogen and progesterone.
- Life events and drugs which increase hormone exposure, such as oral contraceptives, pregnancy, and fertility treatments may increase risk of meningioma recurrence. However, data is heterogenous.
- Contrasted MRI is not safe in pregnancy, but can be safely done while breastfeeding without interruption.

INTRODUCTION

Biologic differences are prevalent throughout many areas of medicine. In oncology, these variances present a unique set of considerations affecting epidemiology, treatment, and outcomes. This has become increasingly evident as more is understood about primary brain tumors. In clinical practice, the treatment of female individuals with brain tumors has an added layer of complexity in the consideration of not only hormonal factors but also pregnancy and family planning. There has been an emphasis on the need for special consideration of sex and biology in neuro-oncology. This review will focus on the biologic sex disparities present in brain tumors and not on gender differences as gender is considered a social construct.

Epidemiology in Brain Tumors

Brain tumors encompass over a hundred different tumor types ranging from grade 1 to grade 4 and from benign to malignant.[1] Specific brain tumor types may have variable

Department of Neurology, Malnati Brain Tumor Institute at the Robert H. Lurie Comprehensive Cancer Center, The Feinberg School of Medicine/Northwestern University, 675 North Saint Clair Street, Suite 20-100, Chicago, IL 60611, USA
* Corresponding author.
E-mail address: lauren.singer@nm.org

Neurol Clin 41 (2023) 331–342
https://doi.org/10.1016/j.ncl.2022.10.005 neurologic.theclinics.com

frequency depending on age, race, or sex (male vs female). For example, gliomas as a whole are more common in male than female individuals. Specifically, astrocytomas and oligodendrogliomas are about 1.3 times the incidence in male versus female individuals.[2] Glioblastoma or glioblastoma multiforme (GBM), the most common primary brain malignancy in adults, is more common in male than female individuals by approximately 1.6 times the incidence.

Beyond the sex-differentiated incidence, there is also evidence that sex plays a role in disease outcomes. Data systematically obtained from the National Cancer Institute's Surveillance, Epidemiology, and End Results program (which includes every state except Ohio) as well as from the Ohio Brain Tumor Study showed that in 5600 adult patients receiving standard of care treatment, the female patients had statistically significantly improved survival as compared with their male counterparts.[3] This analysis was performed using sex-specific Cox proportional hazard models and adjusted for the extent of resection, age, and performance status. Additionally, this female survival advantage was maintained even within an isocitrate dehydrogenase (IDH) wild-type subset of patients. The results of this analysis suggest that female survival advantage in GBM is independent of treatment, age, Karnofsky Performance Status, or *IDH1/2* mutation status.[3] There are various hypotheses attempting to explain the biology behind this survival advantage which we will explore further within the glioma section of this article herein.

In contrast to GBM, meningiomas are more commonly found in female individuals. This distinction is seen specifically in non-malignant meningiomas at a rate of 2.3 times higher in female individuals. Based on the Central Brain Tumor Registry of the United States 2013 to 2017 data, female individuals had 2.8 times the incidence of grade 1 meningiomas as compared with male individuals (111,469 vs 39,166).[2] There was still a female predominance within grade 2 meningiomas at approximately 1.4 times the incidence in female versus male individuals, but this female predominance was largely lost in grade 3 meningiomas. Beyond the women predilection, this divergent incidence in males versus females was impacted by age. The incidence rate ratios were lowest between males and females in individuals <20 years old (where incidence rates for males and females were approximately equal), and the highest from age 35 to 54 years, with a 3.29 times higher incidence rate in female individuals. This age-related sex difference in meningioma incidence suggests potentially a hormonal component that will be explored further in the meningioma section of this review.

Female individuals also have a slightly higher incidence of pituitary adenomas and vestibular schwannomas by a rate of 1.2 and 1.1 times compared with men.[1] Conversely, ependymomas and embryonal germ cell tumors have a predilection in males at an increased rate of approximately 1.4 times compared with female individuals. Germ cell tumors, for example, have a greater than the double propensity to occur in male individuals as compared with female.[2] For these rare tumors, the biology of these differences will not be explored herein, where the focus will be primarily be on gliomas and meningiomas.

Glioma: Survival Differences

Although the incidence of glioma is higher in male individuals, studies show that female have an overall better prognosis. The median survival of GBM has been reported as 17.5 months in male individuals as compared with 20.4 months in female.[4] For diffuse astrocytoma, the 5-year survival is estimated at 46.6% as compared with 42.2% for male.[5] One study directly reviewed the survival of male and female individuals with malignant gliomas subdivided by age.[6] In this study, a higher risk of death was shown in females aged 0 to 9 (male-to-female HR 0.93). However, in ages 10 to 69, female individuals showed decreased hazard of death, with most notable differences in the age group of 20 to 39 years (HR 10–29 1.36, HR 30–39 1.29). This was true across all types of gliomas, including oligodendroglioma and astrocytoma.

Additional studies have stratified survival based on molecular markers, showing that even when accounting for known prognostic molecular markers, females continue to demonstrate prolonged survival. One such study found that among IDH wild-type cases, female individuals had a median survival of 25.5 months as compared with 15.0 months in males.[3] These data ultimately showed that the women survival advantage in GBM exists independent of known molecular prognostics. This has prompted further inquiries into the biologic differences across genders which may confer improved prognosis.

Glioma: Biologic Differences

The biologic differences between the male and female sex have been hypothesized to be related to immune, metabolic, and physiologic variations.[7] During development, sexual differentiation leads to differences in cellular and systemic biology. However, these differences go beyond hormonal influences and instead are related to the biology of tumor cells. At a molecular level, the GBM transcriptome is determined by cell cycle signaling for males and integrin signaling for females.[8] Integrins serve as adhesion molecules and receptors for the extracellular matrix, which gives structure and support to cells.[9] This promotes the remodeling of the extracellular matrix, contributing to proliferation and resistance to immune destruction and various drugs. Integrins also allow for the communication of signals between cancer cells and within the microenvironment, which can ultimately promote the malignant proliferation of cancer cells.

To elucidate the role of the cell cycle and integrins in GBM, sex-specific subgroups are based on transcriptome data.[8] With the use of Joint and Individual Variation Explained data, molecular signatures among male and female individuals were further elucidated, showing that the female-specific component accounted for 33.6% of the variability in the female transcriptome. Subsequently, several male and female clusters were identified, which were defined by 293 and 283 genes, respectively, with 167 unique genes in the female clusters. One specific female cluster (fc3) showed improved median survival regardless of IDH mutational status (1172 days) as compared with its male counterpart (cluster mc5 620 days). This demonstrated that sex, rather than IDH mutational status, was responsible for improved survival in certain populations. Based on the analysis distinguishing transcripts, the female-specific transcripts revealed integrin-signaling pathway as the most significant pathway that separated GBM pathways among male and female individuals. Specifically, six of the nine genes in this pathway were downregulated in the fc3 cluster. This suggests that individuals in the fc3 cluster with an overall decreased integrin-signaling pathway had prolonged survival. Thus, this pathway may be integral to the development of GBM and survival differences are seen.

Moreover, specific biologic responses to various mutations and drivers vary between genders and may plan an important role in tumorigenesis. Tumor protein p53 (TP53) and retinoblastoma (RB) are tumor suppressor genes most commonly mutated across all cancers, including GBM.[10] These genes have been shown to have sex-driven differences in behavior. For example, male astrocytes have been demonstrated to grow faster and have increased malignant transformation in the setting of TP53 mutation.[11] It has also been demonstrated that cell death in male GBM patients was associated with TP53 activity.[12] Alternatively, cell death in female patients was associated with MYC proto-oncogene, a gene that affects transcription, and thus, survival and cell growth in cancer cells.[12,13] Interestingly, when both RB and TP53 are inactivated, there is an equivalent tumorigenic transformation between males and females.[14] However, inactivation of RB tumor suppressor is seen in greater incidence in men along with higher proliferation rates. These differences seen between sexes may contribute to prevalence and survival variations between sexes.

It is furthermore believed that sex hormones may play a role in malignant gliomas. These data are supported by reports that there is an increased risk of disease progression during pregnancy in females with malignant gliomas. Specifically, in one study looking at 23 patients who became pregnant after diagnosis with primary glioma, 44% of those with grade 2 or 3 gliomas showed progression during or immediately after pregnancy.[15] It has been hypothesized that this may be due to increased levels of growth factors, including placental growth factor, which have been shown to promote angiogenesis.[16] Additionally, anti-estrogen drugs, such as tamoxifen, have been shown in some studies to reduce the growth of gliomas.[17] However, as trends in female survival and responsiveness to treatment do not vary with age despite the hormone levels fluctuating, it remains unclear what exact role hormones play in the regulation of gliomas.

Two well-established prognostic markers for glioma are IDH mutational status and O6-methylguanine-DNA methyltransferase (MGMT) methylation status. IDH mutations often confer a better prognosis whereas MGMT methylation is associated both with improved survival and higher response rates to temozolomide (TMZ)—both prognostic and predictive.[18] One study looking at sex differences in these markers showed that although IDH mutations are more common in males, MGMT methylation is more common in women (53%) as compared with men (41%).[19] This study went on to demonstrate that MGMT methylation was associated with longer survival in female patients but not male patients ($P = .003$ vs $P = .603$). These data may further support the overall prolonged survival seen in females with GBM.

Molecular markers have become of particular interest in the study of gliomas; particularly, the GBM data show that grade 2 and grade 3 gliomas that harbor epidermal growth factor receptor (EGFR) amplifications, whole chromosome 7 gain and whole chromosome 10 loss, or telomerase reverse transcriptase (TERT) promoter mutations have molecular characteristics that align with GBM, regardless of IDH mutational status.[20] The EGFR gene allows for transcription of a cell membrane protein which binds several ligands allowing for signaling pathways that promote cell growth and survival.[21] Alternatively, TERT is involved in telomerase development and ensures chromosomal stability in cancer cell division.[22] When analyzing genome-wide assays for the source of glioma risk, EGFR amplification was significantly associated with the risk of glioma in males whereas TERT mutation was associated with the risk of glioma in females.[23] To further support this evidence, another genome-wide assay identified a single nucleotide polymorphism (SNP) in chromosome 7p11.2 in male subjects, which is close in proximity to EGFR.[24] This same study identified SNP in region 3p21.31 in females to correspond to increased risk of glioma. The significance of these molecular targets identifies not only potential screening tools but also potential therapeutic agents.

Glioma: Differential Treatment Considerations

The standard of care for the treatment of GBM remains a maximal safe resection followed by radiation and chemotherapy ± tumor treating fields (Optune).[25,26] The chemotherapy of choice is an alkylating agent (TMZ). One study showed that based on MRI analysis, females showed greater response to treatment with standard-of-care radiation plus TMZ.[8] This response was associated with a longer survival rate and may, in part, account for the prolonged survival reported among females with GBM. As previously discussed, MGMT methylation is more common in women and does portend an improved response to TMZ, thus, further corroborating data regarding survival and response to standard of care. This datum is of particular importance when treating newly diagnosed females with GBM, especially those who are MGMT methylated, as this datum suggests that the current standard of care may potentially confer a prolonged survival rate in females compared with males.

The toxicity of chemotherapy must also be considered before treatment. One of the main toxicities of TMZ is hematologic, including leukopenia and thrombocytopenia.[27] One study demonstrated that females have a higher risk of hematologic toxicity.[28] This emphasizes the importance of regular hematologic monitoring in females receiving TMZ. This should not, however, be a deterrent to using the medication as first-line therapy.

More recently, clinical trials and research have been aimed toward considering the unique biology of each tumor to optimize therapeutic options. As the integrin-signaling pathway was previously identified as being downregulated in female GBM patients, agents blocking this pathway could confer a variable response in men versus women. However, cilengitide, an anti-angiogenic agent targeting the integrin cell pathway, has thus far shown conflicting responses in the clinical trial.[29] Of note, this trial did not stratify results based on gender.[30] This further emphasizes the need for trials that consider an individualized approach to treatment based on unique data such as molecular markers.

Meningioma

Meningiomas are the most common primary brain tumor, accounting for approximately 39% of all brain tumors.[2] Interestingly, the incidence of meningioma has increased among fertile and menopausal women during the last 30 years. Although this may have been attributed to higher imaging rates, the incidence among males has been stationary.[31] Thus, the female-to-male ratio has been increasing over the last couple of decades reaching 3.5:1, with the highest peak during reproductive years.[32]

It has been hypothesized that hormonal factors may play a role in the higher incidence in females. With the increase, the use of exogenous hormones has been increasing with an increase in incidence seen in females.[3] Hormonal receptors are seen in meningiomas with up to 30% expressing estrogen and 70% expressing progesterone.[33,34] It is still not entirely clear how both exogenous and endogenous hormones might influence the incidence and growth of meningiomas, and the results of numerous studies have been heterogenous.

The data surrounding oral contraceptive (OC) use and meningioma risk have been controversial and somewhat contradictory, ranging from protective effect to increased risk. A recent study found that progesterone-only OC users had a significantly shorter time to meningioma recurrence, specifically in premenopausal females with grade 1 tumors.[35] Another study found that long-term progestin treatment was associated with an increased risk of multiple meningiomas.[36]

Similarly, studies involving hormone therapy (HRT) have shown varying results. One study showed an increase in the risk of meningioma in postmenopausal women who used HRT (odds ratio 2.2) with an overall increased frequency of meningioma in women who used HRT (865/100,000) as compared with women who did not (366/100,000).[37] Meanwhile, others found that estrogen-only therapy, as compared with progesterone–estrogen therapy, was associated with a higher risk of meningiomas

(RR 1.42 vs 0.97).[38,39] However, additional studies have shown a range of impacts from no significant association to slightly protective tendencies.[40–42] Drugs targeting hormonal pathways have been studied as possible treatments. Thus far, inhibition of estrogen and progesterone receptors has not been shown to have a convincing significant effect on the natural history of meningioma.[43,44]

The use of cyproterone acetate (CPA), an anti-progesterone and androgen medication, has been shown to increase the risk and growth of meningiomas. A study looking at the need for surgical resection of meningiomas in individuals treated with CPA-containing drugs showed a correlation between prior use of CPA and younger age at the time of resection.[45] Furthermore, there was a specific correlation between CPA dose and duration (median age between CPA initiation and resection 5.5 years). It went on to demonstrate the risk of multiple meningiomas in CPA exposure. The use of CPA was not associated with the progression of meningiomas to higher-grade meningioma. These data have been validated by additional studies showing increased incidence and growth and increased risk of meningioma development.[46]

Fertility treatments pose a special consideration in women as it relates to exogenous hormones. During fertility treatments, high-dose exogenous estrogen and progesterone are used, which may increase the risk of meningioma given previously discussed data surrounding hormone receptors. One study looking at women who received fertility treatments showed younger mean age at diagnosis (51.8 vs 57.3).[47] This same study demonstrated that women who underwent fertility treatments were more likely to have multiple meningiomas (OR 4.97). Interestingly, other studies have shown no relation between fertility medications and the risk of meningioma development.[42] As fertility treatments are becoming increasingly prevalent, more research is needed in this patient population.

Similarly, pregnancy is a unique variable in women that may affect the risk of meningioma growth given hormonal changes. In one study of 17 women, it was shown that meningiomas can increase in size during pregnancy, only to regress after delivery.[48] The increase in size was postulated to be due to increasing hemodynamic demands in the form of increased blood flow to the tumor bed rather than hormonally-driven proliferation. Specifically, in premenopausal women under 50, meningioma is increased in relation to the number of live births.[49] Meanwhile, other studies showed no association between meningioma and parity.[50] Interestingly, one case-control study even demonstrated a protective effect with pregnancy, increasing with parity and age at first pregnancy.[41] Despite controversial data, women with meningiomas are often advised that pregnancy is a potential risk factor for recurrence.[51]

Other hormonal considerations include breastfeeding and menopause, which can uniquely alter hormonal composition in women. One study showed that breastfeeding for at least 6 months could offer protection against meningioma with decreased risk (OR 0.78).[42] Regarding menopause, literature has been controversial, similarly to other data regarding hormonal influences. In some cases, meningioma was shown to increase after menopause.[52] Interestingly, other studies have shown that there is only increased risk in postmenopausal women who use HRT.[50] Other studies show that menopausal women have decreased risk of developing meningiomas (RR 0.58).[53] Overall, more recent studies demonstrate that menopause, including age at menopause, is not associated with meningioma risk.[49] As more data emerge, additional studies will be needed to evaluate the unique effects of sex and hormones on meningiomas.

Special Considerations with Pregnancy and Brain Tumors

Female patients present a unique consideration in oncology when it comes to conception and pregnancy and lactation/nursing. This is especially true in the cohort of women of reproductive age. On diagnosis, one of the first considerations is the future effects on women, including family planning. Before starting chemotherapy, all women should be offered the opportunity to undergo fertility preservation in the form of egg retrieval. Conception is recommended during treatment to avoid pregnancy due to the risk of fetal malformation in the setting of DNA-altering chemotherapy or other medical and investigational agents. Additionally, on stopping chemotherapy, it is generally recommended to wait 6 months before trying to conceive.[54]

When considering treatment of primary brain tumors, the potential side effects of treatment must also be included. Specifically, several agents commonly used in the treatment of brain tumors, including cytotoxic and anti-angiogenic agents, can cause premature ovarian failure. Alkylating cytotoxic agents, such as temozolomide, can cause irreversible ovarian damage, which ultimately leads to infertility and potentially premature ovarian failure.[55] The severity of the dysfunction often depends on the total dose and age at the time of therapy.[56] Because of this, many patients are often offered fertility preservation before starting chemotherapy. Another commonly used drug, bevacizumab, has anti-angiogenic properties which may temporarily or permanently affect fertility. Unlike with temozolomide, this damage may be transient and resolved with drug clearance.[57] However, prolonged use may lead to more permanent infertility.

Moreover, consideration of imaging must be taken when it comes to female brain tumor patients. Standard of care tumor surveillance for patients is done with MRI and most commonly with gadolinium-based contrast agents. Non-contrasted MRI has been demonstrated to be safe in pregnancy without adverse outcomes to the fetus as long as it is done on a 3.0 T scanner or less.[58] As gadolinium is water-soluble, it can cross the placenta and enter fetal circulation and is teratogenic at high and repeat doses.[59] Unique reactions to contrast agents in pregnancy, including fetal bradycardia and preterm labor, have been demonstrated.[60] Although there have been some retrospective studies evaluating the long-term safety of gadolinium exposure, the data are limited as there is no direct comparative study assessing individuals who get MRI as compared with the control group who does not get MRI. Thus, it is not recommended to do contrast-enhanced studies except in cases of emergency or if it significantly improves fetal or maternal outcomes.[59] During breastfeeding, MRI with gadolinium-based contrast may be obtained.[61] Although it is excreted in breast milk, data suggest less than 0.04% of the contrast dose is found in breast milk and an extremely small amount is absorbed by the baby.[62] Thus, while it was previously recommended not to breastfeed for 24 hours after receiving gadolinium-based contrast, there are no documented contraindications to continuing breastfeeding after MRI.

These considerations extend beyond diagnosis and chemotherapy, but also to symptomatic treatment. Often, individuals will experience seizures at diagnosis or during the course of their illness trajectory, necessitating the use of antiseizure medications (ASM). Women pose a unique consideration when it comes to choosing an ASM due to the risk of teratogenicity.[63] The side effects range from developmental delay and dysmorphism to neural tube defects and cardiac abnormalities. The most common offending agents include valproic acid carbamazepine. As many females may remain on these agents even after completion of chemotherapy, it is paramount to consider these effects before initiating treatment.

SUMMARY

There are intrinsic biologic differences when it comes to sex in oncology. Although there is a plethora of data on many solid organ cancers, data in neuro-oncology are just emerging. The differences between male and female individuals in oncology are thought to be due to more than just hormones, but rather due to innate biological differences in cancer cells as well as how cancer cells interact with "host" cells. These interactions influence our understanding of these tumors and, ultimately, how to treat them. It is important to account for these biologic differences when considering the prognosis and therapeutic options. Moreover, women present a unique set of concerns in the setting of conception and pregnancy that must be considered throughout diagnosis and treatment. As we continue to learn more about biologic differences in neurology, and particularly, in oncology, it is important to continue to consider these distinctive factors to provide individualized care for patients. As our understanding of these differences continues to grow, this could inform future clinical trials, and as a result, differential treatment planning based on the patient's sex.

CLINICS CARE POINTS

- While gliomas are more common in male than female individuals, females have an overall improved survival with treatment with standard of care.
- Meningiomas are more commonly found in female individuals.
- Sex differences in gliomas are a result of molecular, hormonal, and biologic differences at the cellular level.
- Unique GBM transcriptomes have been identified in female with integrin established as the predominant signaling pathway.
- Among individuals with gliomas, MGMT methylation is more commonly seen in female individuals and is associated with prolonged survival.
- Many meningiomas express hormone receptors, including estrogen and progesterone.
- Life events and drugs which increase hormone exposure, such as oral contraceptives, pregnancy, and fertility treatments may increase the risk of meningioma recurrence. However, data are heterogenous.
- Several commonly used chemotherapeutic agents can lead to premature ovarian failure.
- Contrasted MRI is not safe in pregnancy but can be safely done while breastfeeding without interruption.

CONFLICTS OF INTEREST

L. Singer has no conflicts of interest. D. Primdahl has no conflicts of interest. P. Kumthekar has had advisory roles at Biocept, Enclear, Affinia Therapeutics. P. Kumthekar served on advisory boards/advised Orbus Therapeutics, Berg, Bioclinia Sintetica, Novocure, Janssen, Angiochem, Celularity, Mirati and SDP Oncology and received research funding from Novocure, Switzerland, Genetech. P. Kumthekar holds European Patent 3,307,327, August 12, 2020 and US Patent Pending 15/737,188.

REFERENCES

1. WHO Classification of Tumours Editorial Board. WHO Classification of Tumours: Central Nervous System Tumours. 5th edition. World Health Organization; 2021.
2. Ostrom QT, Patil N, Cioffi G, et al. CBTRUS statistical report: primary brain and other central nervous system tumors diagnosed in the United States in 2013-2017. Neuro Oncol 2020;22(12 Suppl 2):IV1–96.
3. Ostrom QT, Rubin JB, Lathia JD, et al. Females have the survival advantage in glioblastoma. Neuro Oncol 2018;20(4):576.

4. Gittleman H, Ostrom QT, Stetson LC, et al. Sex is an important prognostic factor for glioblastoma but not for nonglioblastoma. Neurooncol Pract 2019;6(6): 451–62.
5. Gittleman H, Boscia A, Ostrom QT, et al. Survivorship in adults with malignant brain and other central nervous system tumor from 2000-2014. Neuro Oncol 2018;20(suppl_7):VII6–16.
6. Wang GM, Cioffi G, Patil N, et al. Importance of the intersection of age and sex to understand variation in incidence and survival for primary malignant gliomas. Neuro Oncol 2022;24(2):302–10.
7. Massey SC, Whitmire P, Doyle TE, et al. Sex differences in health and disease: A review of biological sex differences relevant to cancer with a spotlight on glioma. Cancer Lett 2021;498:178–87.
8. Yang W, Warrington NM, Taylor SJ, et al. Sex differences in GBM revealed by analysis of patient imaging, transcriptome, and survival data. Sci Transl Med 2019;11(473). https://doi.org/10.1126/SCITRANSLMED.AAO5253/SUPPL_FILE/AAO5253_TABLES_S1_TO_S12.
9. Su CY, Li JQ, Zhang LL, et al. The Biological Functions and Clinical Applications of Integrins in Cancers. Front Pharmacol 2020;11:1435.
10. Sun T, Plutynski A, Ward S, et al. An integrative view on sex differences in brain tumors. Cell Mol Life Sci 2015;72(17):3323.
11. Rockwell NC, Yang W, Warrington NM, et al. Sex- and Mutation-Specific p53 Gain-of-Function Activity in Gliomagenesis. Cancer Res Commun 2021;1(3): 148–63.
12. Colen RR, Wang J, Singh SK, et al. Glioblastoma: imaging genomic mapping reveals sex-specific oncogenic associations of cell death. Radiology 2015;275(1): 215–27.
13. Casey SC, Baylot V, Felsher DW. The MYC oncogene is a global regulator of the immune response. Blood 2018;131(18):2007–15.
14. Sun T, Warrington NM, Luo J, et al. Sexually dimorphic RB inactivation underlies mesenchymal glioblastoma prevalence in men. J Clin Invest 2014;124(9): 4123–33.
15. Yust-Katz S, De Groot JF, Liu D, et al. Pregnancy and glial brain tumors. Neuro Oncol 2014;16(9):1289–94.
16. McNamara MG, Mason WP. Antiangiogenic therapies in glioblastoma multiforme. Expert Rev Anticancer Ther 2012;12(5):643–54.
17. Couldwell W, Hinton D, Surnock A, et al. Treatment of recurrent malignant gliomas with chronic oral high-dose tamoxifen. Clin Cancr Res 1996;2(4):619–22. https://pubmed.ncbi.nlm.nih.gov/9816211/.
18. Yang P, Zhang W, Wang Y, et al. IDH mutation and MGMT promoter methylation in glioblastoma: results of a prospective registry. Oncotarget 2015;6(38): 40896–906.
19. Schiffgens S, Wilkens L, Brandes AA, et al. Sex-specific clinicopathological significance of novel (Frizzled-7) and established (MGMT, IDH1) biomarkers in glioblastoma. Oncotarget 2016;7(34):55169.
20. Brat DJ, Aldape K, Colman H, et al. cIMPACT-NOW update 3: recommended diagnostic criteria for “Diffuse astrocytic glioma, IDH-wildtype, with molecular features of glioblastoma, WHO grade IV. Acta Neuropathol 2018;136(5):805–10.
21. Xu H, Zong H, Ma C, et al. Epidermal growth factor receptor in glioblastoma. Oncol Lett 2017;14(1):512.

22. Dratwa M, Wysoczańska B, Łacina P, et al. TERT—Regulation and Roles in Cancer Formation. Front Immunol 2020;11. https://doi.org/10.3389/FIMMU.2020.589929.
23. Ostrom QT, Coleman W, Huang W, et al. Sex-specific gene and pathway modeling of inherited glioma risk. Neuro Oncol 2019;21(1):71–82.
24. Ostrom QT, Kinnersley B, Wrensch MR, et al. Sex-specific glioma genome-wide association study identifies new risk locus at 3p21.31 in females, and finds sex-differences in risk at 8q24.21. Sci Rep 2018;8(1):1–15.
25. Stupp R, Mason WP, van den Bent MJ, et al. Radiotherapy plus concomitant and adjuvant temozolomide for glioblastoma. N Engl J Med 2005;352(10):987–96.
26. Stupp R, Taillibert S, Kanner A, et al. Effect of tumor-treating fields plus maintenance temozolomide vs maintenance temozolomide alone on survival in patients with glioblastoma: a randomized clinical trial. JAMA 2017;318(23):2306–16.
27. Gerber DE, Grossman SA, Zeltzman M, et al. The impact of thrombocytopenia from temozolomide and radiation in newly diagnosed adults with high-grade gliomas. Neuro Oncol 2007;9(1):47.
28. Gupta T, Mohanty S, Moiyadi A, et al. Factors predicting temozolomide induced clinically significant acute hematologic toxicity in patients with high-grade gliomas: a clinical audit. Clin Neurol Neurosurg 2013;115(9):1814–9.
29. Matteoni S, Abbruzzese C, Villani V, et al. The influence of patient sex on clinical approaches to malignant glioma. Cancer Lett 2020;468:41–7.
30. Stupp R, Hegi ME, Gorlia T, et al. Cilengitide combined with standard treatment for patients with newly diagnosed glioblastoma with methylated MGMT promoter (CENTRIC EORTC 26071-22072 study): a multicentre, randomised, open-label, phase 3 trial. Lancet Oncol 2014;15(10):1100–8.
31. Bhala S, Stewart DR, Kennerley V, et al. Incidence of benign meningiomas in the United States: current and future trends. JNCI Cancer Spectr 2021;5(3). https://doi.org/10.1093/JNCICS/PKAB035.
32. Klaeboe L, Lonn S, Scheie D, et al. Incidence of intracranial meningiomas in Denmark, Finland, Norway and Sweden, 1968-1997. Int J Cancer 2005;117(6):996–1001.
33. Commins DL, Atkinson RD, Burnett ME. Review of meningioma histopathology. Neurosurg Focus 2007;23(4):E3.
34. Hsu DW, Efird JT, Hedley-Whyte ET. Progesterone and estrogen receptors in meningiomas: prognostic considerations. J Neurosurg 1997;86(1):113–20.
35. Harland TA, Freeman JL, Davern M, et al. Progesterone-only contraception is associated with a shorter progression-free survival in premenopausal women with WHO Grade I meningioma. J Neurooncol 2018;136(2):327–33.
36. Peyre M, Gaillard S, de Marcellus C, et al. Progestin-associated shift of meningioma mutational landscape. Ann Oncol Off J Eur Soc Med Oncol 2018;29(3):681–6.
37. Blitshteyn S, Crook JE, Jaeckle KA. Is there an association between meningioma and hormone replacement therapy? J Clin Oncol 2008;26(2):279–82.
38. Benson VS, Kirichek O, Beral V, et al. Menopausal hormone therapy and central nervous system tumor risk: large UK prospective study and meta-analysis. Int J Cancer 2015;136(10):2369–77.
39. Benson VS, Pirie K, Green J, et al. Hormone replacement therapy and incidence of central nervous system tumours in the Million Women Study. Int J Cancer 2010;127(7):1692–8.

40. Korhonen K, Raitanen J, Isola J, et al. Exogenous sex hormone use and risk of meningioma: a population-based case-control study in Finland. Cancer Causes Control 2010;21(12):2149–56.
41. Lee E, Grutsch J, Persky V, et al. Association of meningioma with reproductive factors. Int J Cancer 2006;119(5):1152–7.
42. Claus EB, Calvocoressi L, Bondy ML, et al. Exogenous hormone use, reproductive factors, and risk of intracranial meningioma in females. J Neurosurg 2013; 118(3):649.
43. Ji Y, Rankin C, Grunberg S, et al. Double-blind phase III randomized trial of the antiprogestin agent mifepristone in the treatment of unresectable meningioma: SWOG S9005. J Clin Oncol 2015;33(34):4093.
44. Goodwin JW, Crowley J, Eyre HJ, et al. A phase II evaluation of tamoxifen in unresectable or refractory meningiomas: a Southwest Oncology Group study. J Neurooncol 1993;15(1):75–7.
45. Champeaux-Depond C, Weller J, Froelich S, et al. Cyproterone acetate and meningioma: a nationwide-wide population based study. J Neurooncol 2021;151(2): 331–8.
46. Hage M, Plesa O, Lemaire I, et al. Estrogen and Progesterone Therapy and Meningiomas. Endocrinology 2022;163(2).
47. Shahin MN, Magill ST, Dalle Ore CL, et al. Fertility treatment is associated with multiple meningiomas and younger age at diagnosis. J Neurooncol 2019; 143(1):137.
48. Lusis EA, Scheithauer BW, Yachnis AT, et al. Meningiomas in pregnancy: a clinicopathologic study of 17 cases. Neurosurgery 2012;71(5):951–61.
49. Wigertz A, Lönn S, Hall P, et al. Reproductive factors and risk of meningioma and glioma. Cancer Epidemiol Biomarkers Prev 2008;17(10):2663–70.
50. Michaud DS, Gallo V, Schlehofer B, et al. Reproductive factors and exogenous hormone use in relation to risk of glioma and meningioma in a large European cohort study. Cancer Epidemiol Biomarkers Prev 2010;19(10):2562–9.
51. Owens MA, Craig BM, Egan KM, et al. Birth desires and intentions of women diagnosed with a meningioma. J Neurosurg 2015;122(5):1151.
52. Cowppli-Bony A, Bouvier G, Rué M, et al. Brain tumors and hormonal factors: review of the epidemiological literature. Cancer Causes Control 2011;22(5): 697–714.
53. Schlehofer B, Blettner M, Wahrendorf J. Association between brain tumors and menopausal status. J Natl Cancer Inst 1992;84(17):1346–9.
54. Tang M, Webber K. Fertility and pregnancy in cancer survivors. Obstet Med 2018;11(3):110.
55. Molina JR, Barton DL, Loprinzi CL. Chemotherapy-induced ovarian failure. Drug Saf 2012;28(5):401–16.
56. Chapman RM. Effect of cytotoxic therapy on sexuality and gonadal function. Semin Oncol 1982;9(1):84–94.
57. Imai A, Ichigo S, Matsunami K, et al. Ovarian function following targeted anti-angiogenic therapy with bevacizumab (Review). Mol Clin Oncol 2017;6(6): 807–10.
58. Greenberg TD, Hoff MN, Gilk TB, et al. ACR guidance document on MR safe practices: Updates and critical information 2019. J Magn Reson Imaging 2020; 51(2):331–8.
59. Guidelines for diagnostic imaging during pregnancy and lactation. Obstet Gynecol 2017;130(4):e210–6.

60. Flanagan E, Bell S. Abdominal Imaging in pregnancy (maternal and foetal risks). Best Pract Res Clin Gastroenterol 2020;44–5.
61. Committee Opinion No. 723: guidelines for diagnostic imaging during pregnancy and lactation: correction. Obstet Gynecol 2018;132(3):786.
62. Gatta G, Di Grezia G, Cuccurullo V, et al. MRI in pregnancy and precision medicine: a review from literature. J Pers Med 2021;12(1).
63. Güveli BT, Rosti RÖ, Güzeltaş A, et al. Teratogenicity of antiepileptic drugs. Clin Psychopharmacol Neurosci 2017;15(1):19.

Sex Differences in Alzheimer's Disease

Neelum T. Aggarwal, MD[a,*], Michelle M. Mielke, PhD[b]

KEYWORDS

- Sex differences • Cognitive decline • Alzheimer's dementia • Risk factors
- Biomarkers

KEY POINTS

- Overall, women are two to three times likelier to develop Alzheimer's dementia than men across all age strata after the age of 65.
- Multiple lifestyle factors are known to impact cognitive decline, and modification of these factors may favorably impact women more than men.
- Compared with men, women may initially present with complaints of verbal memory and word-finding difficulties rather than episodic memory in the early stages of cognitive impairment.
- Sex differences in biomarkers (blood, cerebrospinal fluid, and neuroimaging) may help identify the underlying biological mechanisms of these differences.

INTRODUCTION

Alzheimer's disease (AD) dementia is one of the most common types of dementia in older adults. As the population ages, the number of patients who are concerned about cognitive decline and who have AD is dramatically increasing. Barriers to successful diagnosis and care include the failure to properly diagnose dementia early in the course of AD, underestimation by both health care professionals and the public of the morbidity associated with AD, and the inconsistent use of appropriate medications for treatment. The links between diverse sets of risk factors for cognitive decline and dementia have long been recognized in the literature, and more recently, research interest in potential sex differences in disease risk and prevention has emerged. In this article, the latest epidemiological evidence that supports sex differences in AD, clinical and diagnostic considerations, and the role of co-morbidities associated with AD are reviewed.

[a] Department of Neurological Sciences, Rush Alzheimer's Disease Center, Rush University Medical Center, 1750 West Harrison Street, Suite 1000, Chicago, IL 60612, USA; [b] Department of Epidemiology and Prevention, Division of Public Health Sciences, Wake Forest University School of Medicine, Winston-Salem, NC, USA
* Corresponding author.
E-mail address: neelum_t_aggarwal@rush.edu

Neurol Clin 41 (2023) 343–358
https://doi.org/10.1016/j.ncl.2023.01.001

EPIDEMIOLOGY

An estimated 5.7 million Americans live with AD, and an additional 11.6 million Americans are thought to have mild cognitive impairment (MCI).[1,2] AD is the most common cause of dementia, accounting for 60% to 80% of cases. It is the sixth leading cause of death in the United States. The incidence and prevalence of AD increases dramatically with age; it affects approximately 80% of patients aged ≥75 years. Incidence rates increase from 2 per 1000 at age 65 to 74 to 37 per 1000 at age ≥ 85.[3] By 2050, the number of patients with AD in the United States is projected to triple, with the greatest increase among those aged ≥85 years.[4]

The number of individuals with AD is expected to increase more in women than men over the coming years, which reflects increased longevity for women as well as biological influences.[4] The overall lifetime risk of acquiring AD for those aged 65 is 21.2% for women and 11.6% for men.[1,5] Projected survival varies between 4 and 8 years across studies and is impacted by multiple factors, including age at diagnosis, sex, behavioral features, motor system involvement, and medical comorbidities.[6]

Considerations: Sex-Specific Risk Factors

Sex differences in risk factors fall into two categories.

1. Diseases or conditions that are specific to one sex; and
2. Diseases or conditions that have distinct causes, manifestations, outcomes (morbidity or mortality), or responses to treatments for one sex compared with the other.

Sex-specific risk factors of dementia for women include pregnancy and menopause. For example, multiple studies have reported that a history of preeclampsia is associated with an increased risk of MCI, vascular dementia, and AD.[7–9]

In addition, early menopause (natural or surgery-induced), especially before the age of 45 years, is associated with an increased risk of MCI and dementia.[10–13]

Influence of Sex Hormones

The Women's Health Initiative Memory Study (WHIMS) remains the only randomized, placebo-controlled trial on menopausal hormone therapy for the primary prevention of dementia.[14,15] This study enrolled women > 65 years with a uterus who were randomized to receive oral conjugated equine estrogen (CEE) (0.625 mg/day) plus medroxyprogesterone acetate (MPA) (2.5 mg CEE/MPA) or a placebo, and women without a uterus (n = 4532) were randomized to receive oral CEE (0.625 mg/day) or a placebo. Important results from this study suggested that the risk of all-cause dementia was double in the combined CEE/MPA group compared with the group that received only CEE and that these findings were not modified by smoking, cardiovascular disease (CVD) risk factors, stroke, or statin or aspirin use.

In addition, CVD risk factors did not modify the effects of hormone therapy on a composite measure of global cognitive function. MRI brain imaging also showed that for the WHIMS patients, ischemic brain volume did not differ between the hormone therapy and placebo groups. However, the rates of accumulation of white matter lesions and total brain lesion volumes were higher among women with a history of CVD treated with hormone therapy versus a placebo. More recent randomized clinical trial studies have identified the timing and initiation of menopausal hormone therapy as important factors in cognitive decline, with data suggesting that initiating menopausal hormone therapy within 5 years of menopause does not have detrimental effects on cognition.[16–18] However, long-term menopausal hormone therapy use of 5 or more years may be associated with an increased risk. There continues to be relatively little research investigating the effect of declining male sex hormones on cognitive function with age. However, of the studies conducted, one noted that men experience an approximately 2% to 3% decline in testosterone levels per year after the age of 30.[19]

It remains unclear whether low testosterone levels are associated with the risk of dementia among men.[20] However, androgen deprivation therapy, a common therapy for prostate cancer, has been associated with a risk of cognitive impairment and dementia.[21]

Genetic Contributions

Late-onset AD is a complex genetic disorder with an estimated heritability of 60% to 80%. The strongest genetic risk factor for late-onset AD remains the apolipoprotein E (APOE) genotype. APOE encodes the brain's major cholesterol transporter and has three common alleles: e2 (with an estimated frequency of 8.4% in the population), e3 (77.9%), and e4 (13.7%).[22,23]

APOE e4 is associated with an increased risk of developing AD compared with the e3/e3 genotypes,[24] and each APOE e4 allele reduces the average age of symptom onset by a decade. Female carriers of APOE e4 are at a greater risk than male carriers, particularly those aged 65 to 75 years.[25]

APOE e4 contributes to AD risk via a multitude of mechanisms, including enhanced aggregation and decreased clearance of the amyloid-β polypeptide, increased tau phosphorylation, neuronal hyperexcitability, reduced glucose metabolism, and vascular function, and neurodevelopment differences.[24,25] As APOE represents a risk factor but is not considered a deterministic gene, APOE genotyping is currently not recommended in the clinical evaluation of patients with suspected AD.[26]

The APOE4 allele has, however, been associated with an increased risk of amyloid-related imaging abnormalities (ARIA) in individuals treated with plaque-lowering mAbs (eg, aducanumab),[27] and guidelines regarding the appropriate use of genetic testing in patients considering starting an mAB have been developed.[28]

Other genetic investigations, such as genome-wide association studies, have identified more than 20 additional common genetic variants that modify the risk of late-onset AD.[22,29] These genes converge in biological pathways involving lipid metabolism, immunity, and endocytosis. The effect of each gene on AD risk is small (with an odds ratio [OR] of 0.8 to 0.9 for protective alleles and 1:1 to 1:2 for risk alleles), with no known sex differences; thus, these results are not clinically meaningful.

Finally, polygenic hazard scores that attempt to assess the overall burden of AD risk alleles could theoretically enhance the ability to predict at-risk individuals; however, they are still rarely used, and at this time, no specific sex difference considerations are involved in developing these scores. Likewise, mutations in the amyloid-β precursor proteins presently 1 and 2, which lead to familial early-onset AD, remain rare and do not currently show sex-specific differences.[22]

Sex Differences in Risk Factors

Multiple environmental, behavioral, and lifestyle factors have been associated with AD, and the relationships between many of these risk factors and dementia vary by sex and gender.[30]

Traumatic brain injury is a potentially modifiable risk factor for AD and other neurodegenerative disorders.[31] Many of the adverse psychosocial risk factors for TBI disproportionally affect women, whereas sports and occupations, two of the biggest risk factors for TBI, differentially impact men. There is also evidence that, for any given severity of TBI, women are likely to have poorer outcomes, including Alzheimer's disease-related dementias (ADRD).[32,33]

Women have been reported to have twice the risk of *depression* compared with men, and this worsens during the menopausal transition.[34,35] Some studies have reported that elevated rates of depressive symptoms were associated with a stronger risk of AD in men compared with women.[36,37] However, another study that reported a stronger increase in AD risk for women, late-life depression was also associated with an increased risk of cognitive decline,[38] although it is still unclear whether this constitutes a risk factor or is the consequence of early AD neuropathology in serotonergic and noradrenergic brainstem nuclei.[39]

Conversely, increased years of formal *education*, physical activity (PA), and social engagement across one's lifespan moderate the risk of late-life dementia.[30] Historically, women have had less access to education, so more women are affected by this socioeconomic factor.

Common *neuropsychiatric symptoms* of AD include depression, anxiety, mild apathy, irritability, and sleep disturbances (eg, insomnia or disrupted circadian rhythm).[40] In a meta-analysis, female sex was associated with a higher prevalence and greater severity of depressive symptoms, aberrant motor behavior, and psychotic symptoms in AD dementia, whereas male sex was associated with an increased severity of apathy.[41]

Complaints of *sleep* disturbances in both sexes are commonly seen with neuropsychiatric behavior symptoms and have known sex differences.[42] These sleep disturbances are linked to late-life cognitive decline and AD.[43–45] Observational studies indicate that sleep quality is related to cognitive function in both early and late life, whereas disordered breathing is associated with an increased risk of dementia.[45]

Sleep disruption in patients with AD is a common complaint, and disruption to slow-wave sleep (Stage 3) has been linked to an increase in A beta levels.[45] Women are especially vulnerable to sleep disruption at or around the transition to menopause; however, whether sex differences affect AD risk is still under investigation.[46,47]

Multiple studies have identified a strong association between PA and cognitive function. Participation in PA may reduce the risk of dementia by increasing oxygen saturation and neurogenesis, minimizing vascular risk factors, and reducing inflammation and depressive symptoms.[48]

A meta-analysis of prospective studies in older adults without dementia found that all levels of PA (low, moderate, and high) were associated with protection against cognitive decline compared with none at all.[49] In addition, PA was associated with beneficial effects on the brain's structures.[50] Multiple studies suggest that sex modifies the association between PA and cognition. Older women undergoing aerobic training showed greater cognitive gains than older men,[51,52] and PA maintenance over 10 years predicted fewer declines in multiple cognitive domains among women compared with men in the Health, Aging, and Body Composition study.[53]

Increasing evidence suggests that diet and *nutrient intake* are related to dementia risk. Studies have investigated the effects of a variety of specific nutrients, including B vitamins, antioxidants, and fatty acids, on late-onset dementia.[54] Although many studies have shown a strong association between nutrient deficits and cognitive function, the findings of most randomized controlled trials on single-nutrient supplements have not been positive.[55] Dietary requirements vary by sex, and some studies have reported that a diet low in vitamin B12,[56] western dietary patterns,[57] and high in fat and red meat is associated with an increase in AD in men but not women.[58]

The prevention of dementia through dietary intervention and the analysis of specific dietary patterns may be more effective than traditional therapies to treat dementia once it has emerged. The Mediterranean diet is associated with a lower risk of MCI and AD, and the MIND diet is thought to reduce the incidence of AD and slow cognitive decline in older adults.[59–63] Adherence to other healthy dietary patterns has been shown to have a similar association with cognitive function.[64] This is supported by preliminary cross-sectional data obtained from investigations into dietary patterns pertaining to total cerebral brain volume and white matter hyperintensity volumes.[65]

Cardiometabolic and *cardiovascular* risk factors are an important group of associations that show known sex differences. The risk of developing AD and related forms of dementia is increased in patients with vascular risk factors, and growing evidence suggests that the aggressive treatment of risk factors as early as midlife can attenuate the risk of developing cognitive impairment at an older age.[66,67] In addition, vascular risk factors are associated with a faster rate of cognitive decline after a diagnosis of AD, further emphasizing the importance of adequate treatment.[68]

Several cardiovascular risk factors have been shown to have a strong relationship with cognitive decline and dementia, including hyperlipidemia, hypertension, obesity, and diabetes mellitus.

Several mechanisms are implicated, including disruption to insulin signaling, an increase in the accumulation of advanced glycation end-products, and interference with amyloid-β clearance.[69]

In addition, diabetic women had a higher risk of diabetic complications, myocardial infarction, and coronary artery disease than men in studies that assessed the impact of cardiovascular risk factors on older men and women.[70,71]

Echoing the cognitive studies showing the importance of the timing of hormonal influences and replacement therapy across one's lifespan, similar trends are emerging for cardiovascular risk factors. Studies that have closely evaluated the association between metabolic syndrome and cognitive function across the human lifespan[72] note that midlife hypercholesterolemia, hypertension, and obesity are consistently associated with the risk of late-life dementia.[73,74]

In contrast, there are less consistent relationships between late-life vascular risk factors and late-life cognition or dementia.[75] More specifically, some studies suggest that low blood pressure (BP), low cholesterol, and weight loss are associated with dementia risk in later life.[76–78] These findings are likely due to the effects of the underlying disease process even before a diagnosis is obtained and, in the case of hypotension, of reduced cerebral blood flow. The data regarding potential sex differences in these relationships are also inconsistent. For example, we know that men have a higher prevalence of vascular risk factors and conditions up to about the age of 80. However, a recent study suggested that despite the higher prevalence of these conditions in midlife for men, women who had vascular risk factors were at the greatest risk of cognitive decline.[79]

Over the past few years, efforts of the American Heart Association (AHA) and others involved in clinical trials have focused on the management of BP to prevent cognitive decline and dementia. The AHA published recommendations for the management of vascular cognitive impairment, which include the use of selective serotonin reuptake inhibitors (SSRIs) for the treatment of depression (which can occur with cerebrovascular disease) and the aggressive management of CVD risk factors.[80]

Findings from the Systolic Hypertension in Europe trial noted that aggressive BP management was associated with a reduced risk of developing dementia compared with a placebo.[81] More recently, the SPRINT MIND randomized trial evaluated the cognitive effects of intensively lowering BP (to a systolic BP goal of < 120 mm Hg) versus the traditional BP-lowering goal of <140/90 mm Hg.

In adults aged $\geq$ 50 years without diabetes mellitus or prior stroke, intensive BP lowering significantly reduced the rate of MCI (14.6 versus 18.3 cases per 1,000 person-years; HR of 0.81; 95% confidence interval [CI]: 0.69 to 0.95) as well as the combined rate of MCI or probable dementia (20.2 vs 24.1 cases per 1,000 person-years; HR of 0.85; 95% CI: 0.74 to 0.97).[82]

Furthermore, a brain MRI substudy documented a significant reduction in the development of white matter lesions[82] with this intensive BP control. This study, along with others that evaluated BP reduction, pointed to possible pathways that link vascular dementia to AD (known as mixed dementia), which may further help explain varying patterns in cognitive function between the sexes.[83–85]

Variations in the course of CVD between women and men suggest that the interaction between sex and age is an important consideration relative to cognitive impairment. Finally, the Finnish Geriatric Intervention Study to Prevent Cognitive Impairment and Disability investigated a multimodal diet, PA, cognitive intervention that included vascular risk factor monitoring and showed a decrease in cognitive decline over 2 years in the multidomain intervention group. Presently, the data from this study's outcomes are being examined for potential sex differences through an extension of the study.[86]

Given the association between hyperlipidemia or hypertension and dementia, multiple clinical trials have assessed whether statin or antihypertensive use reduces the risk of cognitive decline and dementia.[87] Although these studies have not systematically examined sex differences in response to therapy through stratified analyses, one study did find that statins were similarly associated with reduced dementia risk for both women and men.[88] Thus, whether there were demonstrable sex differences in responses to therapy could not be determined.

Sex Differences in Clinical Presentation

Individuals with AD present with early and prominent involvement of episodic memory and mild impairment of other cognitive domains. The clinical history is usually suggestive of classic AD features, which include cognitive changes that are slow and progressive and appear insidiously. Frustration over the inability to remember recent information, sleep disturbances, and a family history of a cognitive disorder are all suggestive of AD, and research suggests that there may be some important sex differences in complaints and presentation.

The topic of subjective memory complaints (SMC) has garnered recent attention because older patients so commonly report them, yet physicians are not quite sure whether to take these complaints seriously and evaluate them further. Some studies have shown a higher prevalence of SMC in women compared with men,[89,90] whereas others have noted that SMC may be associated more closely with objective memory performance in women than men.[91]

Before a full cognitive battery, screening with rapid cognitive tests, such as the Mini-Mental State Examination (MMSE) or the Montreal Cognitive Assessment (MoCA), is often administered. The MoCA is increasingly used as a foundation test to assess the capacity for attention, the components of executive function, language, and memory because it can do so in greater detail than the MMSE. One small study of 70-year-old community-dwelling patients found women performed better than men on delayed recall on the MoCA whereas men scored better on visuoconstruction and serial subtraction.[92] Presently, however, there are limited studies regarding sex-specific norms for MoCA scores.

Late-onset AD most commonly manifests as an amnestic disorder characterized by episodic memory with varying degrees of executive language and visual-spatial impairment.[93] Patients often show a gradient of memory impairment, with the greatest deficit being their ability to recall recent events, whereas remote memory is relatively less affected. Patients who undergo memory testing (eg, word lists or story learning) show impaired learning, sudden memory loss, and poor, delayed recall.[94] On average, women perform better on tests of verbal memory and processing speed, whereas men perform better on visual-spatial tests.[95] Sex differences in cognitive testing profiles indicate that women often have more difficulty with language and confrontational naming tests.[96,97] Longitudinally, women may also have difficulty with memory tests and, in particular, delayed recall of verbal information.[98]

Clinical Evaluation

In evaluations to address cognitive concerns, it is important to obtain corroborative information from an additional source, such as a family member or close friend, as patient recall or insight may be limited.

Patients with acquired cognitive impairment that represents a decline from their previous level of performance and that has been objectively corroborated by history and examination but does not interfere with daily function are considered to have MCI.[99]

When cognitive decline interferes with independent function, patients meet the criteria for dementia. Equivalent categories of mild and major neurocognitive disorders are defined in the *Diagnostic and Statistical Manual of Mental Disorders, Fifth Edition*.[100] With advances in the field, these categories represent a continuum of cognitive decline that begins with subjective changes and culminates in dementia.

Laboratory Data

The American Academy of Neurology (AAN) guidelines recommend that the following laboratory tests should be ordered in the routine evaluation of patients with cognitive decline: a complete blood cell count, serum electrolytes, liver, and renal function tests, thyroid function tests, and serum vitamin B_{12}.[26] Additional tests may be appropriate in patients with systemic disorders.

Blood-based tests indicative of AD pathology, including tests of amyloid-beta or phosphorylated tau (P-tau) and neurofilament light (NfL) for neurodegeneration, are now available for clinical use.[101] However, these tests are generally not covered by insurance or Medicare.

The Alzheimer's Association recently released appropriate use recommendations for blood-based biomarkers in AD.[102] It was cautiously stated that these blood-based biomarkers could be used in specialized memory clinics as part of a diagnostic workup of patients with cognitive symptoms, but the results should be confirmed with CSF or PET. Moreover, blood biomarkers should not be used in primary care or in isolation to determine a diagnosis. A primary reason for this is that blood biomarkers have not been adequately examined in older, diverse populations, who typically present in primary care with multiple comorbidities and cognitive impairment. Sex differences in blood biomarker levels have not been systematically examined.

Cerebrospinal Fluid

A low CSF ratio of amyloid-beta 42/40 and elevated levels of P-tau are indicative of AD pathology and can aid in the diagnosis of AD dementia. Lumbar punctures and CSF assays are reimbursable in the United States. In addition, CSF NfL is a promising marker of neurodegeneration but is nonspecific to the type of disease. Studies have not found sex differences in levels of CSF amyloid-beta 42 or P-tau. However, CSF NfL has consistently been reported to be higher for men than for women across the clinical disease spectrum.[103,104]

Neuroimaging

Diagnosis of AD are still based on charting a detailed clinical history of cognitive decline and conducting a clinical evaluation to eliminate any reversible causes. The AAN guidelines support the use of brain imaging, either computed tomography (CT) or MRI, in the initial assessment of dementia to rule out the possibility of space-occupying lesions (ie, neoplasms), stroke, subdural hematomas, or, rarely, normal pressure hydrocephalus.[33] CT and MRI can also inform the differential diagnosis of neurodegenerative disease by identifying characteristic brain atrophy patterns and ischemia for vascular injury.

The main findings on MRI are changes that include atrophy of the hippocampus and medial temporal lobes, temporoparietal cortical atrophy, and ventricular enlargement.[46] Patients may also show varying degrees of white matter hyperintensities on T2-weighted/fluid-attenuated inversion recovery (FLAIR) sequences, which are nonspecific but most often associated with small vessel ischemic disease.[48] Notably, cognitively unimpaired women typically have significantly greater white matter hyperintensities compared with men.[105]

Cortical, but not deep, microbleeds correlate with cerebral amyloid angiopathy and amyloid burden. They can be measured using susceptibility-weighted imaging and extensive white matter lesions on T2-weighted/FLAIR sequences.[106] Men have a higher prevalence of cerebral microbleeds than women from mid-to late-life.[107]

Despite the reported MRI findings and knowledge surrounding structural brain differences in women and men, there are limited longitudinal data on sex differences. Data from large-scale neuroimaging databases suggest that women with MCI have increased total brain volume loss and hippocampal volume loss compared with men.[108] Functional MRI and amyloid PET imaging studies are underway to examine potential sex differences in cognitive function and dementia. However, their use is still limited to clinical research.

Treatment Plan

For both sexes, a comprehensive care plan includes treatment with AD-specific medications and the management of vascular risk factors, sleep and mood disorders, and other comorbid conditions. Acetylcholinesterase inhibitors (AChEIs) remain the mainstay of pharmacologic therapy for AD.[109]

As AD is associated with the loss of cholinergic neurons in the basal forebrain, these medications enhance cholinergic transmission by inhibiting the hydrolysis of acetylcholine in the synaptic cleft.

The typical approach to drug treatment of AD includes the initiation of an AChEI in early AD and the addition of memantine when patients enter the moderate stage of the disease. Memantine, a non-competitive N-methyl-D-aspartate receptor antagonist has been approved for the treatment of moderate to severe AD dementia but has not been found to be beneficial for mild dementia or MCI. Although subtle differences exist in the biological effects of different AChEIs, their efficacy is similar across agents. Of the few studies examining AChEI efficacy and longitudinal treatment effects, some have suggested a sex difference, with men showing a greater chance of responding to treatment than women[110] and a lower rate of progression.[111] The possible sex differences reported in that review were small and showed large individual variations; thus, this subject requires further investigation.

In the past decade, drug discovery has been directed at "disease-modifying drugs" that are able to counteract the progression of AD via neuropathological processes. The amyloid cascade hypothesis suggests that increased amyloid-β (Aβ)42

Table
Summary of sex differences in Alzheimer's dementia

	Women and Females	Men and Males
Age of onset	Increased for all age strata compared with men 65 to 74 75 to 84 85 +	
Symptoms	Increased changes in mood: depression as an early symptom	
Physical examination	No consistent differences	
Cognitive profiles	More difficulty with language, confrontational naming tests, delayed recall of verbal information	
Laboratory findings	Blood-based biomarkers: No consistent differences	CSF biomarkers: NfL increased
Radiographic findings	Neuroimaging biomarkers: Increased total brain atrophy and hippocampal volume loss in MCI Greater white matter hyperintensity volumes	
Treatment	No consistent differences	
Comorbidities	Increased CV risk factor prevalence/ severity > 65 years Increased diabetes Increased depression	

production, decreased degradation, and aggregation leads to synaptic changes that cause deposition of Aβ42 in diffuse plaques. Three main therapeutic intervention strategies aimed at reducing, facilitating clearance, or preventing Aβ aggregation have been tested in clinical trials: and include γ- and β-secretases, or monoclonal antibodies (mAbs) to stimulate clearance of Aβ. Recently two mAB's, aducanumab and lecanemab, have been shown to remove beta-amyloid, with variable effects on clinical cognitive outcomes. Unfortunately, for both trials, no data have been reported regarding potential sex differences in clinical outcomes or adverse event profiles to date. The lack of this type of reporting only adds to the dearth of sex-stratified clinical drug data on efficacy, drug dosing, and the type and rate of adverse events.[112]

SUMMARY

AD impacts both sexes in several unique ways (**Table**). First, women have a higher risk of AD. Second, the clinical risk factor profile for the development of AD differs between men and women. Third, the clinical presentation and cognitive testing profiles also differ between the sexes. Finally, treatment and biomarker (blood, CSF, and neuroimaging) profiles have been shown to differ by sex. Current research efforts are continuing to better define sex differences in AD with the goal of identifying the underlying biological mechanisms of these differences.

FUNDING STATEMENT

Aggarwal Grant funding: 1R01AG073627 5P30AG010161.

DISCLOSURE

The authors have nothing to disclose.

REFERENCES

1. Alzheimer's Association. 2018 Alzheimer's disease facts and figures. Alzheimers Dement 2018;14(3):367–429.
2. Petersen RC, Lopez O, Armstrong MJ, et al. Practice guideline update summary: mild cognitive impairment: report of the guideline development, dissemination, and implementation subcommittee of the american academy of neurology. Neurology 2018;90(3):126–35.
3. Hebert LE, Beckett LA, Scherr PA, et al. Annual Incidence of Alzheimer Disease in the United States Projected to the Years 2000 Through 2050. Alzheimer Dis Assoc Disord 2001;15(4):169–73.
4. Hebert LE, Weuve J, Scherr PA, et al. Alzheimer disease in the United States (2010-2050) estimated using the 2010 census. Neurology 2013;80(19):1778–83.
5. Chêne G, Beiser A, Au R, et al. Gender and incidence of dementia in the Framingham Heart Study from mid-adult life. Alzheimer's Dementia 2015;11(3): 310–20.
6. Brodaty H, Seeher K, Gibson L. Dementia time to death: a systematic literature review on survival time and years of life lost in people with dementia. Int Psychogeriatr 2012;24(7):1034–45.
7. Andolf E, Bladh M, Möller L, et al. Prior placental bed disorders and later dementia: a retrospective Swedish register-based cohort study. BJOG An Int J Obstet Gynaecol 2020;127(9):1090–9.
8. Basit S, Wohlfahrt J, Boyd HA. Pre-eclampsia and risk of dementia later in life: nationwide cohort study. BMJ 2018;363:k4109.
9. Fields JA, Garovic VD, Mielke MM, et al. Preeclampsia and cognitive impairment later in life. Am J Obstet Gynecol 2017;217(1):74.e1–11.
10. Coppus AMW, Evenhuis HM, Verberne GJ, et al. Early Age at Menopause is Associated with Increased risk of Dementia and Mortality in Women with Down Syndrome. J Alzheimers Dis 2010;19(2):545–50.
11. Phung TKT, Waltoft BL, Laursen TM, et al. Hysterectomy, oophorectomy and risk of dementia: a nationwide historical cohort study. Dement Geriatr Cogn Disord 2010;30(1):43–50.
12. Rocca WA, Bower JH, Maraganore DM, et al. Increased risk of cognitive impairment or dementia in women who underwent oophorectomy before menopause. Neurology 2007;69(11):1074–83.
13. Rocca WA, Lohse CM, Smith CY, et al. Association of premenopausal bilateral oophorectomy with cognitive performance and risk of mild cognitive impairment. JAMA Netw Open 2021;4(11):e2131448.
14. Shumaker SA. Conjugated equine estrogens and incidence of probable dementia and mild cognitive impairment in postmenopausal women: women's health initiative memory study. JAMA 2004;291(24):2947.
15. Shumaker SA, Legault C, Rapp SR, et al. Estrogen plus progestin and the incidence of dementia and mild cognitive impairment in postmenopausal women: the women's health initiative memory study: a randomized controlled trial. JAMA 2003;289(20):2651.
16. Espeland MA. Long-term effects on cognitive function of postmenopausal hormone therapy prescribed to women aged 50 to 55 years. JAMA Intern Med 2013;173(15):1429.

17. Gleason CE, Dowling NM, Wharton W, et al. Effects of hormone therapy on cognition and mood in recently postmenopausal women: findings from the randomized, controlled KEEPS–cognitive and affective study. PLoS Med 2015; 12(6):e1001833.
18. Henderson VW, St.John JA, Hodis HN, et al. Cognitive effects of estradiol after menopause: a randomized trial of the timing hypothesis. Neurology 2016;87(7): 699–708.
19. Feldman HA, Longcope C, Derby CA, et al. Age trends in the level of serum testosterone and other hormones in middle-aged men: longitudinal results from the massachusetts male aging study. J Clin Endocrinol Metab 2002; 87(2):589–98.
20. Holland J, Bandelow S, Hogervorst E. Testosterone levels and cognition in elderly men: a review. Maturitas 2011;69(4):322–37.
21. Jayadevappa R, Chhatre S, Malkowicz SB, et al. Association between androgen deprivation therapy use and diagnosis of dementia in men with prostate cancer. JAMA Netw Open 2019;2(7):e196562.
22. Carmona S, Hardy J, Guerreiro R. The genetic landscape of Alzheimer disease. In: Geschwind DH, Paulson HL, Klein C, editors. Handbook of clinical neurology. Elsevier; 2018. p. 395–408.
23. Huang Y, Mahley RW. Apolipoprotein E: Structure and function in lipid metabolism, neurobiology, and Alzheimer's diseases. Neurobiol Dis 2014;72:3–12.
24. Liu C-C, Kanekiyo T, Xu H, et al. Apolipoprotein E and Alzheimer disease: risk, mechanisms and therapy. Nat Rev Neurol 2013;9(2):106–18.
25. Neu SC, Pa J, Kukull W, et al. Apolipoprotein E Genotype and Sex Risk Factors for Alzheimer Disease: a meta-analysis. JAMA Neurol 2017;74(10):1178.
26. Knopman DS, DeKosky ST, Cummings JL, et al. Practice parameter: Diagnosis of dementia (an evidence-based review): Report of the Quality Standards Subcommittee of the American Academy of Neurology. Neurology 2001;56(9): 1143–53.
27. Barakos J, Purcell D, Suhy J, et al. Detection and Management of Amyloid-Related Imaging Abnormalities in Patients with Alzheimer's Disease Treated with Anti-Amyloid Beta Therapy. The Journal Of Prevention of Alzheimer's Disease 2022;9(2):211–20.
28. Cummings J, Rabinovici GD, Atri A, et al. Aducanumab: appropriate use recommendations update. The Journal of Prevention of Alzheimer's Disease 2022;9(2): 221–30.
29. Wightman DP, Jansen IE, Savage JE, et al. A genome-wide association study with 1,126,563 individuals identifies new risk loci for Alzheimer's disease. Nat Genet 2021;53(9):1276–82.
30. Baumgart M, Snyder HM, Carrillo MC, et al. Summary of the evidence on modifiable risk factors for cognitive decline and dementia: a population-based perspective. Alzheimer's Dementia 2015;11(6):718–26.
31. Perry DC, Sturm VE, Peterson MJ, et al. Association of traumatic brain injury with subsequent neurological and psychiatric disease: a meta-analysis. J Neurosurg 2016;124(2):511–26.
32. Hasselgren C, Ekbrand H, Halleröd B, et al. Sex differences in dementia: on the potentially mediating effects of educational attainment and experiences of psychological distress. BMC Psychiatr 2020;20(1):434.
33. Kim S, Kim MJ, Kim S, et al. Gender differences in risk factors for transition from mild cognitive impairment to Alzheimer's disease: A CREDOS study. Compr Psychiatr 2015;62:114–22.

34. Goldstein JM, Holsen L, Handa R, et al. Fetal hormonal programming of sex differences in depression: linking women's mental health with sex differences in the brain across the lifespan. Front Neurosci 2014;8:247.
35. Kessler R. Sex and depression in the National Comorbidity Survey I: Lifetime prevalence, chronicity and recurrence. J Affect Disord 1993;29(2–3):85–96.
36. Dal Forno G, Palermo MT, Donohue JE, et al. Depressive symptoms, sex, and risk for Alzheimer's disease. Ann Neurol 2005;57(3):381–7.
37. Goveas JS, Espeland MA, Woods NF, et al. Depressive symptoms and incidence of mild cognitive impairment and probable dementia in elderly women: the women's health initiative memory study: depression and incident MCI and DEMENTIA. J Am Geriatr Soc 2011;59(1):57–66.
38. Invernizzi S, Simoes Loureiro I, Kandana KG, Arachchige KG, et al. Late-Life Depression, Cognitive Impairment, and Relationship with Alzheimer's Disease. Dement Geriatr Cogn Disord 2021;50(5):414–24.
39. Ehrenberg AJ, Nguy AK, Theofilas P, et al. Quantifying the accretion of hyperphosphorylated tau in the locus coeruleus and dorsal raphe nucleus: the pathological building blocks of early Alzheimer's disease. Neuropathol Appl Neurobiol 2017;43(5):393–408.
40. Geda YE, Schneider LS, Gitlin LN, et al. Neuropsychiatric symptoms in Alzheimer's disease: past progress and anticipation of the future. Alzheimer's Dementia 2013;9(5):602–8.
41. Eikelboom WS, Pan M, Ossenkoppele R, et al. Sex differences in neuropsychiatric symptoms in Alzheimer's disease dementia: a meta-analysis. Alzheimer's Res Ther 2022;14(1):48.
42. Sateia MJ. International classification of sleep disorders-third edition. Chest 2014;146(5):1387–94.
43. Bombois S, Derambure P, Pasquier F, et al. Sleep disorders in aging and dementia. J Nutr Health Aging 2010;14(3):212–7.
44. Ju Y-ES, Lucey BP, Holtzman DM. Sleep and Alzheimer disease pathology—a bidirectional relationship. Nat Rev Neurol 2014;10(2):115–9.
45. Yaffe K, Laffan AM, Harrison SL, et al. Sleep-disordered breathing, hypoxia, and risk of mild cognitive impairment and dementia in older women. JAMA 2011; 306(6):613–9.
46. Bixler EO, Vgontzas AN, Lin HM, et al. Prevalence of sleep-disordered breathing in women: effects of gender. Am J Respir Crit Care Med 2001;163(3):608–13.
47. Ju Y-ES, Ooms SJ, Sutphen C, et al. Slow wave sleep disruption increases cerebrospinal fluid amyloid-β levels. Brain 2017;140(8):2104–11.
48. Ahlskog JE, Geda YE, Graff-Radford NR, et al. Physical exercise as a preventive or disease-modifying treatment of dementia and brain aging. Mayo Clin Proc 2011;86(9):876–84.
49. Sofi F, Valecchi D, Bacci D, et al. Physical activity and risk of cognitive decline: a meta-analysis of prospective studies: physical activity and risk of cognitive decline. J Intern Med 2011;269(1):107–17.
50. Erickson KI, Raji CA, Lopez OL, et al. Physical activity predicts gray matter volume in late adulthood: the cardiovascular health study. Neurology 2010;75(16): 1415–22.
51. Barha CK, Davis JC, Falck RS, et al. Sex differences in exercise efficacy to improve cognition: a systematic review and meta-analysis of randomized controlled trials in older humans. Front Neuroendocrinol 2017;46:71–85.
52. Barha CK, Hsiung G-YR, Best JR, et al. Sex Difference in aerobic exercise efficacy to improve cognition in older adults with vascular cognitive impairment:

secondary analysis of a randomized controlled trial. J Alzheimers Dis 2017; 60(4):1397–410.

53. Barha CK, Best JR, Rosano C, et al. Sex-Specific Relationship Between Long-Term Maintenance of Physical Activity and Cognition in the Health ABC Study: Potential Role of Hippocampal and Dorsolateral Prefrontal Cortex Volume. J Gerontol: Series A 2020;75(4):764–70.
54. Benton D. Neurodevelopment and neurodegeneration: are there critical stages for nutritional intervention? Nutr Rev 2010;68:S6–10.
55. Wald DS, Kasturiratne A, Simmonds M. Effect of folic acid, with or without other B Vitamins, on cognitive decline: meta-analysis of randomized trials. Am J Med 2010;123(6):522–7.e2.
56. Tangney CC, Tang Y, Evans DA, et al. Biochemical indicators of vitamin B12 and folate insufficiency and cognitive decline. Neurology 2009;72(4):361–7.
57. D'Amico D, Parrott MD, Greenwood CE, et al. Sex differences in the relationship between dietary pattern adherence and cognitive function among older adults: findings from the NuAge study. Nutr J 2020;19(1):58.
58. Niu H, Álvarez-Álvarez I, Guillén-Grima F, et al. Prevalencia e incidencia de la enfermedad de Alzheimer en Europa: metaanálisis. Neurologia 2017;32(8): 523–32.
59. Morris MC, Tangney CC, Wang Y, Tangney CC, Wang Y, et al. MIND diet slows cognitive decline with aging. Alzheimer's Dementia 2015;11(9):1015–22.
60. Morris MC, et al. MIND diet associated with reduced incidence of Alzheimer's disease. Alzheimer's Dementia 2015;11(9):1007–14.
61. Scarmeas N, Stern Y, Mayeux R, et al. Mediterranean diet and mild cognitive impairment. Arch Neurol 2009;66(2):216–25.
62. Guasch-Ferré M, Willett WC. The Mediterranean diet and health: a comprehensive overview. J Intern Med 2021;290(3):549–66.
63. Ballarini T, Melo van Lent D, Brunner J, et al. Mediterranean diet, alzheimer disease biomarkers, and brain atrophy in old age. Neurology 2021;96(24): e2920–32.
64. Gu Y, Scarmeas N. Dietary patterns in alzheimers disease and cognitive aging. Curr Alzheimer Res 2011;8(5):510–9.
65. Bowman GL, Silbert LC, Howieson D, et al. Nutrient biomarker patterns, cognitive function, and MRI measures of brain aging. Neurology 2012;78(4):241–9.
66. Barnes DE, Yaffe K. The projected effect of risk factor reduction on Alzheimer's disease prevalence. Lancet Neurol 2011;10(9):819–28.
67. Ritchie K, Ritchie CW, Yaffe K, et al. Is late-onset Alzheimer's disease really a disease of midlife? Alzheimer's Dementia 2015;1(2):122–30.
68. Mielke MM, Rosenberg PB, Tschanz J, et al. Vascular factors predict rate of progression in Alzheimer disease. Neurology 2007;69(19):1850–8.
69. Profenno LA, Porsteinsson AP, Faraone SV. Meta-analysis of alzheimer's disease risk with obesity, diabetes, and related disorders. Biol Psychiatr 2010;67(6): 505–12.
70. Azad NA, Al Bugami M, Loy-English I. Gender differences in dementia risk factors. Gend Med 2007;4(2):120–9.
71. Bairey Merz CN, Shaw LJ, Reis SE, et al. Insights From the NHLBI-Sponsored Women's Ischemia Syndrome Evaluation (WISE) Study. J Am Coll Cardiol 2006;47(3):S21–9.
72. Yaffe K. The metabolic syndrome, inflammation, and risk of cognitive decline. JAMA 2004;292(18):2237.

73. Gustafson DR, Backman K, Waern M, et al. Adiposity indicators and dementia over 32 years in Sweden. Neurology 2009;73(19):1559–66.
74. Tolppanen A-M, Solomon A, Soininen H, et al. Midlife vascular risk factors and alzheimer's disease: evidence from epidemiological studies. J Alzheimers Dis 2012;32(3):531–40.
75. Peltz CB, Corrada MM, Berlau DJ, et al. Cognitive impairment in nondemented oldest-old: Prevalence and relationship to cardiovascular risk factors. Alzheimer's Dementia 2012;8(2):87–94.
76. Alhurani RE, Vassilaki M, Aakre JA, et al. Decline in weight and incident mild cognitive impairment: mayo clinic study of aging. JAMA Neurol 2016;73(4): 439–46.
77. Mielke MM, Zandi PP, Shao H, et al. The 32-year relationship between cholesterol and dementia from midlife to late life. Neurology 2010;75(21):1888–95.
78. Mielke MM, Zandi PP, Sjogren M, et al. High total cholesterol levels in late life associated with a reduced risk of dementia. Neurology 2005;64(10):1689–95.
79. Huo N, Vemuri P, Graff-Radford J, et al. Sex Differences in the association between midlife cardiovascular conditions or risk factors with midlife cognitive decline. Neurology 2022;98(6):e623–32.
80. Hachinski V. Multi-infarct dementia. A cause of mental deterioration in the elderly. Lancet 1974;304(7874):207–9.
81. van Veluw SJ, Zwanenburg JJ, Rozemuller AJ, et al. The spectrum of Mr detectable cortical microinfarcts: a classification study with 7-tesla postmortem MRI and histopathology. J Cereb Blood Flow Metab 2015;35(4):676–83.
82. Kjeldsen SE, Narkiewicz K, Burnier M, et al. Intensive blood pressure lowering prevents mild cognitive impairment and possible dementia and slows development of white matter lesions in brain: the SPRINT Memory and Cognition IN Decreased Hypertension (SPRINT MIND) study. Blood Pres 2018;27(5):247–8.
83. Gilsanz P, Mayeda ER, Glymour MM, et al. Female sex, early-onset hypertension, and risk of dementia. Neurology 2017;89(18):1886–93.
84. Kritz-Silverstein D, Laughlin GA, McEvoy LK, et al. Sex and Age Differences in the Association of Blood Pressure and Hypertension with Cognitive Function in the Elderly: The Rancho Bernardo Study. The Journal of Prevention of Alzheimer's Disease 2017;4(3):1–9.
85. Williamson JD, Launer LJ, Bryan RN, et al. Cognitive function and brain structure in persons with type 2 diabetes mellitus after intensive lowering of blood pressure and lipid levels: a randomized clinical trial. JAMA Intern Med 2014; 174(3):324.
86. Ngandu T, Lehtisalo J, Solomon A, et al. A 2 year multidomain intervention of diet, exercise, cognitive training, and vascular risk monitoring versus control to prevent cognitive decline in at-risk elderly people (FINGER): a randomised controlled trial. Lancet 2015;385(9984):2255–63.
87. Shepardson NE. Cholesterol level and statin use in Alzheimer disease: I. Review of epidemiological and preclinical studies. Arch Neurol 2011;68(10):1239.
88. Lee J-W, Choi E-A, Kim Y-S, et al. Statin exposure and the risk of dementia in individuals with hypercholesterolaemia. J Intern Med 2020;288(6):689–98.
89. Jonker C, Launer LJ, Hooijer C, et al. Memory complaints and memory impairment in older individuals. J Am Geriatr Soc 1996;44(1):44–9.
90. Pérès K, Helmer C, Amieva H, et al. Gender differences in the prodromal signs of dementia: memory complaint and IADL-restriction. A Prospective Population-Based Cohort. J Alzheimers Dis 2011;27(1):39–47.

91. Sundermann EE, Edmonds EC, Delano-Wood L, et al. Sex influences the accuracy of subjective memory complaint reporting in older adults. J Alzheimers Dis 2018;61:1163–78.
92. Engedal K, Gjøra L, Bredholt T, et al. Sex differences on montreal cognitive assessment and mini-mental state examination scores and the value of self-report of memory problems among community dwelling people 70 years and above: the hunt study. Dement Geriatr Cogn Disord 2021;50(1):74–84.
93. McKhann GM, Knopman DS, Chertkow H, et al. The diagnosis of dementia due to Alzheimer's disease: recommendations from the National Institute on Aging-Alzheimer's Association workgroups on diagnostic guidelines for Alzheimer's disease. Alzheimer's Dementia 2011;7(3):263–9.
94. Bondi MW, Edmonds EC, Salmon DP. Alzheimer's Disease: past, present, and future. J Int Neuropsychol Soc 2017;23(9–10):818–31.
95. Siedlecki KL, Falzarano F, Salthouse TA. Examining gender differences in neurocognitive functioning across adulthood. J Int Neuropsychol Soc 2019;25(10): 1051–60.
96. Bayles KA, Azuma T, Cruz RF, et al. Gender differences in language of alzheimer disease patients revisited. Alzheimer Dis Assoc Disord 1999;13(3):138–46.
97. McPherson S, Back C, Buckwalter JG, et al. Gender-related cognitive deficits in alzheimer's disease. Int Psychogeriatr 1999;11(2):117–22.
98. Hebert LE, Wilson RS, Gilley DW, et al. Decline of language among women and men with alzheimer's disease. J Gerontol B Psychol Sci Soc Sci 2000;55(6): P354–61.
99. Jack CR, Bennett DA, Blennow K, et al. NIA-AA research framework: toward a biological definition of Alzheimer's disease. Alzheimer's Dementia 2018;14(4): 535–62.
100. American Psychiatric Association and D, Black W. Diagnostic and statistical manual of mental disorders : DSM-5. 5th ed. Arlington, Va: American Psychiatric Association; 2013.
101. Teunissen CE, Verberk IMW, Thijssen EH, et al. Blood-based biomarkers for Alzheimer's disease: towards clinical implementation. Lancet Neurol 2022;21(1): 66–77.
102. Hansson O, et al. The Alzheimer's Association appropriate use recommendations for blood biomarkers in Alzheimer's disease. Alzheimer's Dementia 2022;alz.12756.
103. Bridel C, van Wieringen WN, Zetterberg H, et al. Diagnostic Value of cerebrospinal fluid neurofilament light protein in neurology: a systematic review and meta-analysis. JAMA Neurol 2019;76(9):1035.
104. Mielke MM, Syrjanen JA, Blennow K, et al. Comparison of variables associated with cerebrospinal fluid neurofilament, total-tau, and neurogranin. Alzheimer's Dementia 2019;15(11):1437–47.
105. Fatemi F, Kantarci K, Graff-Radford J, et al. Sex differences in cerebrovascular pathologies on FLAIR in cognitively unimpaired elderly. Neurology 2018;90(6): e466–73.
106. Greenberg SM, Charidimou A. Diagnosis of cerebral amyloid angiopathy: evolution of the boston criteria. Stroke 2018;49(2):491–7.
107. Graff-Radford J, Aakre JA, Knopman DS, et al. Prevalence and heterogeneity of cerebrovascular disease imaging lesions. Mayo Clin Proc 2020;95(6):1195–205.
108. Lin KA, Choudhury KR, Rathakrishnan BG, et al. Marked gender differences in progression of mild cognitive impairment over 8 years. Alzheimer's Dementia: Translational Research & Clinical Interventions 2015;1(2):103–10.

109. Aisen PS, Cummings J, Schneider LS. Symptomatic and nonamyloid/tau based pharmacologic treatment for alzheimer disease. Cold Spring Harbor Perspectives in Medicine 2012;2(3):a006395.
110. MacGowan SH, Wilcock GK, Scott M. Effect of gender and apolipoprotein E genotype on response to anticholinesterase therapy in Alzheimer's disease. Int J Geriatr Psychiatry 1998;13(9):625–30.
111. Doody RS, Pavlik V, Massman P, et al. Predicting progression of Alzheimer's disease. Alzheimer's Res Ther 2010;2(1):2.
112. Martinkova J, et al. Proportion of women and reporting of outcomes by sex in clinical trials for alzheimer disease: a systematic review and meta-analysis. JAMA Netw Open 2021;4(9).

Sex-Specific Neurocognitive Impairment

Sharlet A. Anderson, PhD[a,*], Maria A. Rossetti, PhD[b]

KEYWORDS

• Cognition • Sex • Gender • Neurocognitive disorders • Neurofeminism
• Intersectionality

KEY POINTS

- Both endogenous and exogenous factors result in sex/gender differences in neurocognitive impairment (NCI) and using a biopsychosocial lens can help better understand the complex drivers of these differences.
- Intersectionality of sex/gender/gender identity and other demographic categorizations is rarely examined in NCI research.
- Methodological (eg, neuropsychological normative data) and conceptual (eg, gender essentialism) challenges are evident in current research practices, though gender/sex differences in cognition have been observed across medical and neurologic conditions.
- Intersectionality of biological, sociopolitical, and environmental influences is necessary to better understand the role of sex/gender in NCI.

INTRODUCTION

Despite the well-established understanding that neurologic diseases impact women and men differ in terms of incidence, prevalence, clinical presentation, and treatment response, research on sex and gender differences in these conditions had been limited until recently.[1] Focus on sex/gender differences in the cognitive aspects of neurologic conditions has been even more scant. A recent large-scale cohort study using pooled data from over 26,000 participants[2] revealed that although women had higher cognitive reserve as measured by global, memory, and executive functioning measures when compared with men they showed significantly faster declines in global cognition and executive functioning, but not in memory. Such findings highlight the continued need for research on this topic. Whereas the exclusion of women/females in research studies leads to problems or questions about generalizability, some argue that focusing on sex/gender differences carries the risk of reinforcing harmful stereotypes and perpetuating inequities in health outcomes.[3] However, approaching the problem by using a

[a] Department of Neurological Sciences, Rush University Medical Center, 1725 West Harrison Street, Professional Office Building 755, Chicago, IL 60612, USA; [b] Department of Neurology, University of Virginia School of Medicine, PO Box 800394, Charlottesville, VA 22908, USA
* Corresponding author.
E-mail address: Sharlet_A_Anderson@rush.edu

Neurol Clin 41 (2023) 359–369
https://doi.org/10.1016/j.ncl.2023.01.003

biopsychosocial lens to better understand the complex drivers of these differences can mitigate potential harms that gender essentialism[4] might create. Both endogenous and exogenous factors that result in sex/gender differences in neurocognitive impairment (NCI) can contribute to the practice of precision medicine. When investigating group differences based on demographics associated with a history of systematized discrimination, it is imperative that the selection of methodologies includes mindful consideration of the possibility of perpetuating long-held stereotypes or biases, even with well-intentioned efforts to highlight disparities in the name of health equity.

History

In a recent progress report on the implementation of the 1993 National Institues of Health (NIH) Revitalization Act and the 2016 mandate for all NIH-funded research to include sex as a biological variable, researchers summarize several efforts that were made to foster the appropriate inclusion of females and women in across the spectrum of research studies, from benchside to bedside.[5] Indeed, at a 2020 workshop conducted by the National Academies of Sciences, Engineering, and Medicine's Forum on Neuroscience and Nervous System Disorders, prominent researchers acknowledged the exclusion of female animals in their past work due to concern that inclusion would require much larger sample sizes and more complex analyses.[6] To explore sex-specific NCI, key terms must first be defined.

Definitions

The terms "sex" and "gender" have often been erroneously used interchangeably in the literature. Sex typically refers to the classification assigned at birth based on primary sex characteristics, the development of which is encoded in DNA and influenced by hormones.[7] Gender refers to sociocultural identities, the experience of which is influenced by societal constructs and the confines of what sex classification means.[8] Sex and gender have traditionally been regarded as binary constructs in research. "Male" and "female" are terms used to classify sex, and "woman" or "man" for gender, with the flawed assumption that all individuals classified as female identify as women and all those classified as male identify as men. In other words, they are cisgender. Transgender is a term that refers to people whose gender identity differs from the sex they were assigned at birth. Intersex individuals are born with a combination of male and female primary sex characteristics. Nonbinary is a term that refers to people whose gender identity does not conform to either the traditional male/men and female/women constructs. The meaning of gender nonconforming varies with context. It is an umbrella term that refers to people whose gender expression (appearance and behavior) does not adhere to societal expectations and stereotypes typically associated with men or women, regardless of one's gender identity (cisgender, transgender, non-binary). Modern genetics and biomarker research affirms the social construct of gender fluidity,[9] which refers to a non-fixed gender identity.[10] The term "sexual and gender minorities" (SGM) refers to not only anyone other than cisgender, but also any sexual orientation other than heterosexual, such as lesbian, gay, bisexual, asexual, and pansexual people. For the current review, the terms used (female/male vs women/men or girls/boys) are matched to the ones used in the original sources. The assumption that all research participants are cisgender excludes individuals who are transgender, intersex, non-binary, and gender-nonconforming.

Nature of the Problem

The exclusion of women has limited the generalizability of results, which perpetuates a system of inequity that sustains disparities in health outcomes. Beyond the exclusion of women, SGM are even more likely to be under-represented in neurosciences research,[11] including studies focused on NCI. Furthermore, the intersectionality of sex/gender/gender identity and other demographic categorizations (ethnicity, race, ability status, age, etc.) can have compounding effects of double disenfranchisement across the lifespan,[12] but is rarely examined in NCI research.

Traditional collection methods for collecting demographic data in clinical research usually offer only binary options for sex (male or female). Based on a survey of Alzheimer's Disease Research Centers funded by the National Institute on Aging conducted by Stites and colleagues,[13] the most common approach has been to employ a single measure of self-reported with binary response choices for sex, either man/woman or male/female. Very few centers included additional measures of gender identity, sexual orientation, or genetically assigned sex. Updated research practices are desperately needed as sex and gender contribute uniquely to health and health outcomes, by impacting genetic, epigenetic, and hormonal systems, as well as behaviors rooted in positional power (or lack thereof) including health care access, risk exposure, and perceived stress, to name a few.[14]

DISCUSSION

Biopsychosocial Framework

Structural and social determinants of health (SSDoH) are an important factor in the incidence, impact, and course of NCI, and likely account for some of the heterogeneity observed in research findings.[15] Madsen and Hamilton[16] note that demographic differences in quality of care and outcome in stroke may be due to situational/contextual factors associated with trust in the medical provider, health literacy, and availability of a health proxy to aid in decision making, as well as unconscious bias in the medical provider.[17] With regard to life roles, it is well established that caregiver stress raises the risk of cognitive decline. However, research shows that male caregivers may experience steeper declines in cognition[18] and higher incident dementia risk[19,20] compared with female caregivers, which suggests that sex may moderate the effect of psychosocial stress on cognitive functioning.[21] Stress-related pathways secondary to specific social roles and circumstances,[22] such as caregiver burden and bereavement, are potential risk factors for cognitive decline or Alzheimer's disease (AD).

A framework for SSDoH data collection using a biopsychosocial model was recently proposed for conceptualizing AD risk factors.[15] It includes seven core domains: social stressors and perceived stress, social support, education, and health literacy, occupation, social positioning, social/built environment/neighborhood, and social identity. The authors note that this framework was derived in part from Fundamental Cause Theory[23] and Ecological Systems Theory.[24,25] These theories are grounded in the construct that stresses associated with socially constructed roles lead to differences in underlying neurologic pathways as well as the behavioral expression thereof, thereby causing health disparities. For example, Wolfova and colleagues[26] found that childhood socioeconomic position was more strongly associated with the rate of cognitive decline later in life in women than in men, and that education was the strongest mediator of that relationship. They suggest that this disparity could be rooted in sex-specific responses to early life stressors and the biological pathways that underlie them, setting the stage for more or less cognitive reserve later in life. Sociocultural theory[27] would assume that if early life stressors and mediators, such as education, were equal in women and men, the disparities in rates of cognitive decline in late life would be less pronounced.

Cognitive Measurement Issues

In the field of neuropsychology, sex-based norms are not widely adopted[28] despite the well-established evidence[29] that when compared with men, women across the life-span have stronger cognitive performance in all cognitive domains and verbal memory in particular,[30–33] with the exception of visuospatial skills. The failure to account for sex/gender differences can lead to under-detection of cognitive impairment and, in turn, delayed diagnosis and compromised access to early interventions for women.[28,34,35] The evolution of work in this area over the past decade shows a shift to acknowledging the importance of improving the diagnostic accuracy of amnestic mild cognitive impairment (MCI) in women. For example, Levine and colleagues[2] used a pooled cohort approach to obtain a very large sample size and reported that women had higher baseline performance on several cognitive measures (global, executive function, memory) than men, but faster decline than men in some areas (not memory) independent of cardiovascular risk factors. However, these interpretations could be an artifact of the kinds of measures used and how the results were classified.

In a 2016 editorial, Sano and Gandy[36] highlighted several issues that may contribute to enduring sex biases in research which were exemplified in a study of verbal memory performance as a function of hippocampal atrophy in men and women using the Alzheimer's Disease Neuroimaging Initiative (ADNI) historical dataset. They showed that the use of cut-scores versus sex-based norms or pooled normative data that does not account for sex can result in the risk of failure to detect the presence of subtle early impairments in verbal memory in women. This could create the illusion that the skill being measured is well preserved in women in earlier stages of disease until a tipping point at which a more drastic decline occurs in later stages of illness. Lastly, the authors also describe how the subtle differences in the definition of cognitive reserve (lifelong advantage in cognition vs hippocampal/brain volume) can have an impact on measurement and defining the earliest stage of change (the starting point) and therefore the magnitude of change over time. In a more recent editorial piece,[37] the authors furthered the argument by stating that research designs should also take into account gonadal hormone status, arguing that different endocrine stages across the lifespan (eg, puberty, menstrual cycle, pregnancy, menopause) may be important contributing factors in sex differences observed in neurologic disorders and pathologies.

The use of cut scores and normative data that are not sex/gender adjusted is not the only problem. Several contextual factors that disproportionately affect women may be the driver of differences/disparities observed in NCI. Failure to include other potential variables that go along with sex/gender can lead to the conclusion that certain differences in women's cognitive skills, development, or decline as compared with men (the default reference group) are solely due to inherent differences in physiology (gender essentialism)[38] rather than the systems that shape them.[15]

Current Evidence

Despite the methodological and conceptual challenges described above, sex/gender differences have been reported in many neurologic disorders affecting cognition. The findings span broadly, covering risk factors for dementia risk at large as well as observations in specific conditions. For example, in a 2021 report[39] delineating broad risk factor domains (biomarkers, socio-demographic, lifestyle, and medical), it was noted that different risk factors were more strongly associated with memory decline in women versus men and that the particular risk factors with stronger associations to memory decline changed across the lifespan. For example, for people in their 40s, genetic/medical risk factors were more strongly associated with memory impairment in women, but for men of the same age, demographic and lifestyles were more strongly associated with memory decline. However, for people in their 60s and 70s women with apolipoprotein E (APOE) e4 form APOEe4+/+ genotype had less decline than women with other genotypes (APOEe4 ± and APOEe4−/−), whereas men with the APOEe4+/+ genotype had the lowest/most memory decline than other genotypes. Sex differences in age-related cognitive decline related to APOE and other factors were observed in a large international study.[40] Their observation that rates of decline differed across nationalities, which highlights the need for further research in risk factors across ethnocultural groups.

Focusing more specifically on modifiable risk factors,[41] reported that in women, there were positive correlations between physical activity and processing speed reserve, and between cognitive activity and memory reserve. This pattern was not observed in men. In addition, APOE status moderated these relationships in women, but not men.

White matter hyperintensity (WMH) burden increases with advancing age, but more so for women after menopause in comparison to men and premenopausal women.[42] This finding begs the question of which physiologic aspects of menopause might be contributing to this observation. However, another salient question is how menopause status was defined and captured. The authors acknowledge limitations in methodology such as assessing menopause status only by self-report, binary classification of pre- or postmenopausal (excluding peri-menopausal), failure to include age and cause of menopause (natural vs surgical such as oophorectomy), duration of hormone replacement therapy, and failure to assess gender identity. The potential psychosocial stressors associated with menopause which could differ based on the age of onset, induced by medical complications, or via gender-affirming surgery, were not discussed.[43]

There is a growing body of work that aims to elucidate the role of sex and gender on cognition in specific neurodegenerative conditions, such as AD, Parkinson's disease (PD), Huntington's disease (HD), and frontotemporal dementia (FTD). For example, a recent meta-analysis examined sex differences in executive, visuospatial, and verbal memory performance of nondemented PD patients. Sex differences were noted for executive functioning skills such that male patients showed greater executive deficits than female patients when compared with controls,[44] and that low baseline semantic fluency was associated with a faster decline in women but not men.[45] Also in PD, men with APOE e4 had poorer cognitive performance in nondemented PD patients.[46]

Hentosh and colleagues[47] investigated sex differences in the natural progression of HD by analyzing a large worldwide longitudinal observational dataset (Enroll-HD). Their findings revealed sex-dependent differences in motor, psychiatric, and cognitive symptoms. Women tended to perform worse on Verbal Fluency, Symbol Digit Modalities Test (SDMT), and Stroop Interference Test, with only the latter being statistically significant for the participant's first visit. Overtime, women performed better on the Stroop Interference Test and SDMT, potentially due to practice effects that were not observed in men. Of note, worsening of verbal fluency scores was observed in men.

In behavioral variant FTD (bvFTD), research shows that women outperform men in measures of executive function and have less neurobehavioral changes (appetite, sleep, and apathy) despite having a higher burden of frontal atrophy. Consistent with data from other neurodegenerative conditions, women with bvFTD have higher behavioral and executive reserve compared with men.[48]

Traumatic brain injury (TBI) findings are inconsistent. In human studies, women seem to have better outcomes than men following moderate or severe injuries, but worse outcomes after mild TBI.[49] This pattern is reversed in animal models. The authors suggest that gender stereotypes may influence the types of symptoms and frequency help-seeking behaviors, which may account for these differences. However, this is not specific to cognition per se.

A recent study of human immunodeficiency virus (HIV)-associated NCI showed that the higher prevalence of NCI in HIV + women versus HIV + men was attributed to lower reading level, a potential proxy for education quality.[50] The authors also posit women's vulnerability to HIV-NCI, particularly for Black women, is strongly related to educational disparities and therefore lower cognitive reserve. Animal model studies presumably eliminate the psychosocial factors that influence human development and behavior. For example, sex-based cognitive differences in HIV-1 Tg26 transgenic mice were found, and these differences were related to hippocampal neurogenesis.[51]

Sex differences in long-term coronavirus disease-2019 (COVID-19) symptoms have been investigated, though studies reporting specific cognitive functions are scant. For example, a recent literature review suggests that females reported neurologic, psychiatric, and cognitive sequelae of COVID-19 more often than men, but only in younger populations.[52] Mechanisms proposed include immunologic response, the role of angiotensin-converting enzyme-2, pre-existing comorbidities, and sociocultural differences in gender role expectations.[53] Poor memory[54,55] and working memory difficulties[55] in females versus males have been reported.

Neurodevelopmental disorders are linked to an increased risk of dementia. Therefore, autism spectrum disorder (ASD) and attention-deficit hyperactivity disorder (ADHD) will be discussed in this context, though NCI typically refers to cognitive changes that occur after some period of "normal" cognitive functioning. Findings have been inconsistent with regard to cognitive sex/gender differences in people with ASD. Among those who are high functioning, females performed better than males on tasks of cognitive flexibility whereas males performed better on tests of attention to detail.[56] The sample was comprised of children between 11 and 17 years of age, though the pubertal stage was not delineated, and hormonal influences on the development of executive functioning were not mentioned. Other studies indicate that outcomes were poorer and that comorbid psychopathology was more likely for females with high-functioning ASD than their male counterparts.[57,58] In these reports, there seems to be a suggestion that there are differences in the manifestation of the disorder itself on the molecular or neuronal level. The possibility of differences in societal expectations for social relatedness and communication (core clinical features of ASD) based on gender role stereotypes is not explored. Gender identity formation is part of a developmental process with a sensitive period preceding puberty, which is influenced of course by societal expectations.[59]

A meta-analysis in 2020 showed that there are more similarities in the cognitive profiles of boys and girls with ADHD, but that differences in the behavioral expression of the disorder (more hyperactivity in boys) lead to girls being underdiagnosed.[60] In a narrative review of gender differences in adults with ADHD, studies consistently showed that women reported a more severe sense of impairment than men, which may be colored by societal expectations of women's capabilities compounded by stereotype threat.[61] If girls' behavioral expression of ADHD is more subtle than boys', and they tend to go undiagnosed more, they may attribute difficulties in life (cognitive, social) to personal shortcomings rather than to the external diagnosis.

Studies have also explored the role of sex and gender differences on cognition in psychiatric conditions such as posttraumatic stress disorder (PTSD) and psychosis. Psychiatric disorders are not traditionally considered to be "organic" disorders. However, more modern research approaches have included some psychiatric disorders in the category of neurodevelopment. For example, premorbid intelligence quotient (IQ) has been associated with outcomes following the first episode psychosis, though women with low premorbid IQ had better cognitive outcomes than men with low premorbid IQ.[62] Social cognition, a domain often overlooked in neurocognitive research, differs in women versus men who are recently diagnosed with schizophrenia.[63] Women who endorse a higher level of PTSD symptoms had steeper rates of decline in learning, working memory, processing speed, and attention.[64] Behavioral issues such as low motivation, disinhibition, and emotional dysregulation were more strongly associated with declines in cognitive skills in men than in women.[48]

SUMMARY

Where do we draw the line between biology, social constructs, and the biological reactions and consequences of society's value of those social constructs? At what point does the biological end and psychological begin? Exactly when do psychological impacts begin to manifest biologically? For example, a person assigned male at birth whose gender identity is a woman (transgender), and whose gender expression is feminine whether in clothing, surgery, and/or hormone treatment may face double disenfranchisement.[38,65] Is this person susceptible to the same changes in stress-related pathways and stress response dysregulation as cisgender people who are gender conforming? The shift from gender identity disorder in fourth edition of the Diagnostic and Statistical Manual of Mental Disorders (DSM-IV) to gender dysphoria in the fifth edition (DSM-V) de-pathologizes the experience of individuals whose gender identity/expression is disparate enough from their sex assigned at birth to consider it a mismatch, but still requires the presence of distress to be labeled as such.[59] This distress might not be present in all individuals who are not cisgender. The complex interactions among biology, socio-political context, and environmental influences on health are captured by a syndemics model of health that goes beyond traditional concepts of comorbidity by examining social and environmental factors that both contribute to and are affected by disease clustering in marginalized populations.[66,67] This approach necessitates the inclusion of structural as well as social determinants of health[15] as key factors in the shift toward personalized and precision medicine.[37] Specific to the experience of women and neurologic diseases, a neurofeminist approach to intersectionality in neurosciences research, which uses a critical lens to examine traditional methods and concepts of sex and gender, may be a fruitful strategy in striving for health equity.[68]

CLINICS CARE POINTS

- Sex and gender are not synonymous, though there is bidirectional influence and considerable overlap.
- Structural and social determinants of health (SSDoH) may account for much more in cognitive health outcomes than has been historically acknowledged.
- Mindful consideration of sex, gender, and SSDoH in methods of cognitive skill measurement is crucial in avoiding the pitfalls of gender essentialism as the basis for discrimination leading to health disparities.

DISCLOSURE

The authors have nothing to disclose.

REFERENCES

1. Attarian H, Brandes J, Dafer R, et al. Sex Differences in the Study of Neurological Illnesses. Behav Neurol 2015;2015:1–2.
2. Levine DA, Gross AL, Briceño EM, et al. Sex differences in cognitive decline among US adults. JAMA Netw Open 2021;4(2):e210169.
3. Mendrek A. Is It Important to Consider Sex and Gender in Neurocognitive Studies? Opinion. Front Psychiatr 2015;6. https://doi.org/10.3389/fpsyt.2015.00083.
4. Gelman SA, Taylor MG. Gender essentialism in cognitive development. Toward a feminist developmental, . psychology. New York, NY: Taylor & Frances/Routledge; 2000. p. 169–90.
5. Arnegard ME, Whitten LA, Hunter C, et al. Sex as a Biological Variable: A 5-Year Progress Report and Call to Action. J Womens Health (Larchmt) 2020;29(6):858–64.
6. National Academies of Sciences E, Medicine, Health, et al. The National Academies Collection: Reports funded by National Institutes of Health. In: Stroud C, Norris SMP, Bain L, editors. Sex differences in brain disorders: emerging transcriptomic evidence: proceedings of a workshop. US: National Academies Press; 2021. Copyright 2021 by the National Academy of Sciences. All rights reserved.
7. Eggers S, Sinclair A. Mammalian sex determination—insights from humans and mice. Chromosome Res 2012;20(1):215–38.
8. Fleming PJ, Agnew-Brune C. Current trends in the study of gender norms and health behaviors. Current Opinion in Psychology 2015;5:72–7.
9. Roselli CE. Neurobiology of gender identity and sexual orientation. J Neuroendocrinol 2018;30(7):e12562.
10. Ainsworth C. Sex redefined. Nature 2015;518(7539):288–91.
11. Mielke MM, Aggarwal NT, Vila-Castelar C, et al. Consideration of sex and gender in Alzheimer's disease and related disorders from a global perspective. Alzheimer's Dementia 2022. https://doi.org/10.1002/alz.12662.
12. Farhadi-Langroudi K, Sargent K, Masuda A. Doubly Disenfranchised: An Acceptance-and Compassion-Based Approach to Being a Minority Within GSM Communities. Mindfulness and Acceptance for Gender and Sexual Minorities: A Clinician's Guide to Fostering Compassion, Connection, and Equality Using Contextual Strategies. 2016:247.
13. Stites SD, Cao H, Harkins K, et al. Measuring Sex and Gender in Aging and Alzheimer's Research: Results of a National Survey. J Gerontol: Series B 2022;77(6):1005–16.
14. Mauvais-Jarvis F, Bairey Merz N, Barnes PJ, et al. Sex and gender: modifiers of health, disease, and medicine. Lancet 2020/08/22/2020;396(10250):565–82.
15. Stites SD, Midgett S, Mechanic-Hamilton D, et al. Establishing a Framework for Gathering Structural and Social Determinants of Health in Alzheimer's Disease Research Centers. Gerontol 2022;62(5):694–703.
16. Madsen TE, Hamilton R. Racial- and Gender-Based Disparities in IV-Alteplase Declination. Looking for Barriers and Biases When Patients Say No 2022;98(16):647–8.
17. Mendelson SJ, Zhang S, Matsouaka R, et al. Race-Ethnic Disparities in Rates of Declination of Thrombolysis for Stroke. Neurology 2022;98(16):e1596–604.

18. Pertl MM, Lawlor BA, Robertson IH, et al. Risk of Cognitive and Functional Impairment in Spouses of People With Dementia: Evidence From the Health and Retirement Study. J Geriatr Psychiatry Neurol 2015;28(4):260–71.
19. Norton MC, Smith KR, Østbye T, et al. Greater Risk of Dementia When Spouse Has Dementia? The Cache County Study. J Am Geriatr Soc 2010;58(5):895–900.
20. Vitaliano PP. An Ironic Tragedy: Are Spouses of Persons with Dementia at Higher Risk for Dementia than Spouses of Persons without Dementia? J Am Geriatr Soc 2010;58(5):976–8.
21. Hidalgo V, Pulopulos MM, Salvador A. Acute psychosocial stress effects on memory performance: Relevance of age and sex. Neurobiol Learn Mem 2019;157: 48–60.
22. Wu-Chung EL, Leal SL, Denny BT, et al. Spousal caregiving, widowhood, and cognition: A systematic review and a biopsychosocial framework for understanding the relationship between interpersonal losses and dementia risk in older adulthood. Neurosci Biobehav Rev 2022;134:104487.
23. Phelan JC, Link BG, Tehranifar P. Social Conditions as Fundamental Causes of Health Inequalities: Theory, Evidence, and Policy Implications. J Health Soc Behav 2010;51(1_suppl):S28–40.
24. Bronfenbrenner U. Ecological systems theory (1992). Making human beings human: Bioecological perspectives on human development, 2005, Sage Publications Ltd, Thousand Oaks, CA, 106–173.
25. Bronfenbrenner U. Ecological systems theory. Six theories of child development: revised formulations and current issues. London, England: Jessica Kingsley Publishers; 1992. p. 187–249.
26. Wolfova K, Csajbok Z, Kagstrom A, et al. Role of sex in the association between childhood socioeconomic position and cognitive ageing in later life. Sci Rep 2021;11(1). https://doi.org/10.1038/s41598-021-84022-1.
27. Hyde JS. Gender Similarities and Differences. Annu Rev Psychol 2014;65(1): 373–98.
28. Sundermann EE, Barnes LL, Bondi MW, et al. Improving Detection of Amnestic Mild Cognitive Impairment with Sex-Specific Cognitive Norms. J Alzheimers Dis 2021;84(4):1763–70.
29. McCarrey AC, An Y, Kitner-Triolo MH, et al. Sex differences in cognitive trajectories in clinically normal older adults. Psychol Aging 2016;31(2):166–75.
30. Kramer JH, Delis DC, Daniel M. Sex differences in verbal learning. J Clin Psychol 1988;44(6):907–15.
31. Aartsen MJ, Martin M, Zimprich D. Gender Differences in Level and Change in Cognitive Functioning. Gerontology 2004;50(1):35–8.
32. Pauls F, Petermann F, Lepach AC. Gender differences in episodic memory and visual working memory including the effects of age. Memory 2013;21(7):857–74.
33. Sundermann EE, Maki PM, Rubin LH, et al. Female advantage in verbal memory: Evidence of sex-specific cognitive reserve. Neurology 2016;87(18):1916–24.
34. Sundermann EE, Biegon A, Rubin LH, et al. Does the Female Advantage in Verbal Memory Contribute to Underestimating Alzheimer's Disease Pathology in Women versus Men? J Alzheimers Dis 2017;56(3):947–57.
35. Sundermann EE, Maki P, Biegon A, et al. Sex-specific norms for verbal memory tests may improve diagnostic accuracy of amnestic MCI. Neurology 2019;93(20): e1881–9.
36. Sano M, Gandy S. Sex differences in cognition. Does the "fairer sex" need a fairer test? Neurology 2016;86(15):1364–5.

37. Biegon A, Sundermann E. Considering Biological Sex in Neurological Research. Front Neurol 2021;12:1139.
38. Şahin Ö, Soylu Yalcinkaya N. The Gendered Brain: Implications of Exposure to Neuroscience Research for Gender Essentialist Beliefs. Sex Roles 2021; 84(9–10):522–35.
39. Anstey KJ, Peters R, Mortby ME, et al. Association of sex differences in dementia risk factors with sex differences in memory decline in a population-based cohort spanning 20–76 years. Sci Rep 2021;11(1). https://doi.org/10.1038/s41598-021-86397-7.
40. Lipnicki DM, Crawford JD, Dutta R, et al. Age-related cognitive decline and associations with sex, education and apolipoprotein E genotype across ethnocultural groups and geographic regions: a collaborative cohort study. PLoS Med 2017; 14(3):e1002261.
41. Pa J, Aslanyan V, Casaletto KB, et al. Effects of Sex, APOE4, and Lifestyle Activities on Cognitive Reserve in Older Adults. Neurology 2022. https://doi.org/10.1212/wnl.0000000000200675.
42. Lohner V, Pehlivan G, Sanroma G, et al. The Relation Between Sex, Menopause, and White Matter Hyperintensities: The Rhineland Study. Neurology 2022. https://doi.org/10.1212/wnl.0000000000200782.
43. Utian WH. Psychosocial and socioeconomic burden of vasomotor symptoms in menopause: A comprehensive review. Health Qual Life Outcome 2005;3(1):47.
44. Curtis AF, Masellis M, Camicioli R, et al. Cognitive profile of non-demented Parkinson's disease: Meta-analysis of domain and sex-specific deficits. Parkinsonism Relat Disord 2019;60:32–42.
45. Cholerton B, Johnson CO, Fish B, et al. Sex differences in progression to mild cognitive impairment and dementia in Parkinson's disease. Park Relat Disord 2018;50:29–36.
46. Tipton PW, Bülbül N, Crook J, et al. Effects of sex and APOE on Parkinson's Disease-related cognitive decline. Neurol Neurochir Pol 2021;55(6):559–66.
47. Hentosh S, Zhu L, Patino J, et al. Sex Differences in Huntington's Disease: Evaluating the <scp>Enroll-HD</scp> Database. Movement Disorders Clinical Practice 2021;8(3):420–6.
48. Illán-Gala I, Casaletto KB, Borrego-Écija S, et al. Sex differences in the behavioral variant of frontotemporal dementia: A new window to executive and behavioral reserve. Alzheimer's Dementia 2021;17(8):1329–41.
49. Gupte R, Brooks W, Vukas R, et al. Sex Differences in Traumatic Brain Injury: What We Know and What We Should Know. J Neurotrauma 2019;36(22):3063–91.
50. Sundermann EE, Heaton RK, Pasipanodya E, et al. Sex differences in HIV-associated cognitive impairment. Aids 2018;32(18):2719–26.
51. Putatunda R, Zhang Y, Li F, et al. Sex-specific neurogenic deficits and neurocognitive disorders in middle-aged HIV-1 Tg26 transgenic mice. Brain Behav Immun 2019;80:488–99.
52. Malorni W. The Long COVID: a new challenge for gender-specific medicine? Italian Journal of Gender-Specific Medicine 2021;7(2):59–60.
53. Jensen A, Castro AW, Ferretti MT, et al. Sex and gender differences in the neurological and neuropsychiatric symptoms of long COVID: a narrative review. Italian Journal of Gender-Specific Medicine 2022;8(1):18–28.
54. Sykes DL, Holdsworth L, Jawad N, et al. Post-COVID-19 Symptom Burden: What is Long-COVID and How Should We Manage It? Lung 2021;199(2):113–9.
55. Matta J, Wiernik E, Robineau O, et al. Association of Self-reported COVID-19 Infection and SARS-CoV-2 Serology Test Results With Persistent Physical

Symptoms Among French Adults During the COVID-19 Pandemic. JAMA Intern Med 2022;182(1):19.
56. Bölte S, Duketis E, Poustka F, et al. Sex differences in cognitive domains and their clinical correlates in higher-functioning autism spectrum disorders. Autism 2011; 15(4):497–511.
57. Howlin P, Goode S, Hutton J, et al. Adult outcome for children with autism. JCPP (J Child Psychol Psychiatry) 2004;45(2):212–29.
58. Holtmann M, Bölte S, Poustka F. Autism spectrum disorders: Sex differences in autistic behaviour domains and coexisting psychopathology. Dev Med Child Neurol 2007;49(5):361–6.
59. van Schalkwyk GI, Klingensmith K, Volkmar FR. Gender identity and autism spectrum disorders. Yale J Biol Med 2015;88(1):81–3.
60. Loyer Carbonneau M, Demers M, Bigras M, et al. Meta-Analysis of Sex Differences in ADHD Symptoms and Associated Cognitive Deficits. J Atten Disord 2021;25(12):1640–56.
61. Williamson D, Johnston C. Gender differences in adults with attention-deficit/hyperactivity disorder: A narrative review. Clin Psychol Rev 2015;40:15–27.
62. Ayesa-Arriola R, Setién-Suero E, Neergaard KD, et al. Premorbid IQ subgroups in first episode non affective psychosis patients: Long-term sex differences in function and neurocognition. Schizophr Res 2018;197:370–7.
63. Navarra-Ventura G, Fernandez-Gonzalo S, Turon M, et al. Gender Differences in Social Cognition: A Cross-Sectional Pilot Study of Recently Diagnosed Patients with Schizophrenia and Healthy Subjects. Can J Psychiatr 2018;63(8):538–46.
64. Roberts AL, Liu J, Lawn RB, et al. Association of Posttraumatic Stress Disorder With Accelerated Cognitive Decline in Middle-aged Women. JAMA Netw Open 2022;5(6):e2217698.
65. Sargent K. Intersecting and Multiple Identities in Behavioral Health. In: Benuto L, Duckworth M, Masuda A, O'Donohue W, editors. Prejudice, Stigma, Privilege, and Oppression. Cham: Springer; 2020.
66. Singer M, Bulled N, Ostrach B, et al. Syndemics and the biosocial conception of health. Lancet 2017/03/04/2017;389(10072):941–50.
67. Singer M, Singer M. Brain Syndemics: Cognitive Deficit, Pathways of Interaction, and the Biology of Inequality. Neurol Neurobiol 2021;1–12. https://doi.org/10.31487/j.nnb.2021.02.03.
68. Duchesne A, Kaiser Trujillo A. Reflections on Neurofeminism and Intersectionality Using Insights From Psychology. Review. Front Hum Neurosci 2021;2021:15.

Sex and Gender Differences in Parkinson's Disease

Roshni Patel, MD, MS[a,b,*], Katie Kompoliti, MD[a]

KEYWORDS

• Parkinson's disease • Sex • Gender • Disparities • Movement disorders

KEY POINTS

- Biological, hormonal, and environmental factors may underlie the epidemiological differences in Parkinson's disease (PD) between sexes.
- Estrogen may have neuroprotective properties, although the therapeutic value of hormone therapy in PD is unclear.
- Motor and nonmotor symptoms of PD differ between sexes.
- Women with PD experience disparities in care including undertreatment with deep brain stimulation and less access to caregiving.
- Less information is known about PD in sexual and gender minorities, and more studies are needed in this area.

INTRODUCTION

Parkinson's disease (PD) is the second most common neurodegenerative disease affecting older adults, and it is approximately twice as common in males compared with females.[1] Reasons underlying the epidemiologic difference between sexes are unknown, although they may be related to biological, environmental, and cultural factors, which we will explore in this article. The clinical differences in PD presentation, characteristics, and progression between sexes will also be reviewed. Finally, we will discuss gender-based disparities in PD and address the paucity of literature about PD in gender-diverse people. For the purposes of this article, sex will refer to a biological characterization with categories of male or female, and gender will refer to a social construction with categories of man or woman.[2]

[a] Rush University Medical Center, 725 West Harrison Street, Suite 755, Chicago, IL, USA; [b] Jesse Brown VA Medical Center, 8542 Damen Pavillion, 820 South Damen Avenue, Chicago, IL 60642, USA

* Corresponding author. Jesse Brown VA Medical Center, 820 S Damen Avenue. Chicago, IL 60612.

E-mail address: Roshnipatel1988@gmail.com

Neurol Clin 41 (2023) 371–379
https://doi.org/10.1016/j.ncl.2022.12.001
0733-8619/23/Published by Elsevier Inc.

The Role of Estrogen in Parkinson's Disease

Hormones, particularly estrogen, may explain some of the sex differences in PD. It is thought that estrogen may have a neuroprotective effect on the brain, although the mechanisms are not entirely understood. Animal studies have demonstrated that estradiol increases the synthesis, release, reuptake, and turnover of dopamine.[1] Estrogen may also protect against oxidative stress, and it may have anti-inflammatory properties.[1] In rat models, estradiol has been shown to promote nigrostriatal dopaminergic neuron survival and mediate adaptive response in surviving neurons. In addition to the possible neuroprotective effects of estrogen, physiologic differences between males and females may exist. For example, females may have a higher ratio of dopamine receptor 1 to dopamine receptor 2 in the striatum,[1] as well as sex differences in the nigrostriatal circuitry.[3]

Estrogen may play a role in modifying PD risk, although the evidence is inconsistent. Lifetime endogenous estrogen exposure can be estimated using factors such as reproductive window and fertility. Some epidemiological studies have suggested that greater age at menopause is associated with reduced PD risk,[4,5] although others have suggested no change in risk.[6–8] Greater fertile life duration and number of pregnancies may be associated with delayed age of PD onset.[5,9] Case-control studies have shown that bilateral oophorectomy[10] and hysterectomy with or without oophorectomy[11] may be associated with an increased risk of PD, which may further suggest a protective role of endogenous estrogen. Interestingly, tamoxifen—an estrogen receptor modulator with agonist action in endometrium, antagonist action in breast and presumed agonist action in the nigrostriatal region—was associated with an increased risk of PD when used by female patients with breast cancer.[12] Common estrogen receptor gene polymorphisms do not seem to contribute to PD susceptibility, although further investigation is needed.[13]

The role of exogenous estrogen in modifying PD risk is also unclear, although it may have some potential. Some observational studies describe a reduced risk of PD with oral contraceptive use,[7] whereas others describe an increased risk[14] or no effect on risk.[15] Type of estrogen may be relevant, with esterified estrogen used in combination with progestin possibly associated with increased PD risk, and no risk associated with conjugated estrogen with progestin.[16] Postmenopausal estrogen may be associated with reduced risk of PD,[8,10,17] although reports are similarly inconsistent.[7,10] Lifetime estrogen exposure may also modify progressive supranuclear palsy risk.[18] Type of estrogen, concomitant progesterone use, dose, duration, and timing of administration varies across a person's reproductive life, which likely accounts for inconsistencies in epidemiological reports. Additional factors include differences in study design and study populations with differing genetic and environmental risk factors.

Estrogen may influence nonmotor symptoms in PD. Patients with low lifetime estrogen exposure had lower dopamine transport availability in the posterior and ventral putamen and required greater changes in monthly levodopa equivalent dose.[19] In a cross-sectional study of nursing home patients with PD, exogenous estrogen use was associated with less cognitive impairment and greater functional independence, although interestingly it was also associated with higher rates of depression.[20] A pilot randomized controlled trial in postmenopausal women with advanced PD demonstrated that estrogen replacement therapy for 8 weeks was safe and well-tolerated, although larger and longer studies are required to understand the effect of estrogen in PD, as well as navigate the complex risk/benefit profile.[21] Indeed, the thrombotic and neoplastic risks of exogenous estrogen may limit its therapeutic value.

Sex Differences in Parkinson's Disease Presentation and Progression

PD prevalence and incidence is higher in males compared with females.[1,22] The sex difference in PD prevalence may be more pronounced in early age groups[23] and may be similar between males and females in advanced age.[24,25] Interestingly, the sex-effect may be lost in genetic cohorts of PD, such as leucine-rich repeat kinase 2 (LRRK2)-associated PD, the most common monogenic form of PD[26] Abnormalities in the LRRK2 protein may cause neurodegeneration through its kinase activity, as well as have downstream effects on alpha-synuclein and neuroinflammation, and *LRRK2* mutation seems to have an equal sex distribution.[26,27] Risk factors for PD may differ between sexes with females having higher rate of coffee consumption (protective factor) and lower rates of head trauma and pesticide exposure (risk factors), and anemia—thought to be a PD risk factor—is more common in females.[28]

Some studies report a delayed age of onset of PD in female patients,[29] yet others report no sex difference.[30] Early motor progression may be similar between sexes,[30,31] although one cohort demonstrated female patients with PD are more likely to develop motor fluctuations within the first year of initiating dopaminergic therapy.[32] Interestingly, female sex was found to be a protective factor for freezing of gait in a longitudinal study of patients with de novo PD[33] but in a meta-analysis, which included PD patients in all disease stages, sex was not a predictor of freezing of gait, although the authors noted that females were markedly underrepresented in intervention trials.[34] Another study reported female sex as risk factor for falling.[35] When adjusted for sex-specific mortality in the general population, mortality among females with PD is similar to or greater than that of males,[24] and survival of males with PD has improved in recent years without similar improvement in females with PD.[36] Medical comorbidities can contribute to symptom burden and functional status. Among a large cohort of Medicare beneficiaries, female patients with PD were found to have higher rates of hip fracture, osteoporosis, and arthritis compared with male counterparts, although this was not associated with a change in survival.[37] Due to the biologic and physiologic differences between sexes, as well as the differences in PD motor manifestations, it has been suggested that physical therapy—a mainstay in the treatment of PD—should be prescribed differently for male and female patients. For example, due to higher prevalence of osteoporosis among female patients with PD, appropriate aerobic and resistance exercises should be used to improve mineral bone density.[38]

Regarding dopaminergic medication, females are more like to develop levodopa-induced dyskinesias and motor fluctuations.[32,39] Pharmacokinetics may account for some of these differences; for example, females achieved a higher maximum plasma concentration of levodopa compared with males in a small cohort of levodopa-naive patients[40] but further pharmacologic investigations are needed. Other factors such as absorption and body mass index may also influence levodopa bioavailability.[41] Impulse control disorders, a common complication of dopamine agonist medication, may also differ between sexes, with males more likely to develop sexual behavior and females more likely to develop compulsive shopping.[42]

In terms of nonmotor symptoms of PD, female patients report higher rates of fatigue, depression, anxiety, constipation, restless leg syndrome and pain,[37,43] and lower rates of anosmia, autonomic dysfunction, apathy, and rapid eye movement sleep behavior disorder.[22,44,45] Self-reported quality of life and psychological distress were worse among female patients with PD.[31] Interestingly, patient-reported disability—but not physician-reported disability—was worse among female patients with PD at initial PD care visit compared with male patients with PD,[31] suggesting a mismatch between patient and provider perspectives. In contrast, female patients with PD in an Australian cohort had less motor symptom burden, better quality of life, and less caregiver reliance compared with male patients with PD after matching for disease duration.[46] There may be gender differences in illness narratives in PD, with women emphasizing the impact of ON/OFF state, "thinking problems" and ability to fulfill domestic responsibilities, and men emphasizing the consequences on their physical appearance and social isolation.[47]

Cognitive profiles differ between sexes in PD. Female patients with PD are generally reported to have less cognitive impairment,[30,48,49] although this has not been consistent across studies.[50] There may be domain-specific sex differences in PD, with female patients having better frontal executive, memory and visuospatial performance compared with male patients.[51,52] In the Parkinson's Progression Markers Initiative, a cohort of patients with de novo PD, male participants had greater generalized brain atrophy and disrupted connectivity on diffusion-weighted MRI compared with female participants. And there were sex differences in focal cortical atrophy patterns, with females having greater atrophy in the left frontal lobe, right parietal lobe, left insular gyrus and right occipital cortex; and males having greater atrophy in bilateral frontal and left insular lobes, right postcentral gyrus, left inferior temporal and cingulate gyrus, and left thalamus.[53] In summary, female patients with PD may experience less global impairment compared with male patients with PD, and sexes differ in terms of brain atrophy and connectivity, as well as, performance within specific domains.

Disparities in Care

Gender-based disparities in PD can be seen in health-care utilization, treatment, and caregiving. Female patients with PD had less outpatient physician contact and higher nursing home and skilled nursing facility utilization compared with male patients with PD.[37] Furthermore, women with PD had a delay in diagnosis and delay in specialist referral compared with men with PD.[54] Exercise patterns may also be different between men and women with PD, which may be explained in part by differences in motivation. For example, one study reported that level of physical activity was explained by the enjoyment of physical activity in women with PD, whereas self-efficacy explained the level of physical activity among men.[55]

In terms of treatment, several studies have demonstrated that women with PD are under-treated with deep brain stimulation (DBS).[56,57] Reasons for this are complex and likely multifactorial. One study cited "personal preference" as reason for female patients with PD declining surgery.[57] In a qualitative study in which DBS candidates were interviewed, women expressed fear of complications more frequently and were more likely to consult friends and relatives before deciding about DBS.[58] Interestingly, one study found that women with PD were underrepresented in DBS referrals but were more likely to be approved for DBS compared with men with PD and had longer disease duration and worse dyskinesia at time of DBS evaluation.[56] Future studies should investigate methods for increasing earlier DBS referrals among women with PD, as well as optimizing patient–provider communication to facilitate decision-making.

In general, women with PD have less caregiver support compared with men. Among homebound participants with PD in an interdisciplinary home visit program, women were more likely to live alone and have no caregiver.[59] In a large longitudinal cohort of participants with PD, women were less likely to have a caregiver compared with men, and were less likely to be accompanied by caregiver at baseline visit. Women had a faster rate to use paid caregiver after controlling for confounders.[60] Future efforts should aim to improve access to caregiving for women with PD.

Women are underrepresented in clinical trials, out of proportion to the sex-based difference in PD prevalence.[61] This may be partially explained by delays in diagnosis and lower referral rate to specialty centers, as well as lack of a caregiver who would help navigate and facilitate the rigors of a clinical trial. Nonetheless, it is important for research consortia to foster diverse recruitment.[62] Recent efforts have been made to innovate recruitment strategies to increase diversity in participation in PD research, such as targeted digital outreach and promotion,[63] and using remote decentralized study designs.[64]

Parkinson's Disease in Gender Diverse People

Unfortunately, very less is known about PD in gender diverse individuals.[65] In general, sexual and gender minorities (SGM) experience inequalities in health care due to discrimination and social and economic marginalization, yet we have few studies about this vulnerable population in neurology.[66] One of the barriers to studying this population is the absence of systematic collection of sexual orientation and gender identity in electronic health records.[67] In a sample of patients from an academic movement disorders center, less than half had sexual orientation or gender identity documented in their chart. Of the patients with documentation available, 4.3% identified as SGM.[68] There are many unanswered questions about SGM PD care, including understanding their access to care, psychosocial factors, caregiver and support systems, and more. Long-term health effects associated with gender-affirming hormone therapies, and their impact on PD risk needs to be delineated. Finally, efforts should be made to improve cultural competency among medical providers and staff to create welcoming environments for their SGM patients.[65]

SUMMARY

The lower prevalence of PD in females is not well understood but may be partially explained by sex differences in nigrostriatal circuitry and possible neuroprotective effects of estrogen. PD motor and nonmotor symptoms differ between sexes, and women experience disparities in care including undertreatment with DBS and less access to caregiving. Our knowledge about PD in gender diverse individuals is limited. Future studies should improve our understanding of the role of hormone replacement therapy in PD, address gender-based inequities in PD care and expand our understanding of PD in SGM and marginalized communities.

CLINICS CARE POINTS

- Female PD patients may develop dyskinesias and motor fluctuations earlier in the disease course, thus should be referred for specialty care and considered for deep brain stimulation when appropriate.
- It is important to treat non-motor symptoms in PD, and female patients may have higher rates of depression, anxiety, fatigue, restless leg syndrome and pain. Though cognitive impairment, autonomimc dysfunction and REM behavior disorder are less common in females, it is still important to screen for these as well.
- Ask female patients with PD about caregiver access and support system, and refer for social work services as appropriate.
- Consider developing a standard process for documenting sexual orientation and gender identity in your electronic health record, to increase recognition of sexual and gender minority populations.

DISCLOSURES AND FUNDING

The authors do not have any commercial or financial conflicts of interest pertinent to the content of this article. No funding was received for this study.

R. Patel has received funding from the Department of Veterans Affairs Center for Innovation for Complex Chronic Healthcare. K. Kompoliti is a consultant to Neurocrine, Kyowa, Amneal, Revance, and Lundbeck and an investigator for Lundbeck, Neurocrine, Emalex, Theravance, Pharma 2B, and Sun pharma.

REFERENCES

1. Cerri S, Mus L, Blandini F. Parkinson's disease in women and men: what's the difference? J Parkinson's Dis 2019;9(3):501.
2. Clayton JA, Tannenbaum C. Reporting sex, gender, or both in clinical research? JAMA 2016;316(18):1863–4.
3. Gillies GE, McArthur S. Independent influences of sex steroids of systemic and central origin in a rat model of Parkinson's disease: a contribution to sex-specific neuroprotection by estrogens. Horm Behav 2010;57(1):23–34.
4. Kusters CDJ, Paul KC, Duarte Folle A, et al. Increased menopausal age reduces the risk of parkinson's disease: a mendelian randomization approach. Mov Disord 2021;36(10):2264–72.
5. Yadav R, Shukla G, Goyal V, et al. A case control study of women with Parkinson's disease and their fertility characteristics. J Neurol Sci 2012;319(1–2):135–8.
6. Nicoletti A, Nicoletti G, Arabia G, et al. Reproductive factors and Parkinson's disease: a multicenter case-control study. Mov Disord 2011;26(14):2563–6.
7. Liu R, Baird D, Park Y, et al. Female reproductive factors, menopausal hormone use, and Parkinson's disease. Mov Disord 2014;29(7):889–96.
8. Currie LJ, Harrison MB, Trugman JM, et al. Postmenopausal estrogen use affects risk for Parkinson disease. Arch Neurol 2004;61(6):886–8.
9. Ragonese P, D'Amelio M, Callari G, et al. Age at menopause predicts age at onset of Parkinson's disease. Mov Disord 2006;21(12):2211–4.
10. Canonico M, Pesce G, Bonaventure A, et al. Increased risk of parkinson's disease in women after bilateral oophorectomy. Mov Disord 2021;36(7):1696–700.
11. Benedetti MD, Maraganore DM, Bower JH, et al. Hysterectomy, menopause, and estrogen use preceding Parkinson's disease: an exploratory case-control study. Mov Disord 2001;16(5):830–7.
12. Avram CM, Brumbach BH, Hiller AL. A report of tamoxifen and parkinson's disease in a US population and a review of the literature. Mov Disord 2021;36(5): 1238–42.
13. Maraganore DM, Farrer MJ, McDonnell SK, et al. Case-control study of estrogen receptor gene polymorphisms in Parkinson's disease. Movement Disord 2002; 17(3):509–12.
14. Yoo JE, Shin DW, Jang W, et al. Female reproductive factors and the risk of Parkinson's disease: a nationwide cohort study. Eur J Epidemiol 2020;35(9):871–8.
15. Lv M, Zhang Y, Chen GC, et al. Reproductive factors and risk of Parkinson's disease in women: a meta-analysis of observational studies. Behav Brain Res 2017; 335:103–10.
16. Lundin JI, Ton TGN, LaCroix AZ, et al. Formulations of hormone therapy and risk of Parkinson disease. Mov Disord 2014;29(13):1631–6.
17. Song YJ, ran Li S, wan Li X, et al. The Effect of estrogen replacement therapy on alzheimer's disease and parkinson's disease in postmenopausal women: a meta-analysis. Front Neurosci 2020;14:157.

18. Park HK, Ilango S, Charriez CM, et al. Lifetime exposure to estrogen and progressive supranuclear palsy: ENGENE-PSP study. Mov Disord 2018;33(3):468–72.
19. Lee YH, Cha J, Chung SJ, et al. Beneficial effect of estrogen on nigrostriatal dopaminergic neurons in drug-naïve postmenopausal Parkinson's disease. Sci Rep 2019;9(1):10531.
20. Fernandez HH, Lapane KL. Estrogen use among nursing home residents with a diagnosis of Parkinson's disease. Mov Disord 2000;15(6):1119–24.
21. Parkinson Study Group POETRY Investigators. A randomized pilot trial of estrogen replacement therapy in post-menopausal women with Parkinson's disease. Parkinsonism Relat Disord 2011;17(10):757–60.
22. Georgiev D, Hamberg K, Hariz M, et al. Gender differences in Parkinson's disease: a clinical perspective. Acta Neurol Scand 2017;136(6):570–84.
23. Pringsheim T, Jette N, Frolkis A, et al. The prevalence of Parkinson's disease: a systematic review and meta-analysis. Mov Disord 2014;29(13):1583–90.
24. Brakedal B, Toker L, Haugarvoll K, et al. A nationwide study of the incidence, prevalence and mortality of Parkinson's disease in the Norwegian population. Npj Parkinsons Dis 2022;8(1):1–8.
25. Moisan F, Kab S, Mohamed F, et al. Parkinson disease male-to-female ratios increase with age: french nationwide study and meta-analysis. J Neurol Neurosurg Psychiatr 2016;87(9):952–7.
26. Gan-Or Z, Leblond CS, Mallett V, et al. LRRK2 mutations in Parkinson disease; a sex effect or lack thereof? A meta-analysis. Parkinsonism Relat Disord 2015; 21(7):778–82.
27. Rui Q, Ni H, Li D, et al. The role of LRRK2 in neurodegeneration of parkinson disease. Curr Neuropharmacol 2018;16(9):1348–57.
28. Savica R, Grossardt BR, Bower JH, et al. Risk factors for Parkinson's disease may differ in men and women: An exploratory study. Horm Behav 2013;63(2):308–14.
29. Haaxma CA, Bloem BR, Borm GF, et al. Gender differences in Parkinson's disease. J Neurol Neurosurg Psychiatr 2007;78(8):819–24.
30. Augustine EF, Pérez A, Dhall R, et al. Sex Differences in Clinical Features of Early, Treated Parkinson's Disease. PLoS One 2015;10(7):e0133002.
31. Abraham DS, Gruber-Baldini AL, Magder LS, et al. Sex differences in Parkinson's disease presentation and progression. Parkinsonism Relat Disord 2019;69: 48–54.
32. Colombo D, Abbruzzese G, Antonini A, et al. The "gender factor" in wearing-off among patients with Parkinson's disease: a post hoc analysis of DEEP study. ScientificWorldJournal 2015;2015:787451.
33. Kim R, Lee J, Kim Y, et al. Presynaptic striatal dopaminergic depletion predicts the later development of freezing of gait in de novo Parkinson's disease: an analysis of the PPMI cohort. Parkinsonism Relat Disord 2018;51:49–54.
34. Tosserams A, Mazaheri M, Vart P, et al. Sex and freezing of gait in Parkinson's disease: a systematic review and meta-analysis. J Neurol 2021;268(1):125–32.
35. Parashos SA, Bloem BR, Browner NM, et al. What predicts falls in Parkinson disease? Neurol Clin Pract 2018;8(3):214–22.
36. Kuusimäki T, Kurki S, Sipilä JOT, et al. Sex-dependent improvement in survival of parkinson's disease patients. Mov Disord Clin Pract 2020;7(5):516–20.
37. Fullard ME, Thibault DP, Todaro V, et al. Sex disparities in health and health care utilization after Parkinson diagnosis: rethinking PD associated disability. Parkinsonism Relat Disord 2018;48:45–50.
38. Rigby BR, Davis RW. Should exercise be prescribed differently between women and men? An emphasis on women diagnosed with parkinson's disease. Front

Physiol 2018;9. Available at: https://www.frontiersin.org/articles/10.3389/fphys.2018.01040. Accessed July 31, 2022.
39. Zappia M, Annesi G, Nicoletti G, et al. Sex differences in clinical and genetic determinants of levodopa peak-dose dyskinesias in Parkinson disease: an exploratory study. Arch Neurol 2005;62(4):601–5.
40. Conti V, Izzo V, Russillo MC, et al. Gender differences in levodopa pharmacokinetics in levodopa-naïve patients with parkinson's disease. Front Med 2022;9. Available at: https://www.frontiersin.org/articles/10.3389/fmed.2022.909936. Accessed December 12, 2022..
41. Bachmann CG, Zapf A, Brunner E, et al. Dopaminergic treatment is associated with decreased body weight in patients with Parkinson's disease and dyskinesias. Eur J Neurol 2009;16(8):895–901.
42. Weintraub D, Claassen DO. Impulse control and related disorders in parkinson's disease. Int Rev Neurobiol 2017;133:679–717.
43. Martinez-Martin P, Falup Pecurariu C, Odin P, et al. Gender-related differences in the burden of non-motor symptoms in Parkinson's disease. J Neurol 2012;259(8):1639–47.
44. Solla P, Masala C, Liscia A, et al. Sex-related differences in olfactory function and evaluation of possible confounding factors among patients with Parkinson's disease. J Neurol 2020;267(1):57–63.
45. Ou R, Lin J, Liu K, et al. Evolution of apathy in early parkinson's disease: a 4-years prospective cohort study. Front Aging Neurosci 2021;12. Available at: https://www.frontiersin.org/articles/10.3389/fnagi.2020.620762. Accessed August 2, 2022.
46. Lubomski M, Louise Rushworth R, Lee W, et al. Sex differences in Parkinson's disease. J Clin Neurosci 2014;21(9):1503–6.
47. Solimeo S. Sex and gender in older adults' experience of Parkinson's disease. J Gerontol B Psychol Sci Soc Sci 2008;63(1):S42–8.
48. Gonzalez-Latapi P, Bayram E, Litvan I, et al. Cognitive impairment in parkinson's disease: epidemiology, clinical profile, protective and risk factors. Behav Sci (Basel) 2021;11(5):74.
49. Oltra J, Segura B, Uribe C, et al. Sex differences in brain atrophy and cognitive impairment in Parkinson's disease patients with and without probable rapid eye movement sleep behavior disorder. J Neurol 2022;269(3):1591–9.
50. Gao L, Nie K, Tang H, et al. Sex differences in cognition among Chinese people with Parkinson's disease. J Clin Neurosci 2015;22(3):488–92.
51. Liu R, Umbach DM, Peddada SD, et al. Potential sex differences in nonmotor symptoms in early drug-naive Parkinson disease. Neurology 2015;84(21):2107–15.
52. Curtis AF, Masellis M, Camicioli R, et al. Cognitive profile of non-demented Parkinson's disease: Meta-analysis of domain and sex-specific deficits. Parkinsonism Relat Disord 2019;60:32–42.
53. Tremblay C, Abbasi N, Zeighami Y, et al. Sex effects on brain structure in de novo Parkinson's disease: a multimodal neuroimaging study. Brain 2020;143(10):3052–66.
54. Saunders-Pullman R, Wang C, Stanley K, et al. Diagnosis and Referral Delay in Women With Parkinson's Disease. Gend Med 2011;8(3):209–17.
55. Urell C, Zetterberg L, Hellström K, et al. Factors explaining physical activity level in Parkinson's disease: A gender focus. Physiother Theor Pract 2021;37(4):507–16.
56. Jost ST, Strobel L, Rizos A, et al. Gender gap in deep brain stimulation for Parkinson's disease. NPJ Parkinsons Dis 2022;8:47.

57. Shpiner DS, Di Luca DG, Cajigas I, et al. Gender Disparities in Deep Brain Stimulation for Parkinson's Disease. Neuromodulation 2019;22(4):484–8.
58. Hamberg K, Hariz GM. The decision-making process leading to deep brain stimulation in men and women with parkinson's disease – an interview study. BMC Neurol 2014;14:89.
59. Nwabuobi L, Barbosa W, Sweeney M, et al. Sex-related differences in homebound advanced Parkinson's disease patients. Clin Interv Aging 2019;14:1371–7.
60. Dahodwala N, Shah K, He Y, et al. Sex disparities in access to caregiving in Parkinson disease. Neurology 2018;90(1):e48–54.
61. Tosserams A, Araújo R, Pringsheim T, et al. Underrepresentation of women in Parkinson's disease trials. Movement Disord 2018;33(11):1825–6.
62. Subramanian I, Mathur S, Oosterbaan A, et al. Unmet needs of women living with parkinson's disease: gaps and controversies. Movement Disord 2022;37(3):444–55.
63. Dobkin RD, Amondikar N, Kopil C, et al. Innovative recruitment strategies to increase diversity of participation in parkinson's disease research: the fox insight cohort experience. J Parkinsons Dis 2020;10(2):665–75.
64. Myers TL, Augustine EF, Baloga E, et al. Recruitment for remote decentralized studies in parkinson's disease. J Parkinsons Dis 2022;12(1):371–80.
65. Lin CYR, Rosendale N, Deeb W. Expanding sexual and gender minority research in movement disorders: More than awareness and acceptance. Parkinsonism Relat Disord 2021;87:162–5.
66. Rosendale N, Wong JO, Flatt JD, et al. Sexual and gender minority health in neurology: a scoping review. JAMA Neurol 2021;78(6):747–54.
67. Baker KE, Streed CG, Durso LE. Ensuring That LGBTQI+ People Count - Collecting Data on Sexual Orientation, Gender Identity, and Intersex Status. N Engl J Med 2021;384(13):1184–6.
68. Patel RA, Stebbins G, Witek N. Sexual orientation and gender identity documentation at an academic movement disorders neurology clinic. Clin Park Relat Disord 2022;7:100164.

Autism in Women

Cesar Ochoa-Lubinoff, MD, MPH[a,*], Bridget A. Makol, PhD[b], Emily F. Dillon, PhD[c]

KEYWORDS

• Female autism • Autism spectrum disorder • Sex differences • Male bias

KEY POINTS

- Autism has long been considered a predominantly male disorder, which may affect identification and diagnosis of women on the spectrum.
- Women with autism may have differences in autism spectrum disorder (ASD) symptom expression compared to men due to social and biological differences and therefore not follow the prototypical male profile of ASD symptoms.
- Women on the spectrum have a unique profile with often more subtle presentations, greater number of co-occurring conditions and later diagnosis, resulting in less access to interventions and support.
- We recommend that clinicians have a higher index of suspicion for ASD in women and provide referrals for psychological diagnostic evaluations, to help support their clinical needs.

According to the Diagnostic and Statistical Manual of Mental Disorders, Fifth Edition classification, autism spectrum disorder (ASD) is a set of behaviorally defined brain-based conditions characterized by social communication impairments and restricted repetitive patterns of interest and behavior (RRBs).[1] ASD is a heterogeneous condition with a wide range of cognitive abilities from intellectual disability (ID) to giftedness, core language abilities from typical or advanced to nonverbal, and motor coordination abilities from typical to motor apraxia. ASD is frequently accompanied by medical and mental health comorbidities such as epilepsy, feeding disorders, constipation, attention-deficit hyperactivity disorder (ADHD), anxiety, and depression, which have the potential to influence ASD presentations. ASD has been reported as more prevalent in men than women since originally described.[2,3] Importantly, the wide variation in symptom expression of ASD and nature of a behavior-defined condition without biomarkers creates diagnostic and treatment challenges, resulting in lower identification and access to services groups with less prototypical autism presentations, particularly for women.

[a] Rush University Medical Center, 1725 West Harrison Street, Suite 710, Chicago, IL 60612, USA; [b] Rush University Medical Center, 1653 West Congress Parkway, 12 Kellogg, Chicago, IL 60612, USA; [c] Rush University Medical Center, 1645 West Jackson Boulevard, Chicago, IL 60612, USA
* Corresponding author.
E-mail address: cesar_ochoa-lubinoff@rush.edu

Neurol Clin 41 (2023) 381–397
https://doi.org/10.1016/j.ncl.2022.10.006

neurologic.theclinics.com

In recent decades, there has been a steady increase in the prevalence of ASD in the United States and the rest of the world.[4,5] Over a hundred genes have been identified in the expression of autism,[6] but no evidence suggests that autism should be more prevalent in specific racial or ethnic groups. The most recent composite Autism and Developmental Disabilities Monitoring Network prevalence estimate (1.85%), using 2016 data, was higher than the previous estimate (1.68%) found using 2014 data.[7] This increased prevalence has led to an explosion of research on autism, ranging from basic science to applied clinical studies. This research has led to more clearly defined diagnostic criteria, better and more systematic diagnostic tools, and broadening of the autism spectrum to include individuals with presentations of high functioning mild ASD and moderate-to-severe ID. The explanation for the global increase in the ASD prevalence is multi-factorial and includes these recent diagnostic changes as well as a significant increase in public and professional awareness and the number of clinicians with expertise in autism diagnosis.

The male-to-female ASD ratio has been reported to be 4 to 5:1 in population prevalence review studies.[8,9] However, the first ASD patient databases and research studies overrepresented men,[10–12] influencing the development of the diagnostic tools and criteria that are used today. The overrepresentation of men in research has reinforced a male bias in the public and even health and school professionals' perception of this condition.[13,14] As discussed in this paper, women with autism can have a different, more subtle, clinical presentation as they may compensate better for their social communication impairments and present with less unusual and intense RRBs.[15,16] As a result, women often have a delayed or missed ASD diagnosis, further increasing the burden of this condition by delaying a diagnostic label that promotes better understanding of ASD-related challenges, reducing access to treatment services, and perpetuating the prevalence gap between men and women. More recent population review studies, which only include studies using high methodological quality with active case ascertainment methods, found lower male-to-female ratios of 3:1[14] or 2.5:1.5 The studies that actively looked for ASD cases, regardless of whether they had already been identified by clinical or educational services, found a lower male-to-female odds ratio of 3.25. The passive studies, which only identify cases that have already been diagnosed, have a larger male-to-female odds ratio of 4.56.[14] One possible explanation for these findings is that there are women in the general population who would meet diagnostic criteria for this condition if evaluated, yet have not been identified due to their unique clinical presentation and the male bias in ASD. These changing ratios may also reflect the broadening of ASD diagnostic criteria over time, allowing more high-functioning women to be identified[17] as well as increasing community awareness and the public health response.[5]

When discussing ASD in females, both biological and sociocultural factors should be considered.[18] Although biological sex is understood as a trait assigned at birth, gender socialization also begins at birth,[19] making it difficult to separate the effects of sex and gender on ASD presentation. Moreover, children typically form their own gender identity between the ages of 3 and 5, meaning that they begin noticing gender socialization and stereotypes in their immediate social contexts at a young age.[19] Importantly, for some children, their gender identity may not match how they are treated and perceived by others. There is very limited research on the effects of biological sex and gender identity on ASD symptoms as separate constructs, or on how ASD symptoms may present in children who fall outside of the "male" and "female" binary. As such, given the scope of this paper, our discussion focuses primarily on individuals who were assigned female sex at birth and who have been socialized to present as female in their sociocultural environments while acknowledging that this is a relatively limited discussion of these concepts. In research cited in this review paper, we describe sex and gender based on how it is reported, including for girls/boys (age 0 to 17) and women/men (age 18 or older). However, studies may have varied in how sex and/or gender was assessed.

The objective of this article is to increase awareness of the male bias in autism and unique sex/gender clinical presentations that contribute to women having a delayed or missed ASD diagnosis. Biological and sociocultural factors contributing to the male/female gap in autism will be explored. Finally, the importance of a timely diagnosis in women is discussed as well as strategies that clinicians can use to promote earlier identification and access to treatment of women with ASD.

NEUROBIOLOGICAL FACTORS

Sex differences in autism provide an opportunity to study causal mechanisms and etiologic models for this heterogeneous condition. At the biological level, sex differentiation originates from the interplay of genetic variations, prenatal environments, and epigenetic effects,[20] all of which are candidate mechanisms for the sex-differential liability of autism.[17,21] The main theoretic models that attempt to explain sexual dimorphism in ASD and the evidence supporting them are presented in this section. These models are unable to explain all sex characteristics and differences and can be seen as complementary to each other.

Extreme Male Brain Theory

The extreme male brain (EMB) theory is an extension of the empathizing-systemizing (E-S) theory of typical sex differences.[22] The E-S theory proposes that, on average, women have a stronger drive to empathize (ie, identify and respond to another person's mental state), whereas men have a stronger drive to systemize (ie, analyze or build a rule-based system). According to the EMB theory, men and women with ASD manifest an extreme profile of the typical male E-S dimensions and a more "masculine" brain type.[23] Further, men may need smaller psychological and physiologic changes to present with ASD than women, potentially explaining sex differences in prevalence rates.

Neuroimaging studies identifying anatomic and functional "male brain" patterns in men and women with ASD provide support for this theory. Infant males on average have a larger brain than females[24] and children with autism tend to have even larger brains early in life.[25] The amygdala in typical control (TC) men tends to be larger than in TC females.[26] Males and female toddlers with ASD have a larger amygdala than TC males.[27] Ypma and colleagues,[28] identified the "male brain" pattern using resting-state functional connectivity, in which TC females had an increased DMN connectivity compared with control males and all study participants with ASD. A functional brain connectivity study demonstrated that women and men with ASD tended to follow the typical male pattern of developmental changes in interhemispheric connectivity.[29]

Steroid hormones and their receptors can act as epigenetic fetal programming influences on early brain development. Through their nuclear hormone receptors, steroids can alter gene expression via direct or indirect influence on multiple epigenetic processes.[30] Animal studies have confirmed that early exposure to androgens (eg, testosterone) has a long-lasting impact in the developing brain, causing sex differences in its anatomy and function and leading to differences in cognition and behavior.[31] Human men present three surges of testosterone levels during life:

between 8 to 24 weeks of gestation reaching puberty levels,[32] soon after birth until 4 to 6 months of age when testosterone levels become undetectable,[33] and puberty. The sex differences in fetal androgen levels have been well documented through amniotic fluid studies.[34] In the Danish Historic Birth cohort study of amniotic fluid samples, increased testosterone and other steroidogenic activity was demonstrated during fetal development for men that were later diagnosed with ASD.[35] Another study found that boys and girls who had been exposed to high levels of testosterone in utero had social, communication, and play patterns commonly associated with ASD.[36]

Female Protective Effect

The multiple threshold liability or female protective model states that multiple genetic factors contribute to the presence of ASD, resulting in a higher genetic threshold for women to manifest ASD relative to men.[37–39] The fact that men show higher rates of ASD than women,[37] and the greater risk of ASD for siblings and co-twins of women with ASD than siblings and co-twins of men with ASD[37,40] supports this theory.

Neuroimaging studies show greater changes in brain anatomy and function among women with ASD compared with female TCs relative to men with similar levels of ASD compared with male TCs. A study using diffusion tensor imaging found that girls and young women with ASD showed white matter (WM) integrity reductions in a distributed network compared with female TCs, whereas no WM integrity differences were found between boys and young men with ASD and without ASD.[41] Deng & Wang[42] analyzed a selective high-quality data subset from an open data resource showing that TC men have a more leftward brain asymmetry than TC women.[42] This study found that girls and young women with ASD presented with more leftward gray matter brain asymmetry compared with girls and young women TCs, whereas there was no difference between boys and young men with ASD and TCs. This interaction pattern is supportive of the female protective effect (FPE) theory by showing greater gray matter changes in women with ASD compared with men with ASD.

Gender Incoherence Theory

The gender incoherence (GI) theory suggests that ASD is associated with androgynous features in both men and women.[43] This theory was originally supported by a study examining serum hormone levels and anthropometry measures supposedly related to androgen influence among 50 adult men and women with ASD and age- and sex-matched TCs.[43] Women with ASD had higher testosterone levels, less feminine facial features, and a larger head circumference than female TCs. Men in the ASD group were found to have similar testosterone levels as TCs yet had less masculine body characteristics (ie, higher 2D:4D ratio on the right hand and a nonsignificant trend for larger head circumference compared with male controls) and voice quality. In the total sample, androgynous facial features were also found to correlate well with ASD traits (measured with the Autism-Spectrum Quotient).

Neuroimaging research studying the relation among ASD, sex, and brain measurements has supported the GI theory by finding a shift toward masculinization patterns in the brains of women with ASD and shift toward feminization patterns in the brains of men with ASD. In a pattern consistent with the GI hypothesis, one study of amygdala connectivity found that ASD is associated with attenuated sex differences in amygdala connectivity.[44] Other studies have found single side GI (ie, shift toward masculinization or shift toward feminization).[45,46]

Sexual dimorphism has been strongly connected to sex steroids exerting permanent organizational effects prenatally and transient activating effects later in life.[47] Sexual differentiation and sexual steroid levels have an important evolutionary role. They affect mating behaviors by influencing male/female physical characteristics.[48] Sexual steroids appear to regulate social recognition, social imitation, nonverbal communication, and social reciprocity and mating behavior through its influence on the development of neuronal circuits. All these social communication functions are affected in ASD.[43] Vasopressin and oxytocin, which are influenced by sex steroids and display sexual dimorphism, have received attention due to their impact in social behaviors.[49] Both have been implicated in the biology of ASD.[50,51]

The theories presented here only partially explain sex differences in ASD. Neuroimaging studies demonstrate that some aspects of typical sex differences in brain structure are preserved in individuals with ASD, whereas others are not. Further, although some neuroimaging findings are supportive of these theories, others are inconsistent, do not support the theories, or are supportive of more than one model.[44,45]

CULTURAL AND SOCIAL FACTORS

In addition to the biological factors that may impact the expression of autism symptoms in women, there are also many social and cultural influences. Although children with large developmental delays may be raised with unique developmental expectations, children with autism without large delays are raised under the same social norms as their developmental peers. Children tend to self-segregate by gender, creating distinct social norms.[19] Furthering this distinction, caregivers typically vary their language by their child's sex, resulting in different developmental outcomes.[52] For example, caregivers of girls are more likely to use social language, label emotions, and discuss emotions than caregivers of boys.[53] Mothers of daughters are more likely to increase their vocalizations with their child across development than mothers of sons, resulting in greater vocalizations among daughters.[54] Further, stereotypical "female" toys in early childhood (eg, kitchen sets, dolls), encourage creative and imaginative play and promote modeling of this play by adults and other children interacting with the child.[52,55] Taken together, girls with ASD who do not have notable cognitive delays may have more socialization in activities that tend to attenuate the appearance of "classic" autism symptoms.

The social expectations typically placed on women may also carry stressors in later childhood, adolescence, and adulthood.[56] Social demands and expectations increase throughout development. Interestingly, traditional male friendships are centered largely around activities (eg, attending concerts, sports games, playing video games) and traditional female friendships are centered largely around the exchange of personal information and emotional support.[19] There is a higher requirement of social skills for these female friendships.[57] Therefore, although women with ASD may have more social skill support in early childhood, they also require higher-level social skills to form and maintain friendships into adolescence and adulthood.[56] Additionally, as social awareness increases during adolescence, many young women with ASD begin to recognize and report feelings of "otherness" and difference from their typically developing peers.[58,59]

Emerging research has found that many individuals with ASD engage in "camouflaging" or behaviors that are intended to mask the features of ASD in social situations (ie, social communication differences and repetitive behaviors).[60] Camouflaging is motivated by the desire to connect with others, avoid rejection, and assimilate through strategies such as deliberately copying others' body language and facial expressions, mimicking others' speech patterns, and suppressing repetitive body movements.[60] Although camouflaging is not unique to women with ASD, women report using camouflaging from an earlier age, across more situations, and more frequently than do men.[61] The increased social demands placed on women may lead to increased use of camouflaging techniques, and greater stress and feelings of overwhelm within social interactions. Regardless of sex, use of camouflaging among adults with ASD is associated with higher self-reported symptoms of generalized anxiety, social anxiety, and depression.[62]

An additional component of social and cultural factors is the clinical interpretation of ASD symptoms by caregivers, teachers, and clinicians participating in developmental screening.[63] Autism symptoms in girls and women may not raise concerns about this condition due to the raters' reliance on gender stereotypes and a male biased understanding of ASD. For example, social withdrawal may be interpreted as shyness in a female but be considered a red flag for ASD in a male. In preschoolers with ASD, parents and teachers reported greater pre-diagnostic concerns about these conditions in boys than in girls.[64]

COMORBIDITIES

ASD is a heterogenous condition. Twin studies have suggested that autism has high heritability (more than 80%).[65] Given that the monozygotic concordance rates are never 100%, this heritability occurs in the context of environmental risks and gene–environment interplay.[66] Genetic testing is recommended to individuals with an ASD diagnosis to investigate potential causes of autism. ASD has a range of medical comorbidities that are observed at higher rates than in the general population and have significant developmental, psychological, and physical health sequela. These include higher rates of genetic (eg, Down syndrome, Fragile X syndrome), neurologic (eg, epilepsy, cerebral palsy, macrocephaly), gastrointestinal (eg, chronic constipation, gastroesophageal reflux), sleep (eg, insomnia), metabolic, and allergic (eg, asthma) disorders.[67,68] Approximately 12% to 20% of individuals with ASD may have a diagnosis of epilepsy.[69,70] Epilepsy onset in autism typically occurs during infancy or adolescence and is associated with developmental regression in approximately 25% of cases (eg, Landau-Kleffner syndrome[69]).[69] Emerging research is investigating shared environmental and genetic causes between these two conditions. For example, the *excitation-inhibition balance theory* purports that dysfunction of excitatory and inhibitory circuits in various brain regions may contribute to shared developmental mechanisms.[71] Although it has long been known that individuals with ASD frequently experience sensory sensitivities that impact eating behaviors, there is growing research on unique gastrointestinal physiology within the gut-brain axis among individuals with ASD. For example, mechanisms such as altered feeding behaviors, reduced gut permeability, and increased biodiversity of the gut microbiome, may lead to the onset of GI symptoms such as chronic diarrhea, constipation, abdominal pain, and gastroesophageal reflux.[72]

Although additional research on sex differences in medical comorbidities is needed, there is growing evidence that women have higher rates of epilepsy, metabolic disorders, endocrine/reproductive health disorders (eg, irregular puberty onset), gastrointestinal disorders, and sleep disorders compared with men with ASD and women without ASD.[73–76] Overall, these findings suggest that women with ASD are more likely to have poorer health outcomes, perhaps due to their higher genetic load leading to co-morbid disorders. Research investigating sex/gender differences in medical comorbidities and the biological basis for ASD and its common comorbidities may lead to novel treatments that reduce symptoms or even prevent comorbidities from developing.

ID was previously reported as being present in approximately 70% of ASD cases and has more recently been reported as being present in 30% of cases.[77] This changing rate no doubt reflects the recent broadening of the autism spectrum to include individuals with higher cognitive functioning; even so, the more recent prevalence rate may be an underestimate given that intellectually disabled individuals are under-included in ASD research. Relatedly, women have been identified as having higher rates of co-occurring ID than men.[8] Yet again, it is unclear whether this reflects an ascertainment bias in research in which women with typical or above intellectual functioning are under-represented as opposed to a true difference in rates of ID across sex and gender.[17,78]

One meta-analysis estimating the prevalence of comorbid mental health disorders in ASD across the lifespan found higher rates of comorbidities among individuals with ASD than in the general population.[79] The eight most common comorbid mental health diagnoses included ADHD (28%), anxiety disorders (20%), sleep-wake disorders (13%), disruptive/impulse control/conduct disorders (12%), depressive disorders (11%), obsessive-compulsive disorder (9%), bipolar disorders (5%), and schizophrenia spectrum disorders (4%). On average, women with ASD have been found to have higher rates of comorbid mental health symptoms and diagnoses than men, particularly for anxiety, depression, disordered eating, and borderline personality disorder.[79–82] One study found that having a former or initial diagnosis of anxiety or ADHD delays a more appropriate diagnosis of ASD, with a stronger effect for women.[83] Mood or anxiety difficulties, which are more common among women than men in the general population, may be normalized among women, preventing an in-depth investigation of social communication deficits contributing to emotional challenges. Another study found that over one-third of individuals with ASD (47% of women and 27% of men) in the Netherlands Autism Register had one previous mental health diagnosis removed after receiving a diagnosis of ASD,[81] suggesting that earlier diagnoses represented a missed or delayed ASD diagnosis and even more so for women. The overall higher rates of mental health comorbidities among women with ASD can be interpreted as reflecting a truly higher risk for comorbidity, the many barriers that women face to receiving an accurate ASD diagnosis, and/or a greater mental health burden experienced among women with ASD. Overall, these findings suggest that medical providers who have concerns about female patients' social functioning when several comorbidities are present should consider whether an additional ASD diagnosis may provide a more straightforward and comprehensive explanation of presenting concerns and, consequently, facilitate referrals to assessment services that can establish diagnostic clarity.

SEX DIFFERENCES IN CORE SYMPTOM PRESENTATION

A popular quote that has been attributed to autism self-advocate, Dr Stephen Shore, summarizes the heterogeneity within ASD well: "If you've met one person with autism, you've met one person with autism." Although core symptom criteria include social communication deficits and RRBIs, ASD presentations fall across a broad spectrum that ranges from very mild to severe. Further, even though sex differences in symptom presentations are often present, these differences represent averages, and it is unclear whether the range of symptoms on the spectrum varies across sex/gender. Relatedly, given individual differences in ASD expression, there is no simple sex dichotomy in ASD presentation nor a "female autism phenotype" that can be used to form diagnoses.[13] Sex differences in core ASD symptoms are described below.

Social Communication and Social Interaction

Studies of social communication differences are often confounded by study samples that underrepresent women, and by variations in intelligence or language ability.[84] Given the nuances and complexities of social communication, it is imperative to account for cognitive variability. For example, when intellectual functioning was matched in a sample of adolescents with ASD, sex variations in specific social language components were observed.[85] This study's findings suggested small but consistent differences in which women with ASD demonstrated deficits in social communication skills when compared with TC women, but outperformed men with ASD.[85] Of interest, there were some skills, such as use and knowledge of emotional vocabulary, in which women with and without ASD demonstrated equitable skills (both above men), suggesting that there may be some skills preserved by sex.[85] These small differences may have real impacts on children with autism. In unstructured conversations, women with ASD often make more positive first impressions on others than do men.[86] Further, word choices can have an impact on diagnostics. Cola and colleagues, 2022[87] found specific word choices in verbally fluent children were related to their scores on the diagnostic assessment, the Autism Diagnostic Observation Schedule, Second Edition (ADOS-2).[87] Girls used more "socially-focused" words, specifically regarding friends, than boys despite the samples being matched for intellectual functioning and autism symptom severity. Further, use of these words corresponded to greater ratings of social communication skills. Therefore, equal levels of clinician- and parent-rated autism severity may result in different scores on diagnostic assessments due to sex differences in language use.

Interestingly, when studies use parent-report of social communication and social interaction, they often find no major sex differences.[88,89] However, sex-specific social communication profiles may be more subtle than what can be captured in parent-report measures.

Women with ASD may present as less socially impaired due to their higher social communication abilities. Relative to men with ASD, women with ASD have been shown to have greater expressive social behaviors (eg, reciprocal conversation, sharing of information), more friends, participate in more social groups, and be more aware of exclusion and take steps to reduce exclusion (eg, camouflaging[13,64]).[13,64] Despite having more friendships, women with ASD have been shown to have unique social difficulties relative to men. For example, women may be more skilled in initiating relationships but have difficulty maintaining them or be more likely to experience subtle peer rejection that is poorly understood.[64,90]

Restricted and Repetitive Behaviors

RRBs can include repetitive or unusual motor movements as well as an intense interest in topics or items that range from typical child interests (eg, trains, animals) to atypical interests (eg, patent numbers, flags from around the world). Although there are many facets of RRBs, sex differences are not consistently found in self- or parent-reported number of circumscribed interests (CI). In their review, van Wijngaarden-Cremers and colleagues[78] found that women have lower rates of RRBs and interests.[78] However, the specific topics of CI may vary by sex.[88] CIs may be the most informative RRB to consider as they are more specific to autism and corresponded to eye tracking measures of attention, detail focus and perseveration.[16] Women on the spectrum have been described as having more "random" CIs[64] and thus have less interest associated with the prototypical autism or queried in traditional autism assessments.[64]

Parents often report that, relative to sons on the spectrum, daughters on the spectrum have CIs that are more in line with typically developing peers and that these interests are often associated with positive social interactions.[15,64,91] For example, a girl with ASD may have CIs that are viewed as a common interest for her peer group (eg, pop music band). She may share this interest with her friends, plan social events to watch the band play, or even form a club or online group surrounding the band.

Although this interest is more intense and encompassing than it would be for typically developing girls, she can use it to seek connection socially and thus experience less social impairment as a result of her RRBs than her male counterparts (eg, boy who repetitively talks about airplanes).

Of interest, in some studies, parents report sex differences in repetitive behaviors that are not corroborated by teachers.[89] This may suggest some evidence of female camouflaging of more obvious autism symptom behaviors when outside of the home.[88]

DIAGNOSTIC CHALLENGES

The sex/gender gap between the studies using high methodological quality with active case ascertainment methods and passive methodology studies suggests an under-recognition of ASD in women. A predictive model based on population data estimated that 39% more women should be diagnosed with ASD.[92] Some have suggested that many of the tools designed to assess ASD may not be sensitive enough to capture a female autism presentation and as a result require women to reach a higher diagnostic threshold.[17] However, recent research found that men and women may not vary on their autism severity scores on gold standard measures (eg, ADOS-2[93]) [93] with only small differences when differences are observed.[94] This may suggest that the current diagnostic measures are appropriate for identifying autism in women, when women are referred for evaluation, highlighting the importance of timely evaluation referrals. For additional information on tools that medical providers can use to screen for ASD across the lifespan, see Allison and colleagues[95] and Sappok and colleagues.[96]

IMPORTANCE OF TIMELY DIAGNOSIS

The importance of timely ASD diagnosis is particularly relevant to women. As with any medical condition, timely diagnosis can result in more positive outcomes and reduce the burden caused by a condition. Perhaps most importantly, earlier diagnosis leads to earlier intervention. A meta-analysis investigating improvements in social communication outcomes in children with ASD found that interventions delivered between three and 4 years of age had the largest positive impact on child development, with intervention effectiveness reducing by age eight.[97] Further, social communication skills in infancy predict social skills in middle childhood,[98] highlighting the importance of early intervention for improving outcomes throughout development. Timely diagnosis also allows caregivers to develop effective strategies for managing their child's unique challenges.[99] When an ASD diagnosis is made later in development, it can provide individuals with an increased understanding of their experiences as well as relief that their challenges are not the result of personal failures but instead the unique way in which their brain works. Further, diagnosis empowers individuals to seek appropriate medical treatments (eg, psychotherapy, psychopharmacology) and join community organizations in which they can share their experiences with similar individuals and obtain crucial social support, strategies, and resources.

The harm of late diagnosis for women is significant. Women who receive a later diagnosis describe being labeled as "shy," "rude," and "lazy" throughout their childhood and an emotional and physical toll from years of trying to "appear normal" by masking, compensating, and imitating "neurotypical" social behaviors.[58] Further, given these women's, as well as their families', teachers', and peers', poor understanding of the source of their social challenges, they report persistent social rejection, reduced educational or career obtainment, and elevated rates of victimization including bullying and sexual abuse. The importance of the diagnosis of ASD among women is highlighted and discussed in detail in Bargiela and colleagues,[58] and Leedham and colleagues.[59]

SPECIFIC SUPPORT FOR WOMEN ON THE SPECTRUM

Although all individuals with ASD generally benefit from support in developing social communication skills, specific treatment recommendations should be informed by the individual's needs. Standard supports often include recommendations for applied behavior analysis (ABA) to target adaptive skill development in young children or cognitive behavior therapy (CBT) for verbally fluent individuals who want to address social challenges, anxiety, and depression, among other needs. Group therapies are often the default for support with social communication skills given that they provide a social context in which to practice social skills. Although there is limited research on health service use, no major sex differences have been found. Nevertheless, a survey of service use in adolescent girls indicated that they use more psychiatry and general emergency room services than do boys.[100] The greater reliance on emergency room services may imply that women with ASD are not having their needs met in routine care and thus do not seek services until difficulties reach the level of a crisis. Additionally, the greater proportion of women in psychiatric care may speak to the higher rates of mental health comorbidities among women with ASD.

In addition to most social skills groups being developed for the prototypical expression of autism, which may better support the needs of men with ASD, these groups will have a predominately male membership, due to the nature of recruitment. For some women, the lack of other women may not be an issue. However, there may still be benefits in having other women in a group, especially for topics related to social skills such as dating, sexual activity, and consent. A more gender-balanced group could offer advantages to all group members to generalize social skills practice and to discuss differences if and as they arise.

General. Clinicians could consider offering a female-specific social skill group which may delve into topics more relevant for women or somewhat gender-specific, such as social expectations, later diagnosis, and a discussion of use, limitations and risks of camouflaging behaviors.

Although not specific to woman, there are additional areas that are common needs for those on the spectrum that should continue to be considered for teens and adults on the spectrum. These include but are not limited to how and when to disclose an ASD diagnosis, sexual and gender identity, general dating and navigating preferences in sexual preferences, and contraception. Some individuals may be more comfortable discussing these topics in a single-sex social group, which could be considered in recruiting and forming appropriate clinical groups.

Comorbid mental health conditions. Women with ASD are likely to have one or more co-occurring condition(s).[101] Therefore, interventions focused on social challenges as well as comorbidities may be more helpful for women with autism. Social skill groups have been found to improve social skills among individuals with ASD and anxiety, yet less so for people with ASD and ADHD.[102,103] Psychopharmacology can be used as an adjunct to psychological interventions to address conditions like anxiety, depression, and ADHD, leading to significant improvements in developmental trajectories and functioning.

Intellectual functioning. Women with intellectual disabilities or other cognitive impairments are more likely to have increased RRBs and a more similar expression of autism to their male peers. For these women, gender-specific supports may be less imperative.

Support for medical testing. One final consideration for clinicians when seeing women on the spectrum should be genetic testing as recommended by the American Academy of Genetics and the American Academy of Pediatric Neurology.

SUMMARY

The active ascertainment population studies have identified a higher proportion of women with ASD (2.5 to 3:1)[14] than was previously documented with passive studies (4 to 5:1).[8,9] The public and often medical professional's male-biased understanding of ASD makes it less likely for parents and caregivers to appropriately identify signs of ASD in women and seek timely evaluations. The male bias in ASD extends to diagnostic criteria and tools, which have developed based on nearly a century of research predominantly focused on men. There is evidence that even clinicians specialized in ASD are more hesitant to diagnose women with ASD than men with similar presentations. However, in the last few years, there is increased awareness of ASD in women and their participation in research has increased.

Women with ASD often have a missed or delayed diagnosis, which increases the burden of this condition by delaying and preventing access to services, leading to less desirable developmental trajectories. Relative to the "prototypical" ASD that is more aligned with a male presentation, the clinical presentation of women is often characterized by more subtle social communication deficits, less intense and unusual RRBs, and the presence of compensatory mechanisms (eg, camouflaging) that may mask otherwise noticeable ASD symptoms. The frequent presence of mental health comorbidities (eg, ADHD, anxiety, depression) also contribute to diagnostic delays and misdiagnosis as well as highlight the heightened emotional challenges experiences by women on the spectrum.

Below are a set of strategies clinicians may use to better support female patients for whom they have concerns about a possible ASD diagnosis.

CLINICS CARE POINTS

- When possible, gather self- and collateral-report (eg, parents and romantic partner) of social functioning. Women with autism spectrum disorder (ASD) may use compensatory strategies (eg, mimicking others' facial expressions, using social language in an appropriate yet scripted manner) at the time of the evaluation that masks their social communication differences.
- Explicitly ask women if they use camouflaging strategies in their daily social interactions. As examples, ask whether women deliberately copy others' body language in conversation, force themselves to make eye contact despite intense discomfort or distress, or actively suppress repetitive finger, hand, or body movements.
- When considering whether signs of ASD are present, including social communication difficulties and restricted and repetitive behaviors (RRBs), mentally compare women with typically developing women, not with expectations of ASD.
- Consider the quality of play and other social skills in girls. If developmental social milestones are "met," inquire about whether these skills appear as frequently and flexibly used as when they are observed in typically developing children (ie, across people, contexts, and objects). Follow up with parents about the details of each skill. For example, girls may have more "character toys" to play with but will still demonstrate repetitive play and language.
- When inquiring about RRBs, provide parents with examples across typically gendered activities, such as "Does your child line up trains or dolls?" or "Is she more interested than others in dinosaurs or boybands?" to prompt parents to think more inclusively when

answering. Even when interests appear developmentally appropriate, consider their quality and intensity.

- Given the high rates of co-occurring diagnoses and the increased risk of miss-diagnosis among women, consider whether ASD provides a more straightforward and comprehensive explanation in complex cases with multiple mental health comorbidities.
- To ensure comprehensive care, provide psychiatry referrals to evaluate and treat mental health comorbidities.
- When in doubt, use standardized tools for ASD screening that are less prone to subjective biases about ASD symptoms. See Allison and colleagues[95] and Sappok and colleagues[96] for ASD screening tools that can be used across the lifespan.
- Provide women with identified social communication deficits and/or RRBs with referrals to evaluators with expertise in working with women on the spectrum.

DISCLOSURE

All authors declare that they have no conflicts of interest.

REFERENCES

1. American Psychiatric Association. Diagnostic and Statistical Manual of Mental Disorders (DSM-5-TR).; 2013.
2. Kanner L. Autistic disturbances of affective contact. Nervous Child 1943;2(3): 217–50.
3. Frith U. Asperger and his syndrome. Autism Asperger Syndr 1991;14:1–36.
4. Baio J, Wiggins L, Christensen DL, et al. Prevalence of autism spectrum disorder among children aged 8 years - autism and developmental disabilities monitoring network, 11 Sites, United States, 2014. MMWR Surveill Summ 2018; 67(6):1–23.
5. Zeidan J, Fombonne E, Scorah J, et al. Global prevalence of autism: A systematic review update. Autism Res 2022;15(5):778–90.
6. Larson E, Spring-Pearson S, Sarkar A, et al. SFARI Gene Q4/2021 Report.; 2021. https://gene.sfari.org/sfari-gene-release-notes-for-q4-2021https://gene.sfari.org/sfari-gene-release-notes-for-q4-2021
7. Maenner MJ, Shaw KA, Baio J, et al. Prevalence of autism spectrum disorder among children aged 8 years - autism and developmental disabilities monitoring network, 11 Sites, United States, 2016. MMWR Surveill Summ 2020;69(4):1–12.
8. Fombonne E. REVIEW ARTICLES Epidemiology of Pervasive Developmental Disorders. 2009. http://www.dds.ca.gov/Autism/docs/AutismReport2003.pdf.
9. Christensen DL, Braun KVN, Baio J, et al. Prevalence and characteristics of autism spectrum disorder among children aged 8 years - autism and developmental disabilities monitoring network, 11 sites, United States, 2012. MMWR Surveill Summ 2018;65(13):1–23.
10. Luyster R, Gotham K, Guthrie W, et al. The autism diagnostic observation schedule - Toddler module: A new module of a standardized diagnostic measure for autism spectrum disorders. J Autism Dev Disord 2009;39(9):1305–20.
11. Klin A, Saulnier CA, Sparrow SS, et al. Social and communication abilities and disabilities in higher functioning individuals with autism spectrum disorders: the vineland and the ADOS. J Autism Dev Disord 2007;37(4):748–59.
12. Via E, Radua J, Cardoner N, et al. Meta-analysis of gray matter abnormalities in autism spectrum disorder: should asperger disorder be subsumed under a

broader umbrella of autistic spectrum disorder? Arch Gen Psychiatry 2011; 68(4):409–18.
13. Lai MC, Lin HY, Ameis SH. Towards equitable diagnoses for autism and attention-deficit/hyperactivity disorder across sexes and genders. Curr Opin Psychiatry 2022;35(2):90–100.
14. Loomes R, Hull L, Mandy WPL. What is the male-to-female ratio in autism spectrum disorder? a systematic review and meta-analysis. J Am Acad Child Adolesc Psychiatry 2017;56(6):466–74.
15. Hiller RM, Young RL, Weber N. Sex differences in pre-diagnosis concerns for children later diagnosed with autism spectrum disorder. Autism 2016;20(1): 75–84.
16. Harrop C, Green J, Hudry K. Play complexity and toy engagement in preschoolers with autism spectrum disorder: Do girls and boys differ? Autism 2017;21:37–50. SAGE Publications Ltd.
17. Lai MC, Lombardo Mv, Auyeung B, et al. Sex/gender differences and autism: setting the scene for future research. J Am Acad Child Adolesc Psychiatry 2015;54(1):11–24.
18. Strang JF, van der Miesen AIR, Caplan R, et al. Both sex- and gender-related factors should be considered in autism research and clinical practice. Autism 2020;24(3):539–43.
19. Maccoby EE. Gender and Group Process: A Developmental Perspective. Current Directions in Psychological Science 2002;11(2):54–8.
20. McCarthy MM, Wright CL. Convergence of sex differences and the neuroimmune system in autism spectrum disorder. Biol Psychiatry 2017;81(5):402–10.
21. Baron-Cohen S, Lombardo Mv, Auyeung B, et al. Why are autism spectrum conditions more prevalent in men? Plos Biol 2011;9(6):e1001081.
22. Baron-Cohen S, Richler J, Bisarya D, et al. The systemizing quotient: An investigation of adults with Asperger syndrome or high-functioning autism, and normal sex differences. Philosophical Trans R Soc B: Biol Sci 2003;358(1430): 361–74.
23. Lawson J, Baron-Cohen S, Wheelwright S. Empathising and systemising in adults with and without Asperger syndrome. J Autism Dev Disord 2004;34(3). https://doi.org/10.1023/B:JADD.0000029552.42724.1b.
24. Gilmore JH, Lin W, Prastawa MW, et al. Regional gray matter growth, sexual dimorphism, and cerebral asymmetry in the neonatal brain. J Neurosci 2007; 27(6):1255–60.
25. Courchesne E, Campbell K, Solso S. Brain growth across the life span in autism: Age-specific changes in anatomical pathology. Brain Res 2011;1380:138–45.
26. Good CD, Johnsrude I, Ashburner J, et al. Cerebral asymmetry and the effects of sex and handedness on brain structure: a voxel-based morphometric analysis of 465 normal adult human brains. Neuroimage 2001;14(3):685–700.
27. Schumann CM, Barnes CC, Lord C, et al. Amygdala enlargement in toddlers with autism related to severity of social and communication impairments. Biol Psychiatry 2009;66(10):942–9.
28. Ypma RJF, Moseley RL, Holt RJ, et al. Default Mode Hypoconnectivity Underlies a sex-related autism spectrum. Biol Psychiatry Cogn Neurosci Neuroimaging 2016;1(4):364–71.
29. Kozhemiako N, Vakorin V, Nunes AS, et al. Extreme male developmental trajectories of homotopic brain connectivity in autism. Hum Brain Mapp 2019;40(3): 987–1000.

30. Nugent BM, McCarthy MM. Epigenetic underpinnings of developmental sex differences in the brain. Neuroendocrinology 2011;93(3):150–8.
31. Phoenix CH, Goy RW, Gerall AA, et al. Organizing action of prenatally administered testosterone propionate on the tissues mediating mating behavior in the female guinea pig. Endocrinology 1959;65(3):369–82.
32. Baron-Cohen S, Wheelwright S. The empathy quotient: an investigation of adults with asperger syndrome or high functioning autism, and normal sex differences. J Autism Dev Disord 2004;34(2):163–75.
33. Smail PJ, Reyes FI, Winter JSD, et al. The fetal hormonal environment and its effect on the morphogenesis of the genital system. In: Pediatric Andrology. Netherlands: Springer; 1981. p. 9–19.
34. Dawood MY, Saxena BB. Testosterone and dihydrotestosterone in maternal and cord blood and in amniotic fluid. Am J Obstet Gynecol 1977;129(1):37–42.
35. Baron-Cohen S, Auyeung B, Nørgaard-Pedersen B, et al. Elevated fetal steroidogenic activity in autism. Mol Psychiatry 2015;20(3):369–76.
36. Auyeung B, Taylor K, Hackett G, et al, Open Access RESEARCH. Foetal Testosterone and Autistic Traits in 18 to 24-Month-Old Children. Mol Autism 2010;1(1): 11. Available at: http://www.molecularautism.com/content/1/1/11.
37. Werling DM, Geschwind DH. Sex differences in autism spectrum disorders. Curr Opin Neurol 2013;26(2):146–53.
38. Zhao X, Leotta A, Kustanovich V, et al. A unified genetic theory for sporadic and inherited autism. Proc Natl Acad Sci 2007;104(31):12831–6.
39. Robinson EB, Lichtenstein P, Anckarsäter H, et al. Examining and interpreting the female protective effect against autistic behavior. Proc Natl Acad Sci 2013;110(13):5258–62.
40. Hallmayer J, Cleveland S, Torres A, et al. Genetic heritability and shared environmental factors among twin pairs with autism. Arch Gen Psychiatry 2011; 68(11):1095–102.
41. Lei J, Lecarie E, Jurayj J, et al. Altered Neural Connectivity in Women, But Not Men with Autism: Preliminary Evidence for the Female Protective Effect from a Quality-Controlled Diffusion Tensor Imaging Study. Autism Res 2019;12(10): 1472–83.
42. Deng Z, Wang S. Sex differentiation of brain structures in autism: Findings from a gray matter asymmetry study. Autism Res 2021;14(6). https://doi.org/10.1002/aur.2506.
43. Bejerot S, Eriksson JM, Bonde S, et al. The extreme male brain revisited: Gender coherence in adults with autism spectrum disorder. Br J Psychiatry 2012;201(2): 116–23.
44. Lee JK, Andrews DS, Ozturk A, et al. Altered Development of Amygdala-Connected Brain Regions in Men and Women with Autism. J Neurosci 2022; 42(31):6145–55.
45. Floris DL, Lai MC, Nath T, et al. Network-specific sex differentiation of intrinsic brain function in men with autism. Mol Autism 2018;9(1). https://doi.org/10.1186/s13229-018-0192-x.
46. Lai MC, Lombardo Mv, Suckling J, et al. Biological sex affects the neurobiology of autism. Brain 2013;136(9):2799–815.
47. Hines M, Constantinescu M, Spencer D. Early androgen exposure and human gender development. Biol Sex Differ 2015;6:3.
48. Evans S, Neave N, Wakelin D. Relationships between vocal characteristics and body size and shape in human men: An evolutionary explanation for a deep male voice. Biol Psychol 2006;72(2):160–3.

49. Insel TR. The Challenge of Translation in Social Neuroscience: A Review of Oxytocin, Vasopressin, and Affiliative Behavior. Neuron 2010;65(6):768–79.
50. CARTER C. Sex differences in oxytocin and vasopressin: Implications for autism spectrum disorders? Behav Brain Res 2007;176(1):170–86.
51. Sala M, Braida D, Lentini D, et al. Pharmacologic rescue of impaired cognitive flexibility, social deficits, increased aggression, and seizure susceptibility in oxytocin receptor null mice: A neurobehavioral model of autism. Biol Psychiatry 2011;69(9):875–82.
52. Morawska A. The Effects of Gendered Parenting on Child Development Outcomes: A Systematic Review. Clin Child Fam Psychol Rev 2020;23(4):553–76.
53. Piira T, Champion GD, Bustos T, et al. Factors associated with infant pain response following an immunization injection. Early Hum Dev 2007;83(5): 319–26.
54. Sung J, Fausto-Sterling A, Garcia Coll C, et al. The Dynamics of Age and Sex in the Development of Mother-Infant Vocal Communication Between 3 and 11 Months. Infancy 2013;18(6):1135–58.
55. Boe JL, Woods RJ. Parents' Influence on Infants' Gender-Typed Toy Preferences. Sex Roles 2018;79(5–6):358–73.
56. Mandy W. Social camouflaging in autism: Is it time to lose the mask? Autism 2019;23(8):1879–81.
57. Dean M, Harwood R, Kasari C. The art of camouflage: Gender differences in the social behaviors of girls and boys with autism spectrum disorder. Autism 2017; 21(6):678–89.
58. Bargiela S, Steward R, Mandy W. The Experiences of Late-diagnosed Women with Autism Spectrum Conditions: An Investigation of the Female Autism Phenotype. J Autism Dev Disord 2016;46(10):3281–94.
59. Leedham A, Thompson AR, Smith R, et al. 'I was exhausted trying to figure it out': the experiences of women receiving an autism diagnosis in middle to late adulthood. Autism 2020;24(1):135–46.
60. Hull L, Petrides Kv, Allison C, et al. Putting on My Best Normal": Social Camouflaging in Adults with Autism Spectrum Conditions. J Autism Dev Disord 2017; 47(8):2519–34.
61. Cook J, Hull L, Crane L, et al. Camouflaging in autism: a systematic review. Clin Psychol Rev 2021;89. https://doi.org/10.1016/j.cpr.2021.102080.
62. Hull L, Levy L, Lai MC, et al. Is social camouflaging associated with anxiety and depression in autistic adults? Mol Autism 2021;12(1):13.
63. Lai MC, Szatmari P. Sex and gender impacts on the behavioural presentation and recognition of autism. Curr Opin Psychiatry 2020;33(2):117–23.
64. Hiller RM, Young RL, Weber N. Sex Differences in autism spectrum disorder based on dsm-5 criteria: evidence from clinician and teacher reporting. J Abnorm Child Psychol 2014;42(8):1381–93.
65. Ronald A, Hoekstra RA. Autism spectrum disorders and autistic traits: A decade of new twin studies. Am J Med Genet B: Neuropsychiatr Genet 2011;156(3): 255–74.
66. Corrales M, Herbert M. Autism and environmental genomics: synergistic systems approaches to autism complexity. In: Amaral D, Dawson G, Geschwind DH, editors. Autism Spectrum Disorders. Oxford University Press; 2011. p. 875–92.
67. Al-Beltagi M. Autism medical comorbidities. World J Clin Pediatr 2021;10(3): 15–28.

68. Jones KB, Cottle K, Bakian A, et al. A description of medical conditions in adults with autism spectrum disorder: A follow-up of the 1980s Utah/UCLA autism epidemiologic study. Autism 2016;20(5):551–61.
69. Besag F. Epilepsy in patients with autism: links, risks and treatment challenges. Neuropsychiatr Dis Treat 2017;14:1–10.
70. Lukmanji S, Manji SA, Kadhim S, et al. The co-occurrence of epilepsy and autism: A systematic review. Epilepsy Behav 2019;98:238–48.
71. Bozzi Y, Provenzano G, Casarosa S. Neurobiological bases of autism-epilepsy comorbidity: a focus on excitation/inhibition imbalance. Eur J Neurosci 2018; 47(6):534–48.
72. Bjørklund G, Pivina L, Dadar M, et al. Gastrointestinal alterations in autism spectrum disorder: What do we know? Neurosci Biobehav Rev 2020;118:111–20.
73. Angell AM, Deavenport-Saman A, Yin L, et al. Sex Differences in Co-occurring Conditions Among Autistic Children and Youth in Florida: A Retrospective Cohort Study (2012–2019). J Autism Dev Disord 2021;51(10):3759–65.
74. Kassee C, Babinski S, Tint A, et al. Physical health of autistic girls and women: a scoping review. Mol Autism 2020;11(1). https://doi.org/10.1186/s13229-020-00380-z.
75. Simantov T, Pohl A, Tsompanidis A, et al. Medical symptoms and conditions in autistic women. Autism 2022;26(2):373–88.
76. DaWalt LS, Taylor JL, Movaghar A, et al. Health profiles of adults with autism spectrum disorder: Differences between women and men. Autism Res 2021; 14(9):1896–904.
77. Thurm A, Farmer C, Salzman E, et al. State of the Field: Differentiating Intellectual Disability From Autism Spectrum Disorder. Front Psychiatry 2019;10. https://doi.org/10.3389/fpsyt.2019.00526.
78. van Wijngaarden-Cremers PJM, van Eeten E, Groen WB, et al. Gender and age differences in the core triad of impairments in autism spectrum disorders: a systematic review and meta-analysis. J Autism Dev Disord 2014;44(3):627–35.
79. Lai MC, Kassee C, Besney R, et al. Prevalence of co-occurring mental health diagnoses in the autism population: a systematic review and meta-analysis. Lancet Psychiatry 2019;6(10):819–29.
80. Duvekot J, van der Ende J, Verhulst FC, et al. Factors influencing the probability of a diagnosis of autism spectrum disorder in girls versus boys. Autism 2017; 21(6):646–58.
81. Kentrou V, Oostervink M, Scheeren AM, et al. Stability of co-occurring psychiatric diagnoses in autistic men and women. Res Autism Spectr Disord 2021;82. https://doi.org/10.1016/j.rasd.2021.101736.
82. Rydzewska E, Hughes-McCormack LA, Gillberg C, et al. Prevalence of sensory impairments, physical and intellectual disabilities, and mental health in children and young people with self/proxy-reported autism: Observational study of a whole country population. Autism 2019;23(5):1201–9.
83. Rødgaard EM, Jensen K, Miskowiak KW, et al. Autism comorbidities show elevated female-to-male odds ratios and are associated with the age of first autism diagnosis. Acta Psychiatr Scand 2021;144(5):475–86.
84. Rivet TT, Matson JL. Review of gender differences in core symptomatology in autism spectrum disorders. Res Autism Spectr Disord 2011;5(3):957–76.
85. Sturrock A, Yau N, Freed J, et al. Speaking the same language? a preliminary investigation, comparing the language and communication skills of women and men with high-functioning autism. J Autism Dev Disord 2020;50(5): 1639–56.

86. Cola ML, Plate S, Yankowitz L, et al. Sex differences in the first impressions made by girls and boys with autism. Mol Autism 2020;11(1). https://doi.org/10.1186/s13229-020-00336-3.
87. Cola M, Yankowitz LD, Tena K, et al. Friend matters: sex differences in social language during autism diagnostic interviews. Mol Autism 2022;13(1):5.
88. Sutherland R, Hodge A, Bruck S, et al. Parent-reported differences between school-aged girls and boys on the autism spectrum. Autism 2017;21(6):785–94.
89. Mandy W, Chilvers R, Chowdhury U, et al. Sex Differences in autism spectrum disorder: evidence from a large sample of children and adolescents. J Autism Dev Disord 2012;42(7):1304–13.
90. Head AM, McGillivray JA, Stokes MA. Gender differences in emotionality and sociability in children with autism spectrum disorders. Mol Autism 2014;5(1). https://doi.org/10.1186/2040-2392-5-19.
91. Harrop C, Jones D, Zheng S, et al. Circumscribed interests and attention in autism: the role of biological sex. J Autism Dev Disord 2018;48(10):3449–59.
92. Barnard-Brak L, Richman D, Almekdash MH. How many girls are we missing in ASD? An examination from a clinic and community based sample. Adv Autism 2019. Published online March 11.
93. Kaat AJ, Shui AM, Ghods SS, et al. Sex differences in scores on standardized measures of autism symptoms: a multisite integrative data analysis. J Child Psychol Psychiatry 2021;62(1):97–106.
94. Kalb LG, Singh V, Hong JS, et al. Analysis of race and sex bias in the autism diagnostic observation schedule (ADOS-2). JAMA Netw Open 2022;5(4):e229498.
95. Allison C, Auyeung B, Baron-Cohen S. Toward Brief "Red Flags" for autism screening: the short autism spectrum quotient and the short quantitative checklist in 1,000 cases and 3,000 controls. J Am Acad Child Adolesc Psychiatry 2012;51(2):202–12.e7.
96. Sappok T, Heinrich M, Underwood L. Screening tools for autism spectrum disorders. Adv Autism 2015;1(1):12–29.
97. Fuller EA, Kaiser AP. The effects of early intervention on social communication outcomes for children with autism spectrum disorder: a meta-analysis. J Autism Dev Disord 2020;50(5):1683–700.
98. Greenslade KJ, Utter EA, Landa RJ. Predictors of pragmatic communication in school-age siblings of children with ASD and low-risk controls. J Autism Dev Disord 2019;49:1352–65.
99. Zeng W, Magaña S, Lopez K, et al. Revisiting an RCT study of a parent education program for Latinx parents in the United States: Are treatment effects maintained over time? Autism 2022;26(2):499–512.
100. Tint A, Weiss JA, Lunsky Y. Identifying the clinical needs and patterns of health service use of adolescent girls and women with autism spectrum disorder. Autism Res 2017;10(9):1558–66.
101. Wodka EL, Parish-Morris J, Annett RD, et al. Co-occurring attention-deficit/hyperactivity disorder and anxiety disorders differentially affect men and women with autism. Clin Neuropsychol 2022;36(5):1069–93.
102. White SW, Albano AM, Johnson CR, et al. Development of a cognitive-behavioral intervention program to treat anxiety and social deficits in teens with high-functioning autism. Clin Child Fam Psychol Rev 2010;13(1):77–90.
103. Antshel KM, Polacek C, McMahon M, et al. Comorbid ADHD and anxiety affect social skills group intervention treatment efficacy in children with autism spectrum disorders. 2011. Available at: www.jdbp.org.

Neurology of Systemic Disease

Selected Topics with a Focus on Women

Faten El Ammar, MD[a], Zachary B. Bulwa, MD[b,*]

KEYWORDS

- Sex differences • Neuroinfectious disease • COVID-19 • Paraneoplastic
- Cardiac arrest • Neurologic prognosis

KEY POINTS

- Acute and chronic outcomes of the neurologic complications of infectious disease may be partially explained by sex differences in immune responses.
- Women of reproductive age and pregnant women have unique risks to infectious pathogens in that they may be transmitted vertically to their fetus in utero or during childbirth leading to congenital abnormalities.
- Recognition of paraneoplastic neurologic disorders, especially those in women, is critical in that they may herald the diagnosis of an occult ovarian or breast malignancy.
- There seem to be sex differences in the neurologic outcomes of survivors of cardiac arrest, however, current data are conflicting.

INTRODUCTION

The breadth of systemic disease with neurologic complications is vast. In this article, we selected topics in which there was evidence of sex differences in epidemiology, clinical presentation, treatment approaches, or outcome, highlighting conditions with more recent findings. We review the sex differences in neurologic presentation and outcome of infectious disease, including Severe Acute Respiratory Syndrome Coronavirus 2 (SARS-CoV-2), Human Immunodeficiency Virus (HIV), and congenital infections of the central nervous system with a special focus on Zika virus. We then describe the clinical presentation, diagnosis, and treatment of the most common paraneoplastic neurologic disorders associated with ovarian and breast cancer. Finally, we highlight the conflicting data regarding the relationship between sex and neurologic outcome in survivors of cardiac arrest.

[a] Neurosciences Intensive Care Unit, Department of Neurology, University of Illinois Chicago, 912 South Wood Street, Chicago, IL 60612, USA; [b] Department of Neurology, Northshore University Healthsystem, 1000 Central Suite, Suite 880, Evanston, IL 60201, USA
* Corresponding author.
E-mail address: zbulwa@northshore.org

Neurol Clin 41 (2023) 399–413
https://doi.org/10.1016/j.ncl.2022.10.007

DISCUSSION

Sex Differences in Neuroinfectious Disease

Sex differences, the differential biological susceptibility to and immunogenic response between women and men, to various infectious diseases have an impact on preventive and treatment strategies, and ultimately outcomes. Until the last decade, there was sparse literature evaluating the impact of sex differences on outcomes in infectious diseases, especially on neurologic complications. Recent pandemics have accentuated the need for further study to elucidate the mechanisms that differentiate clinical outcomes among women and men.

Severe acute respiratory syndrome coronavirus 2

No systemic disease has recently had a larger societal impact than severe acute respiratory syndrome coronavirus 2 (SARS-CoV-2) since it first emerged in Wuhan, China, in late 2019. Several months later, coronavirus disease 2019 (COVID-19), the variety of clinical syndromes associated with SARS-CoV-2, was declared a pandemic. Millions of individuals have now died as a result of COVID-19 worldwide with widespread socioeconomic impact on survivors.

SARS-CoV-2 is a coronavirus transmitted through infected respiratory fluids. COVID-19 most closely resembles an influenza-like illness with fever, myalgias, fatigue, cough, and other respiratory symptoms. However, neurologic complications can be the initial presentation of COVID-19.[1] Furthermore, in patients hospitalized with COVID-19, neurologic manifestations are exceedingly common and are associated with in-hospital mortality.[2] In a multicenter cohort including 13 countries across four continents, 82% of patients (n = 3083) either had self-reported neurologic symptoms or clinically objective neurologic signs.[2] The most common self-reported symptoms were headaches (37%) and anosmia or ageusia (26%). The most common clinically objective neurologic signs or syndromes were acute encephalopathy (49%), coma (17%), and stroke (6%).[2] Other, more rare and acute neurologic manifestations of COVID-19 include viral encephalitis, acute necrotizing hemorrhagic encephalopathy, acute disseminated encephalomyelitis, myelitis, Guillain-Barré syndrome, and myositis.[3]

Exploration of sex differences in COVID-19 was emphasized from the early months of the pandemic.[4] Global Health 50/50, an independent research initiative aiming to advance action and accountability for gender equality in global health, has been tracking sex-disaggregated data and is the largest database of such COVID-19 data. As of its November 2021 update, women made up a roughly equal percentage of cases as men (49% vs 51%), but women were responsible for fewer hospitalizations (45% vs 55%), fewer intensive care unit (ICU) admissions (47% vs 63%), and fewer deaths attributable to COVID-19 (43% vs 57%).[5]

Sex differences specific to neurologic manifestations of COVID-19, especially critical neurologic manifestations such as stroke, likely contribute to a portion of these differential outcomes. A multicenter study in the early phases of the COVID-19 pandemic in the Spring of 2020 in Chicago found that in 83 patients with acute stroke, women had better outcomes: lower mortality (13% vs 38%, $P = .02$), lower mRS at discharge (OR 0.53, 95% CI = 1.03–2.09), and were more likely to be discharged home (33% vs 12%, $P = .04$) when adjusting for age, race, ethnicity, and vascular risk factors.[6] In a pooled analysis of 30 health care organizations including 149,410 COVID-19 patients with laboratory confirmation of SARS-CoV-2 RNA or antibodies, 1618 patients (1.1%) had a diagnosis of stroke;[7] 47% of patients (n = 762) were women and were older and more likely to be of the Black race. In a propensity score matched sample of 634 men and 634 women, balanced by covariates, mortality was lower in women (11.7% vs 15.8% $P = .04$).[7]

Sex differences in other neurologic manifestations in the acute phase of COVID-19 have also been reported. In a study of 12 European hospitals including 417 patients with mild to moderate COVID-19, 86% (n = 357) reported olfactory dysfunction and 88.0% (n = 342) reported gustatory dysfunction.[1] Using the short version of the Questionnaire of Olfactory Disorders-Negative Statements to assess olfactory and gustatory dysfunction on quality of life, women were impacted significantly more by their hyposmia or anosmia ($P < .001$) or gustatory dysfunction ($P = .001$).[1]

As the pandemic lengthened, a post-COVID-19 syndrome emerged. On 6 October, 2021, the World Health Organization released a clinical case definition of post-COVID-19 (also known as long COVID).[8] Symptoms of long COVID should be diagnosed no earlier than 4 weeks after known acute COVID-19. General symptoms may include fatigue, post-exertional malaise, shortness of breath, digestive issues, and changes in menstrual cycles. Neurologic symptoms include cognitive changes with inattentiveness and difficulty processing, headache, sleep disturbances, myalgias, dysgeusia, anosmia, depression, and anxiety.[9]

Although men have demonstrated worse outcomes in the acute phase of COVID-19, women have been reported to have worse outcomes from long COVID-19.[10] In their systemic review, Sylvester and colleagues reported that not only were women more likely to have long COVID (OR = 1.22; 95% CI 1.13–1.32), but were more likely to have otolaryngologic (OR = 2.28 95% CI: 1.94–2.67), psychiatric or mood (OR = 1.58; 95% CI: 1.37–1.82), and neurologic (OR = 1.30; 95% CI 1.03–1.63) symptoms.[10] Within the neurologic category of long COVID-19 symptoms, cognitive impairment, headache, myalgias, and sleep disturbance were more commonly reported in women compared with men.[11]

Our collective understanding of the mechanisms underlying sex differences in acute and long COVID-19 outcomes is evolving. Patient age and comorbidities aside, sex differences in immune responses, and perhaps angiotensin-converting enzyme-2 (ACE2) receptor expression, the primary point of entry into cells for SARS-CoV-2, are partly responsible for these findings. Women were found to have a robust T-cell activation compared with men associated with reduced acute COVID-19 severity, whereas men were found to have higher levels of innate immune activation via interleukin-8 and interleukin-18, which was associated with increased acute COVID-19 severity.[12] This has led to the hypothesis that increased adaptive immune responses through T-cell activation are responsible for improved outcomes in women with acute COVID-19, but create vulnerabilities to long COVID-19.[11]

The ACE2 gene is located on the X chromosome[13] and ACE2 receptor expression is modulated by sex hormones, specifically estradiol, in animal studies.[14,15] However, the exact role of ACE2 receptor expression in differential sex outcomes remains to be fully elucidated.

Further study is needed to better understand sex differences in the immune response and protein expression in COVID-19. This improved understanding may help to guide antiviral therapies and vaccinations to reduce vulnerabilities to acute and long COVID-19 complications limiting poor outcomes.

Human immunodeficiency virus

Beginning in 1981 and rapidly spreading globally, the HIV and acquired immunodeficiency syndrome (AIDS) pandemic has now claimed an estimated 40 million lives.[16] HIV infects T cells resulting in immunodeficiency, which can progress to AIDS if untreated. HIV is primarily a sexually transmitted infection, but can also be transferred from mother to fetus during pregnancy, childbirth, or through exposure to other bodily fluids. There remains no cure for HIV infection, however, advancement in prevention strategies and treatment has transformed HIV infection into a chronic health condition, with individuals living longer lives with the disease. As of the end of 2021, an estimated 38 million people were living with HIV, the majority living in Africa.[16]

Neurologic complications of HIV are vast, affecting both the central nervous system (CNS) and peripheral nervous system (PNS), and may occur at any time throughout the course of infection. Neurologic complications may be caused by direct viral invasion, immune-mediated effects, opportunistic infections, or adverse reactions to combination antiretroviral therapy.[17] CNS complications include stroke, vasculopathy, meningitis, cognitive disorders, intracranial mass lesions from opportunistic infections, encephalomyelitis, myelitis, and myelopathy. PNS complications include peripheral neuropathy, mononeuritis multiplex, polyradiculoneuropathy, opportunistic radiculitis, plexopathy, motor neuronopathy, neuromuscular syndrome, myasthenia gravis, and opportunistic myositis.[17]

Sex differences in neurologic complications of HIV-positive (HIV+) patients have been reported in HIV-associated neurocognitive disorders (HAND) and stroke.

The classification of HAND includes asymptomatic neurocognitive disorders (ie, those only detected on neuropsychological testing, but not otherwise clinically apparent), mild and moderate cognitive impairment, and HIV-associated dementia, and excludes acute HIV encephalitis, encephalopathy due to other causes, including chronic cognitive impairment due to opportunistic infections.[17] HAND remains common among patients living with HIV, although treatment with combination antiretroviral therapy has shown to impede the progression of cognitive decline.[18] Few studies have been statistically powered to analyze the sex differences among women living with HIV (WLWH) versus men living with HIV (MLWH) compared with HIV-negative (HIV-) patients separated by sex.[19] As a result, the cognitive profiles and specific domains of impairment in women may be concealed by larger male populations in these studies.[19] In the few studies with adequate statistical power to evaluate significant differences among groups, there is evidence of greater cognitive impairment in WLWH, specifically in the domains of memory, motor function, and processing speed.[20–22]

Among 1361 HIV + patients (204 women) and 702 HIV- patients (214 women), HIV-associated cognitive impairment was 1.5 times more common in women versus men (OR = 1.53; 95% CI: 1.13–2.06), however, this difference was not statistically significant after adjusted for reading level.[20] The low reading level demonstrated a significant interaction with odds of cognitive impairment (OR = 2.88; 95% CI: 2.23–3.70) as did depression (OR = 1.55; 95% CI: 1.24–1.94).[20] Interestingly, this association was not associated with educational level, perhaps indicating that educational quality, especially in lower socioeconomic environments, is more important than quantity.[20] Furthermore, this study was biased by significant racial differences by sex with a most of White MLWH compared with a most of Black WLWH.[20] In a study of 1420 patients, including 429 WLWH and 429 MLWH, WLWH showed cognitive impairment in domains of psychomotor and processing speed, attention, and motor skills compared with MLWH and HIV individuals.[21] The Black race was equally represented and depression was controlled for in the study.[21] In a more recent study of cognitive impairment profiles in 1666 patients living with HIV, including 201 WLWH, cognitive domains of learning, memory, and motor skills were more commonly affected in WLWH compared with MLWH.[22]

Several hypotheses have been shaped to explain the sex differences in HAND. WLWH are particularly vulnerable to socioeconomic risk factors including limited education, poverty, early-life trauma, barriers to health care, and depression.[19,23] There may also be a strictly biological basis for the sex differences in cognitive disorders. Despite combination antiretroviral therapy viral suppression, women have elevated biomarkers of inflammation and immune activation compared with men (interferon-γ: 22.4 vs 14.9 pg/mL, P = .05; tumor necrosis factor-α: 11.5 vs 9.5 pg/mL, P = .02; and CD4: 373 vs 323 cells/mm^3, P = .02), despite lower viral loads at baseline (median $\log_{10}$ HIV load 4.93 vs 5.18 copies/mL, P = .01).[24] These data may suggest that chronically elevated immune activation can influence chronic HIV-associated conditions, such as HAND.

Another neurologic manifestation of HIV is cerebrovascular disease. The cause of both vasculopathy and stroke is likely multifactorial including accelerated atherosclerosis through recurrent endothelial injury and prolonged inflammation mediated by exposure to HIV, adverse effects of combination antiretroviral therapies, comorbid drug use, and other comorbidities, including, but not limited to, endocarditis, hypertension, hyperlipidemia, and diabetes.

In a large retrospective cohort of 6298 HIV + patients from San Francisco General Hospital, 144 had undergone cerebrovascular imaging; 14% of these patients (n = 20) had dolichoectatic vessels and 95% (n = 19) of patients with dolichoectatic vessels had at least one associated intracranial aneurysm. Female sex and higher peak viral load were associated with dolichoectatic vessels and aneurysms.[25]

Sex differences were also demonstrated in ischemic stroke patients in the Boston health care system Partners cohort.[26] Women represented 36% of the total person-years in this cohort. The ischemic stroke hazard ratio between WLWH and HIV-women was 2.16 (95% CI: 1.53–3.04), but not for MLWH and HIV-men. This relationship between HIV status and stroke in women remained significant when adjusting for demographics and vascular risk factors. The authors hypothesized that the sex differences for ischemic stroke may be due to a combination of factors including lower risks of stroke in women in the general population, higher levels of immune activation in women compared with men, and/or by use of oral contraceptive or hormone replacement therapy in these younger women.[26]

Congenital infections of the central nervous system

Women of reproductive age and pregnant women carry unique risks in that infections may be passed along to the fetus. The most common pathogens to cause neurologic dysfunction in neonates have been acronymized into 'TORCH': toxoplasmosis, other infections (including, but not limited to, syphilis), rubella, cytomegalovirus, HIV, and herpes simplex virus. Treatment is available for many of these infections, and therefore, appropriate prenatal education, diagnosis, and intervention are critical to reducing risks to the neonate. Neurologic manifestations in the newborn vary by the pathogen.[27–34] The most recent pathogen to be added to the list of congenital infections of the nervous system is Zika virus.

Zika virus

Zika virus is an arthopod-borne virus primarily transmitted via the bite of the Aedes aegypti mosquitos found mostly in tropical climates although they are prevalent in the southern United States. Most individuals infected with the Zika virus are asymptomatic and most symptomatic patients present with a mild febrile illness accompanied by a maculopapular rash, arthralgias, myalgias, conjunctivitis, and headache. Generally, the infection is self-limited and most symptomatic patients do not seek or require medical care. However, in the latest Zika virus epidemic which originated in Brazil in 2014, a unique risk became apparent in pregnant women and women of reproductive age in the congenital syndrome seen in children born to pregnant mothers infected with Zika virus. The congenital Zika syndrome includes, but is not limited to, severe microcephaly, arthogryposis (multiple contractures) hypertonia, and retinal and optic nerve anomalies.[35]

Microcephaly is the most commonly reported neurologic anomaly.[35] From January 1, 2015, to January 7, 2016, the prevalence of microcephaly at birth in 15 Brazilian states with laboratory-confirmed Zika transmission was 2.80 cases (95% CI: 1.86–4.05) per 10,000 live births compared with 0.60 cases (95% CI: 0.22–1.31) per 10,000 live births ($P < .001$) in four states (without laboratory evidence-confirmed transmission).[36] In a study from Colombia, the rates of microcephaly were 9.6 cases per 10,000 live births.[37] In the US Zika Pregnancy Registry of 972 infants born from completed pregnancies to women with laboratory-confirmed Zika virus infection, 5% of infants had birth defects (n = 51).[38]

To date, there is no effective vaccine against the Zika virus. As such, prevention of infection is paramount. Avoidance of travel to endemic areas and protection against mosquito bites should be prioritized in pregnant women and women of reproductive age. Treatment remains supportive care.

Paraneoplastic Neurologic Disorders

Paraneoplastic neurologic disorders (PNDs) encompass immune-mediated syndromes in the setting of occult or remote cancer. The underlying pathophysiology involves cross-reactivity with onconeuronal antibodies targeting tumor antigens. This spectrum of disorders varies in symptomatology depending on the extent of CNS, PNS, neuromuscular junction, or muscle involvement. The incidence of paraneoplastic neurologic syndromes is estimated to be around 1% of all malignancies.[39]

The leading hypothesis in the pathophysiology of PNDs is the expression of neuronal antigens by the tumor which leads to an immune response against the neoplasm that cross-reacts with nervous tissue. The presence of such antibodies is invaluable for the diagnosis of PNDs but is not critical. Antibodies are extensively studied and include anti-Y (PCA1), anti-Hu (ANNA-1), anti-Ri (ANNA-2), ANNA-3, anti-CV2 (CRMP5), anti-Ma2 (Ta), anti-amphiphysin, among many others. The syndromes include, but are not limited to, encephalitides, myelitis, neuropathies (sensory/motor) in addition to the well-described condition of paraneoplastic cerebellar degeneration (PCD).[39] Among women, the most important PND-associated malignancies are ovarian and breast malignancies (**Table 1**).

Ovarian cancer

Paraneoplastic cerebellar degeneration. Patients with PCD experience symptoms consistent with cerebellar dysfunction including vertigo, truncal or appendicular ataxia, dysarthria, nystagmus, and/or dysdiadochokinesia. Cognitive deficits can also develop. The most common antibody isolated in PCD is anti-Yo, also known as anti-CDR2 (cerebellar degeneration protein-2 antibody) previously termed anti-Purkinje antibody. Anti-Yo is suggestive of ovarian, breast, or less commonly, small-cell lung carcinoma, and should prompt a dedicated diagnostic evaluation to uncover a malignancy. Other antibodies associated with PCD are anti-Ri (antineuronal nuclear antibody type 2, ANNA-2), anti-Hu (ANNA-1), anti-Tr, and anti-mGluR1. PCD is uncommonly seronegative.[40]

The pathophysiology of PCD is thought to be secondary to a T-cell-mediated cytotoxic activity against the CDR2 antigen of both ovarian cancer cells and concomitantly Purkinje cells. Tumor burden can be highly variable from only microscopically detected to advanced metastatic disease.[40–42] Cerebrospinal fluid (CSF) may reveal pleocytosis and/or elevated protein, though a normal CSF profile does not rule out PCD. Intracranial imaging to rule out alternative etiologies of cerebellar dysfunction is imperative. Imaging indicative of PCD includes cerebellar atrophy (the most common finding on magnetic resonance imaging), in addition to cerebellar

Table 1
Paraneoplastic Neurologic disorders associated with common malignancies in women

PND	Antibodies
Ovarian Tumors	
Paraneoplastic cerebellar degeneration (PCD)	Anti-Yo, anti-Ri (ANNA-2), anti-Hu (ANNA-1), anti-Tr, Anti-mGluR1
Anti-N-methyl-D-aspartate receptor (anti-NMDAR) encephalitis	anti-NMDAR
Peripheral neuropathy	anti-Yo, anti-NMDAR, anti-Ri, and anti-amphiphysin
Breast Cancer	
Retinopathy	Anti-enolase, anti-recoverin, anti-transducin, anti-carbonic anhydrase II, and anti-arrestin β
Stiff person syndrome (SPS)	Anti-amphiphysin
Opsoclonus–myoclonus syndrome	Anti-Ri, anti-Yo, anti-Hu and anti-Nova-1 and 2
Sensorimotor neuropathy	anti-Hu, anti-Yo and anti-Ri
Enchephalomyelitis	anti-Hu, anti-Ta, anti-Ma

From Zaborowski MP, Spaczynski M, Nowak-Markwitz E, Michalak S. Paraneoplastic neurological syndromes associated with ovarian tumors. J Cancer Res Clin Oncol. 2015;141:99-108. https://doi.org/10.1007/s00432-014-1745-9; Dalmau J, Tüzün E, Wu HY, et al. Paraneoplastic anti-N-methyl-D-aspartate receptor encephalitis associated with ovarian teratoma. Ann Neurol. 2007;61:25-36. https://doi.org/10.1002/ana.21050; Pan Y. Peripheral Neuropathy in Ovarian Cancer. In: Ovarian Cancer - Clinical and Therapeutic Perspectives. 2012. InTech. p. 109-128; Fanous I, Dillon P. Paraneoplastic neurological complications of breast cancer. Exp Hematol Oncol. 2016;5:29. https://doi.org/10.1186/s40164-016-0058-x.

hypometabolism (or less frequently hypermetabolism) on fluorodeoxyglucose (FDG-PET).[40] Post-mortem pathology reveals cerebellar atrophy with Purkinje cell loss.[43]

Treatment of PCD starts with the diagnostic evaluation for an associated malignancy as tumor resection improves neurologic outcomes.[44] This requires imaging limited to the pelvis or chest, abdomen, and pelvis computerized tomography (CT) scans, transvaginal ultrasonography, pelvic MRI, or FDG-PET imaging. In select cases when clinical suspicion is high, invasive diagnostic evaluations are justified via explorative surgery, especially when the benefit outweighs the risk, generally based on the severity the PND warrants. Aside from tumor resection, other therapies that may be beneficial include corticosteroids, intravenous immunoglobulins (IVIg), plasmapheresis, and other forms of immunosuppression including the use of cyclophosphamide.[43] The overall prognosis is generally not favorable, however, using the currently available combination of therapeutic interventions, the best-reported prognosis is often stability of the neurologic dysfunction.[44]

Anti-N-methyl-D-aspartate receptor encephalitis. The first case of anti-N-methyl-D-aspartate receptor (anti-NMDAR) encephalitis was described by Dalmau and colleagues in 2007.[45] The syndrome was first reported as a neuropsychiatric condition manifesting as behavioral disturbance, psychiatric symptoms, amnesia, seizures, dysautonomia, and sometimes, obtundation and coma, leading to mechanical ventilation.[45] Since the initial findings, significant advancements have been made in the understanding of the physiology, tumor relation, and optimal treatment of anti-NMDAR encephalitis.

Teratoma is the most common tumor associated with anti-NMDAR encephalitis.[40] Ovarian mucinous cystadenoma has also been described but is much less common.[46]

Intracranial imaging in anti-NMDAR encephalitis is abnormal in about half of all patients, most notably revealing a hyperintense T2 signal in the hippocampus, corpus callosum, and temporal and frontal lobes. However, in the other half of patients with encephalitis, imaging is unrevealing, yet may be helpful to exclude other forms of encephalitis.[40] Electroencephalography (EEG) tends to be abnormal in most of the patients with anti-NMDAR encephalitis, with diffuse background slowing most commonly seen on continuous EEG monitoring. A unique pattern described in this condition is termed extreme delta brush, which was noted in 7 of 23 patients (30.4%) in its original description.[47] The group that coined this pattern termed it extreme delta brush owing to its resemblance to the well-known delta brush pattern seen in premature infants with slow- and fast-frequency components.[48]

Physiologically, the same mechanism of cross-reactivity explains the activity of anti-NMDAR antibody on receptors expressed in the CNS leading to the neurologic and psychiatric disturbances seen in this encephalitis.[40] This is further exemplified by the clinical improvement that is seen with the decrease in serologic antibody titers and also explains the clinical benefit of plasma exchange as a therapeutic intervention.[49] As in patients with PCD, patients with anti-NMDAR encephalitis benefit from surgical excision of the teratoma, in addition to steroids, IVIg, and/or plasma exchange. In more severe clinical syndromes, other immunosuppressive agents such as rituximab or cyclophosphamide can be employed.[50]

Paraneoplastic peripheral neuropathy associated with ovarian tumors. Another syndrome traditionally described in association with ovarian tumors is peripheral neuropathy. Antibodies that should prompt the search for ovarian tumors are anti-Yo, anti-NMDAR, anti-Ri, and anti-amphiphysin. However, neuropathy in the setting of an ovarian malignancy may not be paraneoplastic as patients may have other risk factors for neuropathy such as adverse effects of chemotherapeutic agents, nutritional deficiencies, and metabolic and endocrine abnormalities.[51] The variability of PNS involvement ranges from a pure motor or sensory neuropathy to mixed sensorimotor neuropathies, autonomic neuropathy, and acute inflammatory demyelinating polyradiculopathy among others.[39]

Breast cancer

The incidence of breast cancer is one in every eight women, making it the most common malignancy in women, leading to significant advances that have revolutionized screening for and treatment of breast malignancy.[52] Antibodies are detected in about two-thirds of paraneoplastic disorders associated with breast cancer and, as such, are not mandatory for diagnosis, nor should their absence be used to exclude PNDs.[43] The following PNDs have been described in association with breast cancer:

- Paraneoplastic retinopathy
- Stiff person syndrome
- Opsoclonus–myoclonus syndrome
- Sensorimotor neuropathy
- Encephalomyelitis
- Paraneoplastic cerebellar degeneration

Retinopathy. Paraneoplastic retinopathy often presents with photosensitivity and decreased visual acuity. The most common antibodies associated with paraneoplastic retinopathy are anti-enolase, anti-recoverin, anti-transducin, anti-carbonic anhydrase II, and anti-arrestin β. Other malignancies are associated with retinopathy, including lung small cell and non-small cell carcinoma, skin, colon, and lymphoma among others.[43]

Stiff person syndrome. A syndrome heavily associated with anti-glutamic acid decarboxylase antibodies in its autoimmune form, stiff person syndrome leads to painful muscle cramps and stiffness. Anti-amphiphysin antibodies are also described in the paraneoplastic form. Although treatment majorly overlaps with the other PNDs, benzodiazepines are a unique cornerstone in treating stiff person syndrome.[53]

Opsoclonus–myoclonus syndrome. Opsoclonus–myoclonus syndrome is often described in association with neuroblastoma. Clinically, this syndrome manifests with rapid, involuntary eye movements (opsoclonus) and myoclonic jerks. The most common antibodies in this syndrome are anti-Ri, anti-Yo, anti-Hu, and anti-Nova-1 and 2.[43] Prognosis is not as severe as other PNDs with recovery described in the most of the patients.[54]

Sensorimotor neuropathy. As in ovarian cancer, breast cancer can be associated with disturbances in the PNS. Antibodies that should prompt dedicated diagnostic evaluation for breast cancer are anti-Hu, anti-Yo, and anti-Ri.[43] The treatment also consists of immunotherapy and tumor-targeted therapy.[55]

Encephalomyelitis. Most commonly limbic encephalitis, paraneoplastic encephalitis is not only associated with breast cancer but also with lung and testicular malignancy, and is most commonly found to be associated with anti-Hu antibodies. Antiepileptic medications have a unique role in seizure prevention. A complicating feature of paraneoplastic encephalomyelitis is dysautonomia.[43]

Cardiac Arrest

Cardiac arrest leads to the interruption of cerebral perfusion and is thus associated with post-cardiac arrest cerebral injury that can widely vary between patients. Neuroprognostication following cardiac arrest relies heavily on clinical examination, especially brainstem reflexes, motor responses, laboratory biomarkers, intracranial imaging, and electrophysiologic data such as EEG and somatosensory evoked potentials (SSEP). Long-term neurologic outcomes can be difficult to predict and physicians caring for cardiac arrest survivors should employ a comprehensive assessment of these tools to most accurately prognosticate.

The cerebral injury that develops following a cardiac arrest is initially attributed to the interruption of cerebral blood flow leading to immediate neuronal injury. The mechanism of injury is that of energy failure given the interruption of aerobic metabolism and depletion of the adenosine triphosphate reserve. This, in turn, disrupts the energy-dependent cellular ionic exchange, leading to intracellular hypernatremia and cytotoxic edema.[56] On neuroimaging, cerebral edema is evident early after a cardiac arrest on MRI and will later become evident on CT imaging with loss of gray–white matter differentiation, sulcal effacement, and in more severe cases of diffuse cerebral edema, evidence of cerebral herniation.

In cardiac arrest survivors, when the return of spontaneous circulation is achieved, an additional mechanism of injury occurs secondary to reperfusion injury, the basis of which resembles other forms of reperfusion injury such as in ischemic stroke with arterial recanalization, and the mechanism of which has been mostly attributed to neuronal excitotoxicity.[56]

The mainstay of ICU management of post-cardiac arrest patients relies on optimizing cerebral and systemic perfusion, ensuring adequate ventilation while preventing hyperoxia, monitoring for and treating post-cardiac arrest ICU complications such as infections or seizures, which can confound the clinical picture and neuroprognostication efforts, and temperature control.[56] Temperature management seems to have the most robust evidence for neuroprotection. Different temperature targets have been studied in randomized controlled trials including the pioneer targeted temperature management target temperature management (TTM) and TTM-2 trials to establish a safe yet effective hypothermia target.[57,58] However, more recent evidence suggests the importance of strict normothermia, with more recent trials attempting to test the effect of fever control and strict normothermia in comparison with hypothermia.[59]

Sex differences in hypoxic-ischemic injury have long been studied in the neonatal population. Sex differences in the neurologic outcome of cardiac arrest survivors have also been investigated yet appear to be more heterogeneous. Studies have shown that estrogen and progesterone are neuroprotective and may decrease cerebral edema by modulating the inflammatory cascade, exerting a protective effect on the neuronal system during reperfusion injury post-cardiac arrest.[60] How these mechanisms translate into a palpable sex difference in cardiac arrest neurologic outcome appears to be less obvious, yet, has gained extensive attention over the past few decades.

An animal model by Mirza and colleagues inducing hypoxic-ischemic encephalopathy (HIE) in mice demonstrated that although the injury was not sex-dependent in the acute phase, female neonates later developed less infarction and seizures 3 days post-injury, in addition to less cerebral atrophy and long-term behavioral deficits.[61] Literature confirms the worse prognosis in male infants compared with female infants following HIE. In fact, male infants suffer from a higher mortality rate, stillbirths, and increased risk of neurologic deficits attributable to HIE including developmental delay, learning disabilities, blindness, and deafness.[62] Underlying the sex differences in neonatal HIE are differential effects of sex hormones between male infants and female infants with testosterone potentially worsening excitotoxicity and estrogen being neuroprotective.[62]

The adult cardiac arrest population has been extensively studied concerning the most important prognostic markers in long-term functional recovery. Sex differences have been identified, yet results have been heterogeneous. In one study of 4875 resuscitated patients, the rate of survival with good neurologic function (defined as a modified Rankin scale $\leq$3) was lower in women compared with men (17.6% vs 31.0%, $P < .001$).[63] In another study of 2300 cardiac arrest survivors, women had poorer functional recovery and worse quality of life compared with men.[64] Similar findings were the result of a recent meta-analysis, such that women had a worse neurologic prognosis following cardiac arrest (OR = 0.62, 95% CI: 0.47–0.83).[65] In contrast, Kotini-Shah and colleagues evaluated 326,138 adults with cardiac arrest from 2013 to 2019. They found that men were less likely to survive hospital admission (OR = 0.75, 95% CI: 0.73–0.77), survive hospital discharge (OR = 0.83, 95% CI: 0.80–0.85), or have favorable neurologic survival compared with women (OR = 0.88, 95% CI: 0.85–0.91).[66] One hypothesis for the heterogenous results may be the neurologic outcomes measures used (modified Rankin scale vs cerebral performance category vs extended Glasgow outcome scale), which may predispose to variable results.

Despite this variability in results throughout the literature, there invariably seem to be sex differences in the neurologic outcome of survivors of cardiac arrest. The basis of this differential prognosis, if better elucidated, has the potential to introduce novel therapeutic interventions in the post-cardiac arrest population.[67,68]

SUMMARY

Sex differences exist within the neurologic complications of systemic disease. Herein, we reviewed the differential impact sex has in shaping our response to the neurologic manifestations of infectious disease and neurologic outcome after cardiac arrest. However, a deeper exploration of these relationships is needed. We highlighted key paraneoplastic presentations associated with malignancy in women to improve early diagnosis. It remains crucial to consider reporting sex-disaggregated data in all fields to better highlight these differences, promoting new avenues for prevention and novel therapeutics.

CLINICS CARE POINTS

- Acute and chronic outcomes of the neurologic complications of infectious disease may be partially explained by sex differences in immune responses.
- Women of reproductive age and pregnant women have unique risks to infectious pathogens in that they may be transmitted vertically to their fetus in utero or during childbirth leading to congenital abnormalities.
- Recognition of paraneoplastic neurologic disorders, especially those in women, is critical in that they may herald the diagnosis of an occult ovarian or breast malignancy.
- There seem to be sex differences in the neurologic outcomes of survivors of cardiac arrest, however, current data are conflicting.

DISCLOSURE

The authors have no conflict of interest or commercial or financial disclosures to declare.

REFERENCES

1. Lechien JR, Chiesa-Estomba CM, De Siati DR, et al. Olfactory and gustatory dysfunctions as a clinical presentation of mild-to-moderate forms of the coronavirus disease (COVID-19): a multicenter European study. Eur Arch Otorhinolaryngol 2020;277:2251–61.
2. Chou SHY, Beghi E, Helbok R, et al. Global Incidence of Neurological Manifestations Among Patients Hospitalized With COVID-19-A Report for the GCS-NeuroCOVID Consortium and the ENERGY Consortium. JAMA Netw Open 2021;4:e2112131.
3. Nath A. Neurologic manifestations of severe acute respiratory syndrome coronavirus 2 infection. Continuum (Minneap Minn) 2021;27:1051–65.
4. The Lancet. The gendered dimensions of COVID-19. Lancet 2020;395:1168.
5. Global Health 50/50. The sex, gender, and COVID-19 project. 2021. 2021. Available at: https://globalhealth5050.org/the-sex-gender-and-covid-19-project/. Accessed July 04, 2022.
6. Trifan G, Goldenberg FD, Caprio FZ, et al. Characteristics of a Diverse Cohort of Stroke Patients with SARS-CoV-2 and Outcome by Sex. J Stroke Cerebrovasc Dis 2020;29:105314.
7. Vahidy FS, Meeks J, Pan A, et al. Abstract 13: Sex differences in mortality among patients with COVID-19 related stroke. Stroke 2021;52:A13.

8. World Health Organization. A clinical case definition of post-COVID-19 condition by a Delphi consensus. 2021. Available at: https://www.who.int/publications/i/item/WHO-2019-nCoV-Post_COVID-19_condition-Clinical_case_definition-2021.1. Accessed July 4, 2022.
9. Centers for Disease Control and Prevention. Long COVID or Post-COVID Conditions. 2022. Available at: https://www.cdc.gov/coronavirus/2019-ncov/long-term-effects/index.html. Accessed July 4, 2022.
10. Sylvester SV, Rusu R, Chan B, et al. Sex differences in sequelae from COVID-19 infection and in long COVID syndrome: a review. Curr Med Res Opin 2022;1–9. https://doi.org/10.1080/03007995.2022.2081454.
11. Jensen A, Castro AW, Ferretti MT, et al. Sex and gender differences in the neurological and neuropsychiatric symptoms of long covid: a narrative review. Ital J Gender-specific Med 2022;8:18–28.
12. Takahashi T, Ellingson MK, Wong P, et al. Sex differences in immune response that underlie COVID-19 disease outcomes. Nature 2020;588:315–20.
13. Salah HM, Mehta JL. Hypothesis: sex-related differences in ACE2 activity may contribute to higher mortality in men versus women with COVID-19. J Cardiovasc Pharmacol Ther 2021;26:114–8.
14. Dalpiaz EPLM, Lamas AZ, Caliman IF, et al. Correction: sex hormones promote opposite effects on ACE and ACE2 activity, hypertrophy and cardiac contractility in spontaneously hypertensive rats. PLoS One 2015;10:e0133225.
15. Gupte M, Thatcher SE, Boustany-Kari CM, et al. Angiotensin converting enzyme 2 contributes to sex differences in the development of obesity hypertension in C57BL/6 Mice. Arterioscler Thromb Vasc Biol 2012;32:1392–9.
16. World Health Organization. HIV. 2022. Available at: https://www.who.int/news-room/fact-sheets/detail/hiv-aids. Accessed July 8, 2022.
17. Grill MF. Neurologic complications of human immunodeficiency virus. Continuum (Minneap Minn) 2021;27:963–91.
18. Sacktor N, Skolasky RL, Seaberg E, et al. Prevalence of HIV-associated neurocognitive disorders in the multicenter AIDS cohort study. Neurology 2016;86:334–40.
19. Rubin LH, Neigh GN, Sundermann EE, et al. Sex differences in neurocognitive function in adults with HIV: patterns, predictors, and mechanisms. Curr Psychiatry Rep 2019;21:94.
20. Sundermann EE, Heaton RK, Pasipanodya E, et al. Sex differences in HIV-associated cognitive impairment. AIDS 2018;32:2719–26.
21. Maki PM, Rubin LH, Springer G, et al. Differences in cognitive function between women and men with HIV. J Acquir Immune Defic Syndr 2018;79:101–7.
22. Rubin LH, Sundermann EE, Dastgheyb R, et al. Sex differences in the patterns and predictors of cognitive function in HIV. Front Neurol 2020;11:551921.
23. Maki PM, Rubin LH, Valcour V, et al. Cognitive function in women with HIV: findings from the Women's Interagency HIV Study. Neurology 2015;84:231–40.
24. Mathad JS, Gupte N, Balagopal A, et al. Sex-related differences in inflammatory and immune activation markers before and after combined antiretroviral therapy initiation. J Acquir Immune Defic Syndr 2016;73:123–9.
25. Edwards NJ, Grill MF, Choi A, et al. Frequency and risk factors for cerebral arterial disease in a HIV/AIDS neuroimaging cohort. Cerebrovasc Dis 2016;41:170–6.
26. Chow FC, Regan S, Feske S, et al. Comparison of ischemic stroke incidence in HIV-infected and non-HIV-infected patients in a US health care system. *J Acquir Immune Defic* Syndr 2012;60:351–8.

27. Patel P. Congenital infections of the nervous system. Continuum (Minneap Minn) 2021;27:1105–26.
28. Bollani L, Auriti C, Achille C, et al. Congenital toxoplasmosis: the state of the art. Front Pediatr 2022;10:894573.
29. World Health Organization. WHO guidelines for the treatment of treponema pallidum (syphilis). 2016. Available at: https://www.who.int/publications/i/item/9789241549714. Accessed July 14, 2022.
30. Arnold SR, Ford-Jones EL. Congenital syphilis: a guide to diagnosis and management. Paediatr Child Health 2000;5:463–9.
31. Winter AK, Moss WJ. Rubella *Lancet* 2022;399:1336–46.
32. Lazzarotto T, Guerra B, Gabrielli L, et al. Update on the prevention, diagnosis and management of cytomegalovirus infection during pregnancy. Clin Microbiol Infect 2011;17:1285–93.
33. Wilmshurst JM, Hammon CK, Donald K, et al. NeuroAIDS in children. Handb Clin Neurol 2018;152:99–116.
34. Rudnick CM, Hoekzema GS. Neonatal herpes simplex virus infection. Am Fam Physician 2002;65:1138–42.
35. Freitas DA, Souza-Santos R, Carvalho LMA, et al. Congenital Zika syndrome: A systematic review. PLoS One 2020;15:e0242367.
36. Kleber de Oliveira W, Cortez-Escalante J, De Oliveira WTGH, et al. Increase in reported prevalence of microcephaly in infants born to women living in areas with confirmed Zika virus transmission during the first trimester of pregnancy - Brazil, 2015. MMWR Morb Mortal Wkly Rep 2016;65:242–7.
37. Cuevas EL, Tong VT, Rozo N, et al. Preliminary report of microcephaly potentially associated with Zika virus infection during pregnancy - Colombia, January-November 2016. MMWR Morb Mortal Wkly Rep 2016;65:1409–13.
38. Reynolds MR, Jones AM, Petersen EE, et al. Vital signs: update on Zika virus-associated birth defects and evaluation of all U.S. Infants with congenital Zika virus exposure—U.S. Zika Pregnancy Registry, 2016. MMWR Morb Mortal Wkly Rep 2017;66:366–73.
39. Rees JH. Paraneoplastic syndromes: When to suspect, how to confirm, and how to manage. J Neurol Neurosurg Psychiatry 2004;75(2):ii43–50.
40. Zaborowski MP, Spaczynski M, Nowak-Markwitz E, et al. Paraneoplastic neurological syndromes associated with ovarian tumors. J Cancer Res Clin Oncol 2015;141:99–108.
41. Peterson K, Rosenblum MK, Kotanides H, et al. Paraneoplastic cerebellar degeneration: I.A clinical analysis of 55 anti–Yo antibody–positive patients. Neurology 1992;42:1931–7.
42. Rojas I, Graus F, Keime-Guibert F, et al. Long-term clinical outcome of paraneoplastic cerebellar degeneration and anti-Yo antibodies. Neurology 2000;55:713–5.
43. Fanous I, Dillon P. Paraneoplastic neurological complications of breast cancer. Exp Hematol Oncol 2016;5:29.
44. Keime-Guibert F, Graus F, Fleury A, et al. Treatment of paraneoplastic neurological syndromes with antineuronal antibodies (Anti-Hu, Anti-Yo) with a combination of immunoglobulins, cyclophosphamide, and methylprednisolone. J Neurol Neurosurg Psychiatry 2000;68:479–82.
45. Dalmau J, Tüzün E, Wu HY, et al. Paraneoplastic anti-N-methyl-D-aspartate receptor encephalitis associated with ovarian teratoma. Ann Neurol 2007;61:25–36.

46. Cho EH, Byun JM, Park HY, et al. The first case of Anti-N-methyl-D-aspartate receptor encephalitis (Anti-NMDAR encephalitis) associated with ovarian mucinous cystadenoma: A case report. Taiwan J Obstet Gynecol 2019;58:557–9.
47. Schmitt SE, Pargeon K, Frechette ES, et al. Extreme delta brush; A unique EEG pattern in adults with anti-NMDA receptor encephalitis. Neurology 2012;79: 1094–100.
48. Whitehead K, Pressler R, Fabrizi L. Characteristics and clinical significance of delta brushes in the EEG of premature infants. Clin Neurophysiol Pract 2016; 2:12–8.
49. Dalmau J, Gleichman AJ, Hughes EG, et al. Anti-NMDA-receptor encephalitis: case series and analysis of the effects of antibodies. Lancet Neurol 2008;7: 1091–8.
50. Dalmau J, Lancaster E, Martinez-Hernandez E, et al. Clinical experience and laboratory investigations in patients with anti-NMDAR encephalitis. Lancet Neurol 2011;10:63–74.
51. Pan Y. Peripheral neuropathy in ovarian cancer. In: Farghaly S, editor. Ovarian cancer - clinical and therapeutic Perspectives. InTech; 2012. p. 109–28.
52. Mcpherson K, Steel CM, Dixon JM. ABC of breast disease. Breast cancer - epidemiology, risk factors, and genetics. BMJ 2000;312:624–8.
53. Murinson BB. Stiff-person syndrome. Neurologist 2004;10:131–7.
54. Klaas JP, Ahlskog JE, Pittock SJ, et al. Adult-onset opsoclonus-myoclonus syndrome. Arch Neurol 2012;69:1598–607.
55. Peterson K, Forsyth PA, Posner JB. Paraneoplastic sensorimotor neuropathy associated with breast cancer. J Neurooncol 1994;21:159–70.
56. Sandroni C, Cronberg T, Sekhon M. Brain injury after cardiac arrest: pathophysiology, treatment, and prognosis. Intensive Care Med 2021;47:1393–414.
57. Nolan JP, Morley PT, Hoek TLV, et al. Therapeutic hypothermia after cardiac arrest: An advisory statement by the Advanced Life Support Task Force of the International Liaison Committee on Resuscitation. Circulation 2003;57:231–5.
58. Nielsen N, Wetterslev J, Cronberg T, et al. Targeted Temperature Management at 33°C versus 36°C after Cardiac Arrest. N Engl J Med 2013;369:2197–206.
59. Dankiewicz J, Cronberg T, Lilja G, et al. Hypothermia versus Normothermia after Out-of-Hospital Cardiac Arrest. N Engl J Med 2021;384:2283–94.
60. Johnson MA, Haukoos JS, Larabee TM, et al. Females of childbearing age have a survival benefit after out-of-hospital cardiac arrest. Resuscitation 2013;84: 639–44.
61. Mirza MA, Ritzel R, Xu Y, et al. Sexually dimorphic outcomes and inflammatory responses in hypoxic-ischemic encephalopathy. J Neuroinflammation 2015; 12:32.
62. Murden S, Borbélyová V, Laštůvka Z, et al. Gender differences involved in the pathophysiology of the perinatal hypoxic-ischemic damage. Physiol Res 2019; 68:S207–17.
63. Mody P, Pandey A, Slutsky AS, et al. Gender-based differences in outcomes among resuscitated patients with out-of-hospital cardiac arrest. Circulation 2021;143:641–9.
64. Nehme Z, Andrew E, Bernard S, et al. Sex differences in the quality-of-life and functional outcome of cardiac arrest survivors. Resuscitation 2019;137:21–8.
65. Lei H, Hu J, Liu L, et al. Sex differences in survival after out-of-hospital cardiac arrest: a meta-analysis. Crit Care 2020;24:613.
66. Kotini-Shah P, Del Rios M, Khosla S, et al. Sex differences in outcomes for out-of-hospital cardiac arrest in the United States. Resuscitation 2021;163:6–13.

67. Noppens RR, Kofler J, Grafe MR, et al. Estradiol after cardiac arrest and cardiopulmonary resuscitation is neuroprotective and mediated through estrogen receptor-β. J Cereb Blood Flow Metab 2009;29:277–86.
68. Ikeda M, Swide T, Vayl A, et al. Estrogen administered after cardiac arrest and cardiopulmonary resuscitation ameliorates acute kidney injury in a sex- and age-specific manner. Crit Care 2015;19:332.

Are America's Caregivers on the Brink of Extinction? The Pandemic Straw that Broke the Nurses' Back

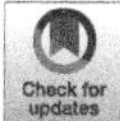

Rachel Elana Norris, MA, MD

KEYWORDS

• COVID-19 • Nursing • Depression • Anxiety • PTSD • Workplace violence

KEY POINTS

- Women comprise majority of the US nursing workforce.
- Nurses experience a higher prevalence of certain neuropsychological disorders than the general public.
- The coronavirus disease 2019 pandemic disproportionately affected health-care workers, particularly nurses.
- Increased prevalence of depression, anxiety, posttraumatic stress disorder, and workplace violence may be contributing to nurses leaving the field.
- Hospital administrators and government agencies must implement policies and practices and adapt the workplace environment to attract and retain nurses.

INTRODUCTION

In March of 2022, The American Nurses Foundation (ANF) published some alarming results of an impact survey of nurses in the United States (US). More than 12,000 nurses participated. More than 50% of those nurses completing the survey planned to leave or were considering leaving their position, an increase of about 20% from the prior year.[1] It was evident from the numerous concerns noted that the emotional and physical stress of working as a nurse throughout the coronavirus disease 2019 (COVID-19) pandemic has taken its toll.

This pandemic has disproportionately influenced health-care workers and particularly bedside nurses. Numerous studies around the globe have demonstrated an increased prevalence of various neuropsychological disorders among nurses during the last 2 years, including depression, anxiety, and other stress-related conditions such as posttraumatic stress disorder (PTSD).[2] This is further exacerbated by

Imagine Healthcare PLLC, 708 W Grand Avenue, Chicago, IL 60654, USA
E-mail address: rachelnorrismd@imaginehealthcare.org

Neurol Clin 41 (2023) 415–423
https://doi.org/10.1016/j.ncl.2022.11.001
0733-8619/23/

workplace violence (WPV) toward nurses, which has been increasing for more than a decade but dramatically increased during the pandemic.[3]

Hospital administrators, government agencies, and the health-care system at large must act judiciously to improve the working conditions for nurses before the next pandemic when a severe nursing shortage would put the health and safety of the US population at high risk.

History

Nursing is this nation's largest health-care profession, with nearly 4.2 million registered nurses (RNs) nationwide.[1] It is historically, and currently, still, a female-dominated profession, with more than 80% of the US RNs being women.[4] Not only do women dominate the profession but they have also historically been its most significant contributors.

Female pioneers in the nursing field, such as Florence Nightingale, made indisputable contributions to both nursing and the health-care profession. Nightingale's approach to caring for patients revolutionized how nurses practiced through her implementation of disease prevention measures, including an emphasis on handwashing and other hygiene practices.

Many might view nurses as the exemplar of Carl Jung's Caregiver archetype: selfless and self-sacrificing, always putting their patients first, making their rounds when they should be eating or taking a much-needed break, as embodied by the "Lady with the Lamp" so famously did nearly 2 centuries ago during the Crimea War. However, even these infinitely selfless caregivers must have a breaking point.

Nightingale, perhaps Jung's quintessential caregiver, would have been appalled by the lack of progress in conditions under which many nurses found themselves during the COVID-19 pandemic: frequently faced with a lack of personal protective equipment, inadequate support, longer shifts due to personnel shortage, inadequate staffing, living in isolation from friends and family, abusive patients and family members, fear of falling ill to the same virus plaguing their patients, watching patients and colleagues succumb to COVID-19, all of which resulted in an excessively stressful workplace environment. Unsurprisingly, many of these issues have been cited as reasons for nurses leaving or planning to leave their positions.[5]

Background

Before the onset of the global COVID-19 pandemic in 2020, there was already a nursing crisis in the US nursing shortages have been a somewhat cyclical societal issue during the last century with various causes. Frequently, the shortage boiled down to either supply or demand.[6] During the Great Depression, for example, increased use of the health-care system led to heightened demand for nurses rather than an actual reduction in the number of nurses. During World War II, the US military ciphered tens of thousands of nurses from the civilian sector to join the war effort. This nursing shortage was very much a supply problem.

The Institute of Medicine published the landmark report "The Future of Nursing" in October 2010. The report called for doubling the number of nurses with doctoral degrees and increasing the percentage of nurses with baccalaureate degrees in the workforce to 80%.[7] According to the most recent workforce survey referenced above conducted by the National Council of State Boards of Nursing, only 64.2% of RNs is educated/trained at the baccalaureate or graduate level.[1] The current nursing workforce falls far short of the report's recommendations, and the situation is projected to worsen. According to The Registered Nurse Workforce Report Card and Shortage

Forecast for the US, a nationwide shortage of RNs is anticipated to persist between 2016 and 2030, with the western and southern states being the most affected.[8]

One factor contributing to the shortage is simply a matter of demographics. The US population is aging; nearly one-third is aged older than 58 years. Both patients and nurses alike are getting closer to retirement age. Nearly half (47.5%) of all RNs is now aged older than 50 years.[9]

Although a significant percentage of the population is close to retirement, research shows that the "choice" to retire is not always voluntary. Between 2010 and 2018, an analysis of data from a high-quality longitudinal survey from the University of Michigan suggests that most of those who hold career jobs in their 50s will get pushed out of those jobs before official retirement age.[10] Senior staff nurses are not immune to this nationwide phenomenon. However, whether these older nurses leave voluntarily or involuntarily, younger nurses can advance by moving into positions that pay more and may offer more fulfillment. These tend to be administrative positions that take them away from the bedside, resulting in fewer nurses left in direct patient care, thereby increasing the workload for those remaining and accelerating burnout and more departures.[6]

The term "burnout" is often used to describe the reason for the mass exodus from bedside nursing. However, the term does not adequately encapsulate the mental health crisis that has plagued the nursing profession since the first human cases of COVID-19 were reported in Wuhan City, China, in December 2019.

The Evidence

Depression

The World Health Organization (WHO) defines depression as "persistent sadness and a lack of interest or pleasure in previously rewarding or enjoyable activities. It can also disturb sleep and appetite. Tiredness and poor concentration are common.[11] According to the latest data from the WHO, approximately 5% of adults worldwide suffer from depression.[12] In the US, 8.1% of adults aged 20 years and older experienced depression in a given 2-week period during 2013 to 2016.[13] The prevalence of depressive symptoms in US adults climbed more than 3-fold higher compared with prepandemic levels.[14]

Depression seems to affect women more than men. Some sources note that women are nearly twice as likely to be diagnosed with depression as men.[15] The reasons are multifactorial and complex and may involve reporting bias but there is also evidence for biological and psychosocial causes. With women representing more than 80% of US nurses, depression in this profession is essentially an epidemic of female caregivers.

Nursing is a stressful, demanding, and taxing profession with higher rates of depression linked to job stress.[16] One study published well before the pandemic showed that nurses experience depressive symptoms at a rate twice as high as individuals in other professions.[17] There is a paucity of data specifically on the prevalence of depressive symptoms of US nurses during the pandemic, however.

In a meta-analysis involving nearly 30 countries, including the US, the authors examined the prevalence of stress, depression, anxiety, and sleep disturbance among nurses during the COVID-19 pandemic.[18] Included were 93 cross-sectional studies of 93,112 nurses demonstrating high proportions of the symptoms mentioned above. The aggregate prevalence of depression was 35% among nurses during the COVID-19 outbreak.[18] This rate is higher than that of the general population in the US and around the globe during the same time frame.

Younger nurses may experience even higher rates of depression than their senior counterparts. In the previously cited survey by the ANF, it was found that, during the pandemic, of nurses aged younger than 35 years, 43% reported feeling depressed. In contrast, about one-fifth of nurses aged older than 55 years reported feeling depressed.[1]

Anxiety

Anxiety may be defined as feeling tense, worried, or having ruminating thoughts, as well as experiencing physical changes such as increased rapid heart rate or blood pressure.[19] According to the WHO, the prevalence of anxiety disorders worldwide is approximately 3.4%.[20] In 2019, before the onset of the pandemic, the prevalence of anxiety in the United States was even higher than global rates at about 8%.[21] As with depression, anxiety disorders are more common among women than men: 4.6% compared with 2.6% at the international level.[20]

Early in the pandemic, the prevalence of anxiety among the US population nearly tripled.[22] In the meta-analysis noted above conducted by Al Maqbali *and colleagues*, the pooled prevalence of anxiety was 37% among nurses.[18] Similar to depression, this rate was significantly higher than the general population.

Again, younger nurses noted even higher rates of anxiety than depression based on the ANF survey, with 66% of nurses aged younger than 35 years reported feeling anxious, although still a significant rate of 35% of nurses aged older than 55 years also reported anxiety.[1]

The prevalence of anxiety and depression, stress, and sleep disturbance was higher during the COVID-19 pandemic than reported during the previous Middle East respiratory syndrome coronavirus (MERS) and severe acute respiratory syndrome (SARS) epidemics.[18] One might postulate that these higher rates could be related to the different natures of the viruses themselves. For instance, although MERS and SARS have a higher fatality rate, COVID-19 is far more infectious, spreading easily from person to person, even in the absence of symptoms. This high infectivity rate changed the way nurses and the population as a whole lived their lives.

Another significant difference between MERS/SARS and COVID-19 is the sheer number of lives lost due to COVID-19. Since 2012, 858 deaths have been attributed to MERS.[23] During the 2003 SARS outbreak, there were 8098 confirmed cases worldwide, with 774 deaths. In the US, only 8 people had laboratory evidence of SARS-associated coronavirus infection.[24]

The most recent statistics reported by the WHO demonstrate more than 615 million confirmed cases of COVID-19 worldwide, with more than 6.5 million deaths.[25] More than 1 million of these deaths were in the US.[26] During the first year of the pandemic, more than 3600 health-care workers in the US lost their lives to the virus; 1 in 3 deaths (32%) were nurses.[23] More US nurses lost their lives to COVID-19 than the entire world population lost to either SARS or MERS. This a shocking statistic and one which cannot be overlooked when discussing the state of mental health of our nurses.

Posttraumatic Stress Disorder

The term “burnout” is often used when citing reasons for nurses leaving the profession. It is worth taking a moment to understand this term better. Based on the International Classification of Diseases 11th Revision (ICD-11) released this year, “burnout” is defined as “a syndrome conceptualized as resulting from chronic workplace stress that has not been successfully managed. Three dimensions characterize it:

- Feelings of energy depletion or exhaustion;
- Increased mental distance from one's job, or feelings of negativism or cynicism related to one's job; and
- Reduced professional efficacy."[27]

Burnout is *not* a medical diagnosis. Moreover, although many nurses may have experienced job burnout before the pandemic, what many have experienced since 2020 is not burnout but rather PTSD.

PTSD can occur in people who have witnessed or experienced a traumatic event. The American Psychiatric Association explains that "people with PTSD have intense, disturbing thoughts and feelings related to their experience that last long after the traumatic event has ended. They may relive the event through flashbacks or nightmares; they may feel sadness, fear, or anger; and they may feel detached or estranged from other people. People with PTSD may avoid situations or people that remind them of the traumatic event, and they may have strong negative reactions to something as ordinary as a loud noise or an accidental touch."[28]

During the COVID-19 pandemic, nurses involved directly with patient care often witnessed not just a single traumatic event but multiple traumatic events, sometimes on the same day. Many witnessed not only the deaths of their patients but also colleagues, family, and friends. Due to visitor restrictions during the pandemic, most patients died without loved ones around them—their nurse was the only one present when they left this earth.

In one study of nurses working in acute care settings during the pandemic in the US, 58.7% were at risk for developing PTSD.[29] A similar study found 47% at risk for PTSD, which, although a lower rate than the study mentioned above, is still higher than veterans of Vietnam, The Gulf War, or Operation Iraqi Freedom, according to the US Department of Veterans Affairs.[30–32]

Although the mental health of nurses worsened during the COVID-19 pandemic, it alone is not to blame for nurses leaving the profession in mass. Other endemic issues have not been comprehensively addressed and have been left to fester within the health-care system for decades. Insufficient staffing and a workplace environment negatively influencing one's health and well-being are 2 of the most common reasons nurses want to leave their current positions.[1] Feeling unsupported by an employer during the pandemic, a lack of trust in an employer, the need for a higher income, and a poor organizational response to COVID-19 are additional reasons for wanting to leave.[1] However, incivility and a complete lack of respect for this nation's largest caregiver group is an epidemic that has infiltrated our hospitals and clinics but is often overlooked.

Workplace Violence

Bullying and incivility toward nurses are something that has likely been around as long as the nursing profession itself. Senior nurses bullying new recruits is seen by some as a rite of passage in the profession. Physicians bullying nurses has become a societal norm exemplified in what seems like nearly every medical drama on television. Although bullying and incivility have no place in any professional environment, WPV is a shocking reality faced by members of the health-care field every day.

The most common health-care environment-based assault is one in which the perpetrator is a member of the public with whom the nurse interacts during the course of their regular duties. This is known as Type II WPV. According to the US Bureau of Labor Statistics 2020 data, nurses experience a high rate of Type II WPV.[31] Reported rates are likely lower than actual rates. The complexities of reporting lead to underreporting, which, in turn, results in underestimating the extent of the problem. Since hospital administration is unaware of the full magnitude of the issue, there may be minimal effort to address it.[33]

Being a hospitalized patient during the pandemic was both physically and psychologically straining, particularly early on when there were still so many unknowns about the virus itself and providers were unsure how to best treat the disease. The fear alone may have been overwhelming, causing patients to act out either verbally or physically toward caregivers. Fever, electrolyte imbalances, hypoxia, and other components of the disease process could lead to delirium, causing patients to behave in ways they usually would not act when healthy. Families and visitors of patients also experienced increased levels of stress.

Nurses' poor mental health, increased workload, inadequate staffing, and lack of support all contributed to an increase in vulnerability, which could exacerbate both WPV and its underreporting.[33,34] For instance, it has been demonstrated that unmet patient health-care needs and requests are a risk factor for Type II WPV. It is possible that these issues were made worse by staffing shortages and reduced hospital capacity during the COVID-19 pandemic.[35]

An alarming 66% of nurses during the pandemic said they experienced increased bullying at work compared with before the pandemic.[36] Incivility and bullying were predominately identified as coming from patients and their families.[1] About 33% of nurses said they had experienced violence in their workplace, and it does not stop at the hospital doors—nearly a quarter of nurses reported bullying outside of work, and 12% reported violence outside of work.[36] This is consistent across different surveys.

DISCUSSION

Numerous measures have already been implemented to address the mental health crisis involving our nation's health-care workers, including those created by individual hospital systems and new organizations born out of the pandemic. Some examples include the following:

- The Lorna Breen Health Care Provider Protection Act—The bill was named after an assistant professor of emergency medicine at Columbia University Vagelos College of Physicians and Surgeons who died by suicide in April 2021. Its purpose is to help create training programs focused on well-being and behavioral health and a national campaign encouraging health-care professionals to seek support and treatment.
- "Don't Clock Out"—Friends and colleagues of Michael Odell, a critical care nurse who died by suicide in January 2022, founded the not-for-profit as a peer support community and mental health resource for nurses.

However, the problem does not seem to be a lack of resources but rather that the resources already in place are not being used. According to one survey, 72% of nurses have access to mental health services but 90% never take advantage of these services.[37] The reasons behind this are multifactorial. The stigma surrounding mental health is a significant deterrent for many to seek help. There might be fears regarding professional licensing if one were to report that they were seeking help for a mental health disorder.

Regarding WPV, there were already several initiatives introduced before the pandemic by various organizations to decrease its prevalence.

- 2015—American Nurses Association (ANA) concluded deliberations and issued a new position statement on incivility, bullying, and WPV.
- 2016—Occupational Safety and Health Administration issued a Request for Information soliciting information on the topic of WPV.

- 2019—H.R. 1309 (Workplace Violence Prevention for Health Care and Social Service Workers Act, 2019) was introduced by US House of Representative Joe Courtney. This bill, if passed, would require a comprehensive WPV prevention plan be developed and implemented by covered employers in the social service and health-care sectors.
- 2019—ANA launched the #EndNurseAbuse campaign to increase awareness of WPV against nurses.

Yet, despite these efforts, bullying and incivility increased dramatically during the pandemic.[36] There is still no current nationwide to protect health-care workers from WPV. Representative Courtney's bill was introduced to the senate in May of 2022 but no further action has been taken.

SUMMARY

The COVID-19 pandemic has drawn attention to many of the inadequacies of the US health-care system. When it comes to addressing critical issues such as the mental health of its largest group of providers, nurses, and ensuring that health-care workers have a safe environment in which to work, most efforts have fallen short. Many nurses are leaving hospital-based careers, whereas some are leaving the field altogether. Hospital administrators and government agencies must implement policies and practices and adapt the workplace environment to attract and retain nurses by focusing on their safety and the intersection of their work demands and mental health to avoid a potential demographic crisis in the next decade. Unless we act quickly and comprehensively to address the issues that matter to nurses, the next pandemic could be far more deadly, not because the virility of the next virus is higher but because we will have fewer caregivers to save us.

DISCLOSURE

The author has no relevant financial or nonfinancial interests to disclose. The author has no conflicts of interest to declare relevant to this article's content. The author certifies that she has no affiliations with or involvement in any organization or entity with any financial interest or nonfinancial interest in the subject matter or materials discussed in this article. The author has no financial or proprietary interests in any material discussed in this article.

REFERENCES

1. Smiley RA, Ruttinger C, Oliveira CM, et al. The 2020 National Nursing Workforce Survey. J Nurs Regul 2021;12(1):S1–96.
2. Sun P, Wang M, Song T, et al. The Psychological Impact of COVID-19 Pandemic on Health Care Workers: A Systematic Review and Meta-Analysis. Front Psychol 2021;12. https://doi.org/10.3389/fpsyg.2021.626547.
3. Ramzi ZS, Fatah PW, Dalvandi A. Prevalence of Workplace Violence Against Healthcare Workers During the COVID-19 Pandemic: A Systematic Review and Meta-Analysis. Front Psychol 2022;13. https://doi.org/10.3389/fpsyg.2022.896156.
4. U.S. Census Bureau. Your Health Care Is in Women's Hands. The United States Census Bureau. Available at: https://www.census.gov/library/stories/2019/08/your-health-care-in-womens-hands.html. Published August 14, 2019.

5. Shah MK, Gandrakota N, Cimiotti JP, Ghose N, Moore M, Ali MK. Prevalence of and Factors Associated With Nurse Burnout in the US. JAMA Netw open 2021; 4(2). https://doi.org/10.1001/jamanetworkopen.2020.36469.
6. The Real History of U.S. Nursing Shortages. Clipboard Health. Available at: https://clipboardhealth.com/real-history-of-us-nursing-shortages. Published April 26, 2022.
7. Medicine I of. The future of nursing: leading change. Advancing Health 2010. Available at: https://nap.nationalacademies.org/catalog/12956/the-future-of-nursing-leading-change-advancing-health.
8. Zhang X, Tai D, Pforsich H, Lin VW. United States Registered Nurse Workforce Report Card and Shortage Forecast: A Revisit. Am J Med Qual 2017;33(3): 229–36.
9. University of St. Augustine for health sciences. The 2021 American nursing shortage: a data study. University of St. Augustine for Health Sciences; 2021. Available at: https://www.usa.edu/blog/nursing-shortage/. Published May 25.
10. Johnson R, Gosselin P. How Secure Is Employment at Older Ages?. 2018. Available at: https://www.urban.org/sites/default/files/publication/99570/how_secure_is_employment_at_older_ages_2.pdf. Accessed March 8, 2022.
11. World Health Organisation. Depression. 2019. Available at: https://www.who.int/health-topics/depression#tab=tab_1. Published November 29.
12. World Health Organisation. Depression. World Health Organization. Available at: https://www.who.int/news-room/fact-sheets/detail/depression. Published September 13, 2021.
13. Products - Data Briefs - Number 303 - February 2018. Available at: https://www.cdc.gov/nchs/products/databriefs/db303.htm. Published 2019.
14. Ettman CK, Abdalla SM, Cohen GH, Sampson L, Vivier PM, Galea S. Prevalence of Depression Symptoms in US Adults Before and During the COVID-19 Pandemic. JAMA Netw Open 2020;3(9):e2019686.
15. Albert P. Why is depression more prevalent in women? J Psychiatry Neurosci 2015;40(4):219–21.
16. Brandford AA, Reed DB. Depression in registered nurses. Workplace Health Saf 2016;64(10):488–511.
17. Letvak S, Ruhm CJ, McCoy T. Depression in hospital-employed nurses. Clin Nurse Specialist 2012;26(3):177–82.
18. Al-Maqbali M, Al-Sinani M, Al-Lenjawi B. Prevalence of stress, depression, anxiety and sleep disturbance among nurses during the COVID-19 pandemic: A systematic review and meta-analysis. J Psychosomatic Res 2021;141:110343.
19. American Psychological Association. Anxiety. American Psychological Association. Available at: https://www.apa.org/topics/anxiety. Published 2022.
20. World Health Organization. Depression and other common mental disorders global health estimates. 2017. Available at: https://apps.who.int/iris/bitstream/handle/10665/254610/WHO-MSD-MER-2017.2-eng.pdf.
21. Daly M, Robinson E. Anxiety reported by US adults in 2019 and during the 2020 COVID-19 pandemic: population-based evidence from two nationally representative samples. J Affective Disord. Published online February 2021. doi:10.1016/j.jad.2021.02.054
22. Panchal N, Kamal R, Muñana C. Aug 21 PCP, 2020. The Implications of COVID-19 for Mental Health and Substance Use - Issue Brief. KFF. Available at: https://www.kff.org/report-section/the-implications-of-covid-19-for-mental-health-and-substance-use-issue-brief/. Published August 21, 2020.

23. Middle East respiratory syndrome coronavirus (MERS-CoV). Available at: www.who.int https://www.who.int/health-topics/middle-east-respiratory-syndrome-coronavirus-mers#tab=tab_1.
24. CDC. SARS. Centers for Disease Control and Prevention. Available at: https://www.cdc.gov/sars/about/fs-sars.html. Published 2019.
25. World Health Organization. WHO COVID-19 dashboard. World Health Organization; 2022. Available at: https://covid19.who.int/.
26. World Health Organization. WHO Coronavirus Disease (COVID-19) Dashboard. Available at: https://covid19.who.int/region/amro/country/us. Published 2020.
27. World Health Organization. Burn-out an "occupational phenomenon": International Classification of Diseases. Available at: www.who.int https://www.who.int/news/item/28-05-2019-burn-out-an-occupational-phenomenon-international-classification-of-diseases#:~:text=%E2%80%9CBurn%2Dout%20is%20a%20syndrome. Published May 28, 2019.
28. Torres F. What is Posttraumatic Stress Disorder (PTSD)? psychiatry.org. Available at: https://psychiatry.org/patients-families/PTSD/What-is-ptsd. Published August 2020.
29. Hernandez JM, Munyan K, Kennedy E, Kennedy P, Shakoor K, Wisser J. Traumatic stress among frontline American nurses during the COVID-19 pandemic: A survey study. Traumatology 2021. https://doi.org/10.1037/trm0000320. Published online August 16.
30. Guttormson JL, Calkins K, McAndrew N, Fitzgerald J, Losurdo H, Loonsfoot D. Critical Care Nurse Burnout, Moral Distress, and Mental Health During the COVID-19 Pandemic: A United States Survey. Heart & Lung 2022;55:127–33.
31. National Center for PTSD. How common is PTSD in Veterans? - PTSD: National Center for PTSD. Va.gov. Available at: https://www.ptsd.va.gov/understand/common/common_veterans.asp.
32. Byon HD, Sagherian K, Kim Y, et al. Nurses' Experience With Type II Workplace Violence and Underreporting During the COVID-19 Pandemic. Workplace Health Saf 2021. https://doi.org/10.1177/21650799211031233. 21650799211031233.
33. Arnetz JE, Hamblin L, Ager J, et al. Underreporting of workplace violence: comparison of self-report and actual documentation of hospital incidents. Workplace Health Saf 2015;63(5):200–10.
34. Byon HD, Sagherian K, Kim Y, Lipscomb J, Crandall M, Steege L. Nurses' experience with type II workplace violence and underreporting during the COVID-19 Pandemic. Workplace Health Saf 2021. https://doi.org/10.1177/21650799211031233. 216507992110312.
35. Najafi F, Fallahi-Koshknab M, Ahmadi F, Dalvandi A, Rahgozar M. Antecedents and consequences of workplace violence against nurses: A qualitative study. Journal of Clinical Nursing 2018;27(1–2):e116–28.
36. Violence. Incivility, & bullying | american nurses association. ANA. Available at: https://www.nursingworld.org/practice-policy/work-environment/violence-incivility-bullying.
37. Beyond burnout nurses suffer from PTSD as spiraling work demands force them to sacrifice their mental well-Being. Available at: https://www.intelycare.com/wp-content/uploads/2022/02/ICRG-%E2%80%A2-Beyond-Burnout-%E2%80%A2-February-2022.pdf.

Challenges Training Women in Neurology

Stasia Rouse, MBChB[a,*], Ashley Raedy, DO[b], Farah Khan, MD[b]

KEYWORDS

- Women training in neurology • Childbearing • Maternity • Caregiver • Implicit bias • Mentorship • Academic role differences • Sexual harassment

KEY POINTS

- Women training in neurology face several different stressors than their male counterparts.
- *Childbearing* can coincide with residency/fellowship that places a lot of pressure on the individual in all spheres of her life including professionally.
- *Maternity* tends to be more complicated for physicians with fertility issues, higher rates of miscarriage and pregnancy complications.
- Women trainees bear the responsibility of the *caregiver* role in their families contributing to fatigue and potential burnout.
- There is *implicit bias* against women neurologists including *sexual harassment* in the work environment affecting assigned leadership *academic roles*, and such missing opportunities often create challenges finding suitable career *mentorship*.

INTRODUCTION

The challenges that current women neurologists in training face remain similar to a certain extent to those experienced by their women neurologists' mentors. The key challenge that often coincides with residency or fellowship is childbearing. This has the potential to prolong training time and delaying graduation. Women neurologists in training face additional challenges of juggling between family responsibilities—as caregivers—and professional roles.

Some are subject to sexual harassment which further erodes their ability to succeed in their professional career. In addition, women physicians in training face difficulties finding a suitable mentor, which leads to an imbalance of leadership roles during training and throughout career development.

[a] Advocate Lutheran General Hospital, 1875 Dempster Street, Parkside Center, Suite 625, Park Ridge, IL 60068, USA; [b] Loyola University Medical Center, 2160 South First Avenue, Maywood, IL 60153, USA

* Corresponding author.

E-mail address: stasia.rouse@aah.org

Neurol Clin 41 (2023) 425–431
https://doi.org/10.1016/j.ncl.2022.12.003

Part 1: Caregiver

Caregiving is an innate quality of nurturing and dedication to others for their well-being most often seen, or expected, in women. It is unclear whether this is due to women historically caring for children and family while men hunt and provide, or whether it is something genetic. In medicine, being a caregiver is a desirable quality as this improves patient outcomes. Women physicians devote more time to their patients and in turn, and patients cared for by women internists have better survival rates and reduced hospital readmission rates compared with those treated by men internists.[1]

However, at what expense are women in medicine providing this desirable type of care? A recent study showed that women physicians often see fewer patients, tend to spend longer time listening to and assessing patients, and overall spend more time on documentation in the electronic medical records. Thus, while working equal amount of time or longer hours than their male counterparts, women physicians have lower patients' volume, lower pay, and unsurprisingly higher burnout rate s.[2]

Not only are women physicians feeling overworked in a professional setting, but they also have to balance between work and personal life. There are expectations for women to care for their family (spouse, children, and pets), with multitude of unseen thankless household tasks and parental duties, ranging from scheduling children's activities and appointments to caring for the household necessities such as cleaning, cooking, laundry, grocery shopping, and errands. In addition, women tend to care for aging parents or sick family members, as well as assume additional tasks of serving on volunteer committees in the community.

The coronavirus disease-2019 pandemic affected the work–home balance of many working physicians, with closure of daycare and online schooling. Although for some parents remote work was a possibility, this was not an option for health care workers. Tele-video visits and virtual meetings were often challenging for physicians with demanding young children. Many working parents, specifically women physicians were left with the choice of working or taking time off to care for their children. The difficulties finding a satisfying work–life balance, especially during the pandemic led to a higher burnout trend among women physicians compared with male colleagues.[3]

Although tasks can be divided among spouses, and although help can be obtained by hiring aids and assistances, full-time working women often have a sense of guilt, feeling that they are insufficiently providing care for their family. In a survey from 2015, when working parents were asked about career advancements, mothers were three times more likely to report difficulty advancing their careers compared with fathers. In the same survey, working mothers were more likely to quit their job for familial reasons compared with working fathers.[4]

Caregiving is an expectation for women who are under constant pressure to leave their careers to provide for their homes. Career interruptions due to maternity leave or to care for children, an ill family member, or an ailing parent often slow professional career advancements.

Part 2: Maternity Considerations

Most agree there is no right time to start a family. That is especially true for women in medical training. A woman's peak reproductive years are in her twenties and thirties, which, on average, are the same years she may be in medical school, residency, fellowship, or early career as a physician. The rigor of medical training across the nation involves countless hours and night calls spent caring for patients, interpreting diagnostic labs and tests, and making thoughtful yet quick diagnostic decisions, all with a level of sleep deprivation, lack of regular exercise, and poor diet. All these factors, compounded over the 4 to 7 years of neurology residency and fellowship training, may lead to delaying childbearing, a higher rate of pregnancy complications, and/or problems with fertility. Almost one in four female physicians is diagnosed with infertility which is nearly twice the rate of the general population.[5]

For women in medical training, starting a family is cumbersome. Women in medicine often wait for much longer than the general population to have children, as they have trouble adapting to longer working hours. This gap does however close once training. In a review of retrospective studies from the 1980s to 2000s by Susan Finch, an increased risk of pregnancy complications and premature labor was observed among physicians. One possible cause is a decrease in intrauterine blood flow mediated by the elevated catecholamine levels during physical and mental stress.[6] Another study assessing pregnancy during medical training showed that demands of training and long work hours were the most common factors in delaying having children.[7] Of all the participants, 25.5% reported fertility issues, 52.5% reported significant workplace barriers to breastfeeding, and 39.4% stated that their job prevented breastfeeding for the desired length of time.[7]

The resident workplace environment significantly impacts one's decision to conceive. Challenges include a busy call schedule, varying perceptions and attitudes of faculty and co-residents or co-fellows, variable maternity leave options, lack of postpartum support such as adequate lactation room provision, and possible negative effect on graduation or eligibility to board examinations. In 2018, *JAMA Surgery* published a national survey of 347 female general surgeons who had one or more pregnancies during residency to assess the perception and experience of general surgery residents. Of the participants, 72.9% witnessed faculty members or other residents making negative comments about pregnant trainees or the concept of childbearing during training. A maternity leave period of 6 weeks or less was reported by 78.4% of respondents. Childcare support was offered (in the form of preferential daycare enrollment, discounted daycare or access to backup childcare services) for only 18.4% of respondents, with 85% stating the childcare support options were not feasible due to lack of consideration of surgical resident's work hours. It was noted that 66.8% responded that additional women mentorship on balancing pregnancy and motherhood would have been helpful.[8] Although surgical residencies may be structured differently than that in neurology, the above study provides insight into a perception of pregnancy during medical training.

A retrospective cohort study from the Mayo Clinic examining the effect of gender and pregnancy for internal medicine (IM) residents on evaluations by peers and faculty, showed lower mean peer evaluation scores for female residents compared with their male colleagues.[9] These implicit biases certainly affect one's medical training experience and can possibly affect future academic prospects and definitely impact one's morale. Neurology residency programs tend to be smaller (averaging 4 to 10 residents per class) than IM programs and have more rigid call schedules; therefore, relying on colleagues for coverage during maternity leave or parental responsibilities becomes more challenging.

Maternity leave policies among residency training programs are inconsistent. In general, longer maternity leave is associated with improved breastfeeding practices, infant well-being, and better satisfaction with parenthood. Yet, several factors force female residents to take only 6 weeks of maternity leave, most importantly financial burden, as well as a professional relationship and concerns about repercussions from colleagues.[10] In supporting physicians' development, and as of July 1, 2022, Accreditation Council for Graduate Medical Education-accredited programs are required to offer 6 weeks of paid leave to residents and fellows for medical, parental, and caregiver leave. This is a positive step toward a more compassionate medical training environment.

Despite a steep increase in women joining neurology residencies,[11] research on the effect of pregnancy during neurology training is sparse and needs further evaluation.

Part 3: Implicit Bias

Despite medical schools graduating more female physicians, and despite more female entering neurology residency, gender-based implicit biases remain inadvertently acquired from culture and education. Patients' assumptions about health care professional, and stereotypical bias toward males as physicians and females as nurses remain common.[12,13] Implicit biases negatively affect women in their medical training and career development, and contribute to women underrepresentation in leadership roles, reduced scholarly activities, lower compensations, and higher burnout.

Part 4: Sexual Harassment

Medical trainees are a vulnerable at-risk group for sexual harassment. Unfortunately, most of the sexual harassments in the medical field are directed toward women,[14] with nearly half of women medical students had experienced incidents of sexual harassment during their training; and likely many more remain unreported,[15] with higher frequency of sexual harassment incidents in work environments with male-dominated leadership.[14] Such offenses vary from jokes to comments, to other more serious offences. The trauma related to sexual harassment causes a disruption in training, both emotionally and physically, and can interfere with work relationships and career advances.

There are avenues of action that are being implemented to enforce a safe work environment for all employees. Title IX of the Educational Amendments of 1972 is a federal law that protects people from discrimination based on sex in education programs and "prohibits sexual harassment in educational institutions."[14] Title IX applies to institutions that receive federal financial assistance from the Department of Education. This law has revolutionized women's rights and has provided crucial protection for women victims of sexual harassment and sex-based discrimination.

Part 5: Academic Role Differences

For years, there has been a discrepancy between men and women in neurology, which used to be a male-dominant specialty. In 2013, women neurologists made up only 26% of the total active neurologists in the United States.[16] Recently, there has been a shift with an increasing number of women entering not only neurology but the field of medicine as a whole. According to the American Medical Association, in the most recent years, women have surpassed men matriculating for medical schools. [17] Yet despite this ongoing shift, fewer women pursue neurology as a career.

There is an increasing gap between academic neurologists with only one in three being women. Among the top 29 ranked neurology departments in the United States, women accounted for only 31% of academicians compared with 69% among men neurologists. [18] The gap widens with seniority and with professional rank. [18] Women neurologists tend to gravitate to the community or private practices, which tend to offer a flexible schedule, including part-time practice opportunities to help balancing work–life schedule, and less stress of scholarly publications. [19]

Part 6: Mentorship

More than 60% of neurology residents attribute their choice of residency to a mentor. Mentorship has been shown to be beneficial at all career levels for both the mentor and the mentee. For mentors, benefits include greater perception of career success, intellectual stimulation, personal satisfaction, less likelihood of burnout, among others. Among some of the benefits of having a mentor include higher job and personal satisfaction, faster rate of promotions, increased professional visibility and networking, positive affect on health and wellbeing, higher faculty retention and decreased burnout. Opportunities for mentorship in neurology can begin as early as the first year of medical school with programs such as Comprehensive Opportunities for Research and Teaching Experience which have resulted in increased academic productivity, guidance on the residency application process and an increased number of students matching into neurology programs. Other mentorship opportunities include the American Academy of Neurology's Student Interest Group in Neurology which has a cohort at most US medical schools.[20]

It is also important to note the lack of data on mentorship for and from underrepresented racial and ethnic minority populations as well as those that identify as lesbian, gay, bisexual, transgender, or queer. These vulnerable groups, similar to women, also face challenges in job obligations while battling stereotypes. The lack of mentorship and sponsorship, in addition to potential harassment, often leads to burnout which contributes to the "leaky pipeline."[20]

Mentorship is also beneficial in tackling "imposter syndrome," in which one has doubts about personal ability, competency, and qualifications despite being accomplished. Imposter syndrome is associated with low motivation to have an academic career, poor career planning, and a lower drive to pursue leadership opportunities.

A key element in bridging the gender gap is by incorporating "women-specific faculty development programs" which address career development, research, promotion, communication, time management, and ethical issues. Specific teaching points include enhanced clinical teaching skills, grant and manuscript writing, development of scientific presentations as well as access to biostatisticians and research stipends. Access to a sponsorship program is also important. Sponsors help advance professional careers by identifying and providing leadership opportunities for women physicians.[20]

Several templates for instituting mentorship programs have been proposed. Key stakeholders include the mentor, mentee, department, institution, and finally social and professional organizations. Mentors should be trained to be effective and mentees should be able to select a mentor that aligns with one's goals. Departments should construct mentorship programs, monitor program's effectiveness, and support mentors through promotion and/or protected time as well as provide an incentive to the mentorship role. On an institutional level, extra-departmental mentors can be beneficial, and resources can be shared among departments. Finally, professional organizations such as Women Mentoring Excellence in Neurology, Women in Neurocritical Care mentorship program, and American Medical Women's Association, among others, may be options for further discourse on the topic and could provide access to variable resources.[20]

Challenges in mentorship for women in neurology include the role of gender concordance. One study showed that 80% of women faculty reported that gender concordance was not a factor in choosing a mentor, emphasizing that male mentors can play important roles in closing the gender gap. In contrast, women residents were more likely to choose same-gender mentors thinking they would be more understanding.[20] Another challenge is the hesitance of men to mentor women in training as an unintended consequence of the #MeToo movement. It can be argued that mentorship is an obligation for physicians to trainees and the fear of a sexual misconduct accusation should not deter men from mentoring women. It is critical for men to continue to mentor women in medicine, whereas remaining aware of gender gaps in clinical and academic achievement.[20]

Neurology has one of the greatest gender disparities in compensation and clinical and academic leadership in part due to a lack of formal mentorship and sponsorship programs. Formal mentorship programs should be available to women, underrepresented racial and ethnic minority physicians, and sex and gender minority physicians to support professional development.

SUMMARY

Empowering and inspiring women neurologists in training is necessary to tackle gender disparities. The best guidance we can provide to women in training in neurology is to support them through guidance, mentorship, and coaching.

Having regular contact sessions with a mentor is mutually beneficial and can lead to creative solutions and camaraderie. Sharing struggles often sheds light on potential solutions in the given scenario but also in the mentor's realm. This process will foster greater workplace satisfaction and decrease burnout. Mentors may be sought in different departments, even different organizations, as sometimes a different perspective is refreshing. Closing the gender pay and promotion gaps is arguably the most effective way to promote career growth of the women in the academic workforce. Further support for colleagues in their childbearing years is essential. The future for women in neurology is bright; we must continue the fight to address gender inequality, eliminate the pay gap, tackle the gender disparity in faculty ranking and promotions, recognize authorship and promote scientific advancement, provide mentorship, promote scientific, and attaining leadership positions.

DISCLOSURE

The authors have no commercial conflict of interest or financial disclosures.

REFERENCES

1. Tsugawa Y, Jena A, Figueroa J, et al. Comparison of Hospital Mortality and Readmission Rates for Medicare Patients Treated by Male vs Female Physicians. JAMA Intern Med 2017;177(2):206.
2. Adams K. Female clinicians spend more time in the EHR, study finds. 2022. Available at: Beckershospitalreview.com; https://www.beckershospitalreview.com/ehrs/female-clinicians-spend-more-time-in-the-ehr-study-finds.html. Accessed 31 August 2022.
3. Khan N, Palepu A, Dodek P, et al. Cross-sectional survey on physician burnout during the COVID-19 pandemic in Vancouver, Canada: the role of gender, ethnicity and sexual orientation. BMJ Open 2021;11(5):e050380. Available at: https://pubmed.ncbi.nlm.nih.gov/33972345/. Accessed 2 September 2022.
4. Parker K. Despite progress, women still bear heavier load than men in balancing work and family. [online] Pew Research Center. 2015. Available at: https://www.pewresearch.org/fact-tank/2015/03/10/women-still-bear-heavier-load-than-men-balancing-work-family/. Accessed 31 August 2022.
5. Stentz NC, Griffith KA, Perkins E, et al. Fertility and Childbearing Among American Female Physicians. J Womens Health (Larchmt) 2016 Oct;25(10):1059–65.
6. Finch SJ. Pregnancy during residency: a literature review. Acad Med 2003;78(4):418–28.

7. Armijo PR, Flores L, Huynh L, et al. Fertility and Reproductive Health in Women Physicians. J Womens Health (Larchmt) 2021;30(12):1713–9.
8. Rangel EL, Smink DS, Castillo-Angeles M, et al. Pregnancy and Motherhood During Surgical Training. JAMA Surg 2018;153(7):644–52.
9. Krause ML, Elrashidi MY, Halvorsen AJ, et al. Impact of Pregnancy and Gender on Internal Medicine Resident Evaluations: A Retrospective Cohort Study. J Gen Intern Med 2017;32:648–53.
10. Stack SW, Jagsi R, Biermann JS, et al. Maternity Leave in Residency: A Multicenter Study of Determinants and Wellness Outcomes. Acad Med 2019;94(11): 1738–45.
11. Gil Tommee C, Nalleballe K, Dandu V, et al. Trends in Demographics of Neurology House Staff in the United States. Cureus 2021;13(9):e17754. Published 2021 Sep 6.
12. Pappas S. Male Doctors, Female Nurses: Subconscious Stereotypes Hard to Budge. 2016. Available at: livescience.com; https://www.livescience.com/55134-subconscious-stereotypes-hard-to-budge.html. Accessed 31 August 2022.
13. Xun H, Chen J, Sun A, et al. Public perceptions of physician attire and professionalism in the US. JAMA Network Open; 2021. p. e2117779. Available at: https://jamanetwork.com/journals/jamanetworkopen/fullarticle/2782564#: ~ :Public Perceptions of Physician Attire and Professionalism in the US. Accessed 31 August 2022.
14. Silver J. Understanding and addressing gender equity for women in neurology. Neurology 2019;93(12):538–49.
15. Binder R, Garcia P, Johnson B, et al. Sexual Harassment in Medical Schools. Acad Med 2018;93(12):1770–3.
16. Joy K. Only 1 in 3 Academic Neurologists Are Women, Study Finds. [online] University of Michigan. 2018. Available at: https://labblog.uofmhealth.org/industry-dx/only-1-3-academic-neurologists-are-women-study-finds. Accessed 31 August 2022.
17. Fall Applicant, Matriculant, and Enrollment Data Tables. 2019. Available at: https://www.aamc.org/system/files/2019-12/2019 AAMC Fall Applicant Matriculant and Enrollment Data Tables.
18. McDermott M, Gelb D, Wilson K, et al. Sex Differences in Academic Rank and Publication Rate at Top-Ranked US Neurology Programs. JAMA Neurol 2018; 75(8):956. Available at: https://jamanetwork.com/journals/jamaneurology/article-abstract/2676799?redirect=true#noi180011r6. Accessed 31 August 2022.
19. West J, Jacquet J, King M, et al. The Role of Gender in Scholarly Authorship. PLoS ONE 2013;8(7):e66212. Available at: https://pubmed.ncbi.nlm.nih.gov/23894278/. Accessed 31 August 2022.
20. Farheen AS, George IC, Singhal D, et al. Current status and future strategies for mentoring women in neurology. Neurology 2021;97(1):30–7. https://search.proquest.com/docview/2548908050.

Printed and bound by CPI Group (UK) Ltd, Croydon, CR0 4YY
03/10/2024
01040470-0003